AF861688

COMPREHENSIVE PRACTICAL

Biology

For A' Levels

COMPREHENSIVE PRACTICAL

Biology

For A'Levels

Salma Siddiqi
B.Sc (Hons.) London
Science Co-ordinator and Senior Lecturer,
Dept. of Biology at Aitchison College
Lahore, Pakistan

FEROZSONS (PVT.) LTD.
RAWALPINDI - LAHORE - KARACHI

ISBN 969 0 01572 9

First Published 1999 by
Ferozsons (Pvt.) Ltd.
60, Shahrah-e-Quaid-e-Azam, Lahore-Pakistan
277, Peshawar Road, Rawalpindi
Mehran Heights, Main Clifton Road, Karachi

Siddiqui, Salma

Comprehensive Practical Biology for A' Levels

Reprinted 2004,2005,2008,2010

Available in the UK
ASG (UK) Limited
10, Melrose Avenue,
Norbury, London, S.W. 16, 4QU, UK
email: asguk@lineone.net

author email: salma.siddiqui42@gmail.com

Designed, Printed and Bound in Pakistan by
Ferozsons (Pvt.) Ltd., Lahore.
email: support@ferozsons.com.pk
www.ferozsons.com.pk

Contents

13 TISSUES, ORGANS AND SYSTEMS

Acknowledgements

In developing a book of this magnitude, I have depended on the constructive advice of several sincere friends. I am indebted to Mr Asad Jamil (Senior lecturer, Aitchison College), who has been most generous in giving his valuable time and for his helpful comments on the text.

A word of special thanks is due to the following colleagues and friends for their help and advice: Mr. Shamim Khan (Principal, Aitchison College), Mr Shakoor Aslam (ex-head of biology department, Aitchison College), Mr Saleem Safdar (Head of biology department, Aitchison College), Ms. Farida Chughtai (Senior biology lecturer, Lahore Grammar School)and Mr. Hamid Khan.

I would like to thank my publishers, Ferozsons Pvt. Ltd., particularly Ms. Farhat Toor, Mr. Asghar Khan, and my editor and now a cherished friend Ms. Iram Nawaz Awan for their encouragement and help during the preparation of this manual.

Finally my husband, Asif and my children; without their tolerance, encouragement and support this book would not have been possible.

SALMA SIDDIQUI

June, 1999

The author and publisher would like to thank the following for their help and assistance in the preparation of this book:

Aitchison College, Lahore for making available their resources;

Dr. Sohail Chughtai, Associate Professor, King Edward Medical College, Lahore;

Dr. Arif Siddiqui, Assistant Professor, Agha Khan Medical College, Karachi.

The title design shows details of pollen grains, DNA structure, heart trace and the circulatory system of the human body.

About the Author

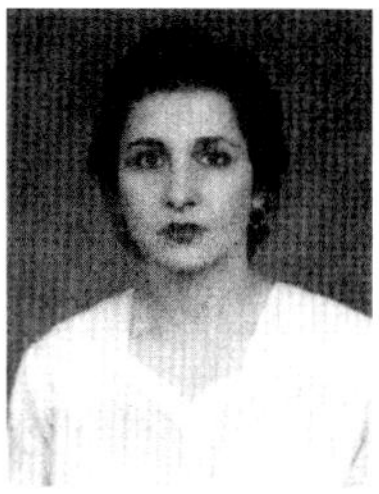

Salma Siddiqui was brought up and educated in London. After graduation, she worked for over ten years as a research biochemist at St. George's Hospital Medical School. She has to date published several research papers in reputed medical journals in England.

After moving back to Pakistan, Ms. Siddiqui joined Aitchison College. There, she helped establish new laboratories, introduced new and modern equipment and teaching aids from England and teaches Senior Cambridge (O'Level) and Higher Senior Cambridge (A'Level) biology. Currently, she is the Curriculum Adviser and Co-ordinator for science at Aitchison College, Lahore.

Salma is currently teaching A level biology at the Lahore College of Arts and Sciences (LACAS) where she is also the Science Co-ordinator and Curriculum Advisor. She regularly trains teachers in using multi-media and information techinology (IT) in teaching. She is the author of **Comprehensive Junior Science for Classes 1 to 5** also a Ferozsons Publications.

She divides her time between teaching, writing and social work.

Reviews & Recommendations

Comprehensive Practical Biology for A'Levels by Salma Siddiqui is an excellent attempt at providing students with materiel for the A'Level biology syllabus, especially in this era of competition. The book not only answers the need of A'Level and HSC biology students in Pakistan, it will also prove very useful to students of South East Asia, the Far East and the Middle East. Although this book was written for students of A'Levels, I now feel that this will be an excellent book of reference for biology teachers and students of medicine and other professional degrees. Using this book has certainly made my life as a biology teacher easier.

A detailed section of plant histology, anatomy, practicals and microscopic photographs and illustrations have been included. Hence the problem faced by students who had to buy and consult several books for references has now been solved.

A separate guide for teachers and technicians has also been added which will help make pre-preparations of different practicals more organised and systematic.

ASAD JAMIL
Senior Lecturer
Department of Biology
Aitchison College

A'Level students at Aitchision College have used *Comprehension Practical Biology* written by Salma Siddiqui as a biology practical manual for several years in an un-published form. This excellent book **also** covers the HSC practical syllabus for biology and provides key facts and essential techniques, with detailed, simple to follow directions for biology students. Diagrammatic representation and electron micrographs of various microscopic slides are also included which will prove to be very useful in developing the understanding of practicals and investigations.

The author has also made a special effort to replace the names of foreign plants with local ones, which used to be a major cause of confusion to both students and teachers. She has worked very hard over a period of several years to develop this book and I applaud her brave effort.

In so doing, she has set precedence for other teachers to come forward and develop books and manuals for our children instead of relying on material written by foreign authors.

SALEEM SAFDAR
Head of Department of Biology
Aitchison College

Salma Siddiqui's book *Comprehension Practical Biology for A'Levels* is an excellent pioneering effort. It covers the biology practical syllabus of all major examination boards. The success of this book, I feel, lies in the inclusion of superb and accurate illustrations and diagrams and in the fact that it caters for the local environment. The book is an invaluable guide for teachers and students alike for the Advanced Level.

FARIDA CHUGHTAI
Senior Lecturer, Biology
Lahore Grammar School

A note for teachers and students

Science is a practical subject.

In my opinion, science without 'practical' is not science! When you actually dissect an animal and see its tissues, organs, systems etc. you will remember it for life whereas learning only from textbooks about what these look like can be daunting. Similarly to read that the liver liberates oxygen when hydrogen peroxide is added to it may not have much impact on you, but when you do this practical yourself you will always remember and recall it. As they say, 'seeing is believing!'

Hence all investigations in this book are devised and planned to help biology students build a bridge between theory that they study in class and practicals that they perform in laboratories.

Teachers and students should be well versed in the **Assessment Objectives of the University of Cambridge Examination Syllabus for the year 2000** especially the section concerning the Biology Practical Course which states:

> **'...it is expected that *practical activities* will underpin the teaching of the whole syllabus'.**

Teachers and students should keep the following points in mind:

(a) Experimental activities should be scientifically devised and planned.

(b) Appropriate practical techniques should be selected and used.

(c) Conclusions and results of the investigation should be precisely and scientifically deciphered, evaluated and imparted.

Preparing for the Biology Practical Exam

The Biology Practical Exam, Paper 6, lasts 2 hours and carries 60 marks. This exam is set and marked by the University of Cambridge Local Examinations Syndicate (UCLES) and consists of investigations which are derived from the Biology A'Level syllabus. However, in all cases full and clear instructions are always given.

Essential Skills needed for successful Practical work.

Students are expected to exhibit the following essential skills required for practical work:

* Follow sequence of given instructions exactly.
* Perform experiments in a methodical and organised way with due respect for safety.
* Use all apparatus, materials and techniques in a suitable way.
* Plan and devise experimental activities scientifically.
* Use and select appropriate practical techniques.
* Determine the authenticity and precision of data and techniques by recognising and assessing errors.
* Interpret and study results derived from the investigation to reach valid conclusions.
* Record data, results, and plans clearly and exactly using tables, graphs etc.

Recording Practical Observations

Students are expected to record practical observations in the following manner:

* Exact and detailed observations and drawings under the microscope (low and high power) of specimens with accurate labelling.
* Apply prior knowledge to experimental results to reach valid conclusions.
* Take measurements precisely within the limitations set by the apparatus.
* Conclusions and results of the investigation should be precisely and scientifically deciphered, evaluated and imparted.
* All information and data, be it numerical or non-numerical be presented in a scientifically and mathematically sound manner.

Additional Information for successful Practical Work

Additional information about the following topics such as materials, equipments, concepts, equations etc. will be invaluable for students:

- Electromagnetic spectrum
- Light microscope, compound microscope, hand lens
- Energy changes such as potential, activation, chemical bond etc.
- Isotopes
- Molecules, atoms, ions, electrons
- Hydrolysis and condensation
- Oxidation and reduction
- Acids, bases, pH, buffers
- Calculation of mean, ratio, percentages
- Construction of graphs
- Calculation of rates of processes
- Use of *t*- and *chi*- squared tests

Preface

The purpose of this book is to provide a detailed selection of practical laboratory investigations suitable for Advanced Level biology students.
Comprehensive Practical Biology covers the course of both the Senior Cambridge and London Boards.
All the investigations presented in this book are arranged in order according to the A'Level syllabus and covers every aspect of the syllabus. This will help the students as well as the teachers to work systematically with their syllabus. The book also aims to train students to understand the principles and applications of biology and make logical deductions and conclusions. It encourages students to interpret and analyse results of their practical work. As students progress through this course, they will develop their knowledge, extend their existing skills and acquire new skills as well.

In compiling this manual I lay little claim to originality. Indeed, most of the practicals have been compiled from previously attempted investigations and from questions and problems featured in past examination papers. However, investigations included here have been modified to make them as effective as possible and were specifically tried and tested by biology students and the staff of Aitchison College over a period of several years.

All illustrations in this book have been paired with step-by-step written explanations. Slides, anatomical drawings, illustrations, tables etc. all have been used profusely to help students get a clear overview of the concepts and structures explained. It also contains an extensive coloured section on histology. Text and corresponding visuals have been systematically placed, hence the student need not flip pages back and forth unnecessarily in order to understand a concept. Wherever necessary, coloured illustrations have been provided. At the end of the manual I have included useful references such as a glossary of biological terms, a technician's guide and an index.

A major drawback in existing practical biology books for A'Levels is that they are written by Europeans, using the flora and fauna of Europe. Such specimens, basic equipment and sometimes even chemicals are difficult to obtain in Pakistan. Neither the climate nor the working conditions in this part of the world are suitable for such experiments and hence results vary and are usually not exact. Most teachers have little or no practical experience of how to overcome these problems and cannot organise practical classes without the help of trained technicians. Sadly, in most schools even of the highest calibre, trained technicians are not available!

Keeping these problems in mind, I scoured every possible source and collected and compiled investigations that are possible to perform in Pakistan, within our limitations. While developing this book I have solved and answered all problems and difficulties that I encountered as a teacher while teaching biology to A'Level students. I now know that any teacher using this book will benefit from my extensive and exhaustive research.
I have used the flora and fauna of Pakistan, mentioning the botanical names of plants and trees as well as the common names in English and local names in Urdu. For example, the botanical name of the *mulberry* tree is *Morus alba* and the local name in Urdu is *shehtoot*.
In so doing, I decided to write my own manual with the needs of the student, teacher and technician constantly in mind.
This book is the fruit of my labour.

SALMA SIDDIQUI
June, 1999

1 Approaching Practical Biology

Approaching Practical Biology

The aim of this manual is to provide an essential selection of practical investigations and questions suitable for Advanced Level biology students in schools and colleges. Whatever the approach and whatever the techniques, the ultimate purpose of laboratory work for the student should be to explore and investigate the world of living things and not merely for the purpose of passing an examination. In this manual all practical investigations are systematically organised to carefully guide the students through the activity, step by step. The manual is designed to enable students to carry out important biology experiments and to gain expertise in particular techniques.
All the investigations included are designed to fit into two periods of 45 minutes each. The time required for microscopic work and dissection will vary according to the aptitude of the students and availability of resources. It is essential that the students should make their own drawings and record their own observations and write up the experiments which they, themselves, carry out.
A list of requirements for each investigation and practical is given at the end of the book in the teacher's and technician's guide.

Some tips before you begin your investigation

1. Read the whole procedure carefully, **before** you arrive in the laboratory.
2. Before beginning any experiment make sure you know the aim of the experiment and exactly what you are expected to do. If you are uncertain it is best to ask and clarify before you begin rather than waste time, chemicals and besides **it could be dangerous.**
3. Avoid wasting time doing unnecessary work, **(time management is vital, learn this now to help you on that particular day!)**
4. If the procedure requires you to wait for any length of time see if you can work on another part, or write up the method etc. whilst waiting for reaction to occur.
5. Accurately record all observations, measurements, timings and any special precautions and alterations in a register. These records would be useful when writing your reports.
6. Tabulate results neatly on a separate sheet of paper or in your register (scraps of paper have a habit of getting lost) so that you don't have to copy them neatly later.
7. Write up your practical reports as soon as possible, otherwise you are likely to forget important details and it is much easier to write up one report than many at a time.

Use and design of controls

A control is often required in investigations to prove that any reactions occurring in the investigation are in fact due to the stated cause and not due to other factors. **In your control only one factor (the factor you are investigating) should be changed, all others should remain constant.** This includes temperature, volume, pH timing etc. The control will then provide reference point of comparison for the main experiment.

Writing practical reports

The report should be written in a detached manner, using only past tense, and in a logical sequence of events under appropriate headings. The headings are as follows:

Title:

This should be a clear statement outlining the aim of the experiment e.g.
'Experiment to see the effect of temperature on enzyme action'.
It should briefly and concisely outline what you intend to find out or prove.

Procedure:

This should be written as a report in the past tense, stating clearly, concisely and precisely what you did, in a logical and detached manner. This report should be so precise that another scientist using this information should be able to carry out the same experiment e.g. 'Five test tubes were labelled 1, 2, 3, 4 and 5. To each, $5cm^3$ of saliva was added...'

Result and observations:

Your data should be presented here in a concise form and be easy to understand. Graphs rather than tables, small tables rather than large ones, and histograms etc. should be presented here. (Your register would be handy here!) If several repeated readings were taken, mean value should be presented. These could be qualitative or quantitative depending on the nature of your experiment, or they could be verbal, stating your observations.

Discussion and conclusion:

This is the most important part of your report. It should be brief and to the point, answering any questions that may arise and/or a confirmation of them. A conclusion, if any, should be added here. Chemical reactions and any theory should be explained here. You could also suggest what to do next to promote your work further. If the desired results were not obtained (as is the case quite often!) do not get discouraged. It is quite normal. **Investigations have to be repeated again and again to get good results.** However, it is important that you **try and explain what went wrong** and how you could overcome the problem to prove/demonstrate the aim of your investigation.

Recording and presenting data

Quantitative Data (also known as numerical data)

Numerical data can be recorded in various ways. It is best to try and present it in a way, which is most accurate and simple to comprehend. There are various ways of presenting numerical data such as: tables, line graphs, histograms, bar charts, pie charts, scatter graphs, pictographs to name a few.

Tables

Raw data (data you have collected) presented in a simple table makes it easier to understand and follow. A table provides a neat and accurate record of your data values **Fig 1.1**.

Time (days)	Height (mm)
0	0
2	1
4	2
6	10
8	22
10	38
12	60
14	80
16	90
18	100
20	108
22	110
24	110
26	110

Fig. 1.1 Table showing Mean Height of Oat Seedlings

1. Each column must be arranged in a logical and meaningful way. Avoid giving unnecessary information and divide each column using clear lines.
2. Quote values to a sensible significant figure.
3. Make sure to add appropriate units of measurements at the **top** of each column, if required, but not with each reading.
4. A table must have a brief descriptive title.
5. Any abbreviations or modifications should be added in footnotes.
6. If several tables are used they should be numbered so they can be quoted in the text.

Line graphs

Line graphs should provide an immediate visual summary of your tabulated data, which should be relatively easy to understand **Fig. 1.2**.

Fig. 1.2 Graph Showing Mean Height of Oat Seedlings

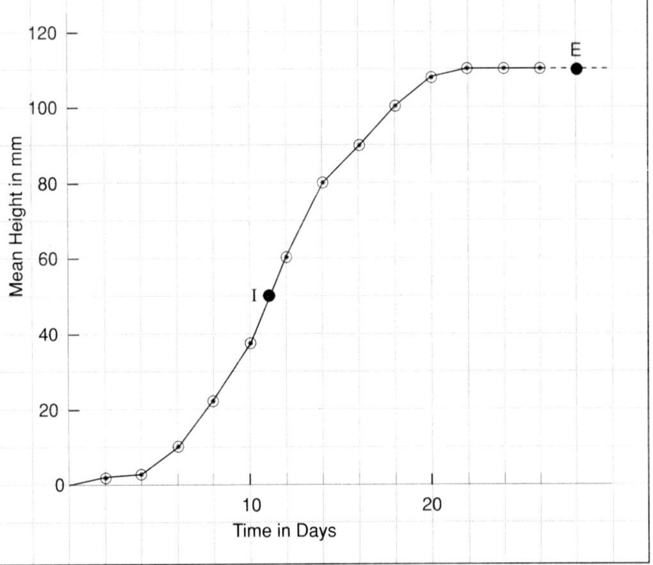

1. Graphs should be **self-contained** – they should contain all the information necessary to convey the appropriate message without referring to the text.
2. Consider the layout and scale of the axis carefully. Most graphs illustrate the relationship between two variables (x and y), and have two axis at right angles.
3. Usually x-axis is the independent variable, and y-axis the dependent variable.
4. When neither variable is determined by the other or where the variables are independent, the axis may be plotted either way round.
5. Each axis must have a descriptive label showing what it represents together with the appropriate unit measurements.
6. Each axis must have a scale with clear reference marks on the axis to show the location of all numbers used. In some cases it may be inappropriate to start the scale at zero. In such cases show the break clearly as —/ /—, just beyond zero.
7. **Remember that the purpose of the graph is to communicate information easily and clearly.** Do not clutter unnecessary information on your graph.
8. A legend can be used to provide explanatory detail.
9. Each point on the graph should be visible either as a cross **x** or a dot with a circle around it ⊙.
10. If there is more than one set of data on the graph, make sure to label each line clearly e.g. you could plot one set of data using circled dots and the other with crosses. You may use different colours for different sets of data, and then add a key on the graph to indicate which colour represents which set of data.
11. The points marked on the graph are a record of the actual observations made and may be joined by a series of straight lines using a ruler, (most accurate!), by a smooth curve or in some cases by a 'line of best fit'.

12. Every graph must have a concise **explanatory title** to establish the content.
13. If several graphs are used they should be clearly numbered so that they can be quoted in the text.
14. Only the points on the graph represent actual data, but estimations of other values can be obtained from reading off co-ordinates at any point on the line. This is called **interpolation** e.g. at **x I**. Similar co-ordinates outside the range of the graph may also be **estimated** by extending the lines on the graph, a technique known as **extrapolation** e.g. at **x E**.

Histogram

The histogram is the most suitable form of data presentation when the number of data points is too few to allow a trend line to be drawn. The x-axis represents continuous values of independent variables grouped together into small classes of equal size e.g. the leaf size of a particular plant **Fig. 1.3**.
The columns are adjacent to each other. Histograms can also be used to represent frequency distributions.

Bar graphs/charts

Bar graphs or charts are drawn when one of the two variables is not numerical (e.g. number of flowers per plants or energy values of different fruits). They should be made up of narrow blocks of equal width, which do not touch. The blocks can be arranged in any order **Fig. 1.4**.

Frequency diagrams

These are drawn when plotting the frequency of distribution with continuous data (e.g. frequency of leaves of different length). The blocks should be drawn in decreasing order or in increasing magnitude and they should be touching.

Pie charts

Pie charts should normally be drawn with sectors in descending order, beginning at noon and proceeding anti-clockwise. If a comparison is to be made between two pie charts however, the second chart should keep the same sequence of segments as the first whatever their relative sizes. Comparison between pie charts can also be made by making the area of the circle proportional to the size of each sample. Preferably pie charts should contain no more than six segments **Fig. 1.5**.

Recording by Drawing

As part of your practical work you are required to study a vast range of biological specimens and tissues, make accurate visual observations, use a microscope and record your observations by drawing. The basic skills can be learned with determination and require no artistic ability, just accurate observations and practice.

A guide to making good biological drawings

Drawing should *prove* useful as a record for future

Fig. 1.3 Histogram of Leaves of Different Length on a Plant

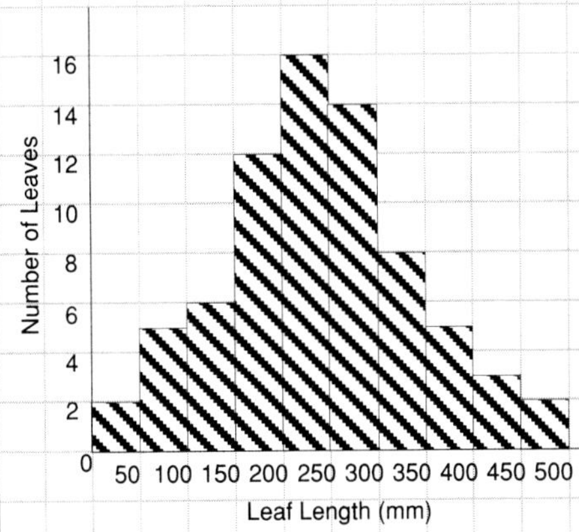

Leaf Length (mm)	Numbers
0–50	2
50–100	5
100–150	6
150–200	12
200–250	16
250–300	14
300–350	8
350–400	5
400–450	3
450–500	2

Fig. 1.4 Bar Chart Showing Energy Values (KJ) Per 100 g of Fresh Fruit

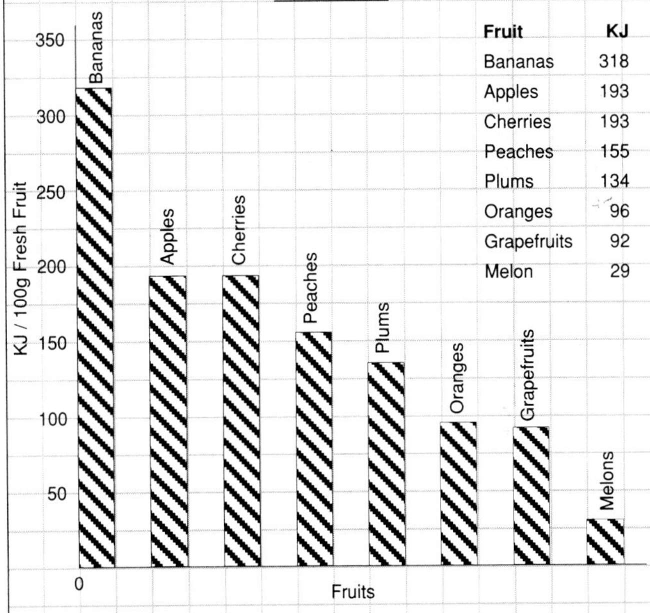

Fruit	KJ
Bananas	318
Apples	193
Cherries	193
Peaches	155
Plums	134
Oranges	96
Grapefruits	92
Melon	29

Fig. 1.5 Table Showing the Number of Arthropods on an Eucalyptus Tree

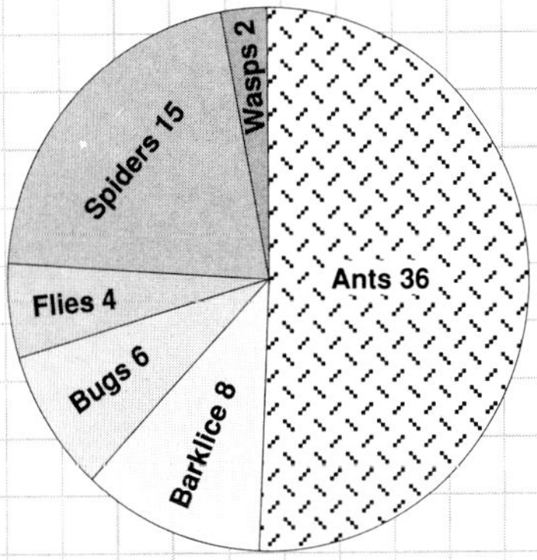

Arthropod	Eucalyptus
Ants	36
Barklice	8
Bugs	6
Flies	4
Spiders	15
Wasps	2

reference, helping you to remember what you have recorded. You are required to **draw** using a microscope as part of the final practical exam, so practice, practice, and practice!

1. Good quality A4 loose, plain paper, kept safely in a boxed folder is best but if you think you will lose your drawings, an interleaf copy would suffice.
2. Always have a good selection of pencils. 2B, B, HB are most useful, as well as a good eraser, ruler and a sharpener. (Pen and ink drawings are only used for posters and project reports.)
3. Drawing should be drawn at a defined magnification. Pretend that you are drawing for someone who has never seen this specimen. They should know exactly what it looks like, and how large it is without seeing the specimen.
4. Start your drawing in the centre of the page. It should take up approximately a third of the space, with ample space on either side for labels.
5. Often you need to draw larger than the original specimen, and then have to specify the exact magnification. If you have difficulty in making a start, measure the specimen, say it is 2cm, then decide how large you want your drawing to be i.e. 5X the specimen so, 2X5 = 10 **Fig. 1.6**.
   Take a ruler and mark out 10cm in the centre of the space, now start by drawing very faint 'construction lines' using a sharp soft pencil, to allow you to get the basic proportions correct before progressing. These can be erased once the drawing is complete.

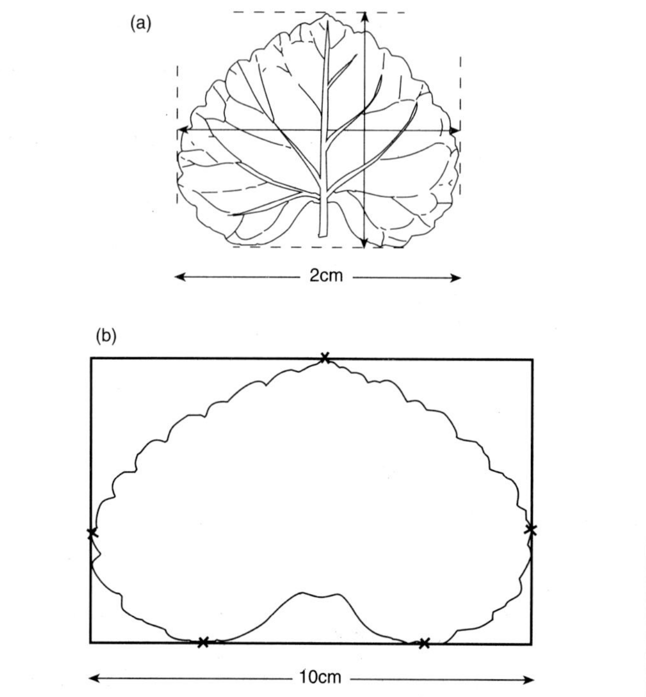

Fig. 1.6 Drawing an object. (a) determine linear dimensions, (b) construct a frame and outline

6. Mark out the main structures in the correct position and proportion. Again if you have trouble in drawing the correct proportions, use the same technique of measuring and multiplying. If the drawing needs to be smaller than the specimen, use the same technique, but divide instead of multiplying. After some practice you will not need to follow this method.
7. Using a soft pencil draw faint, clear, smooth lines. Avoid hesitant fuzzy or broken lines. If you do draw in such a manner make sure to rub these out and go over them in smooth continuos lines. Now add the main structures.
8. Observation is the key to good drawing. Look carefully at how each structure is linked to the main plan of construction **Fig. 1.7**.

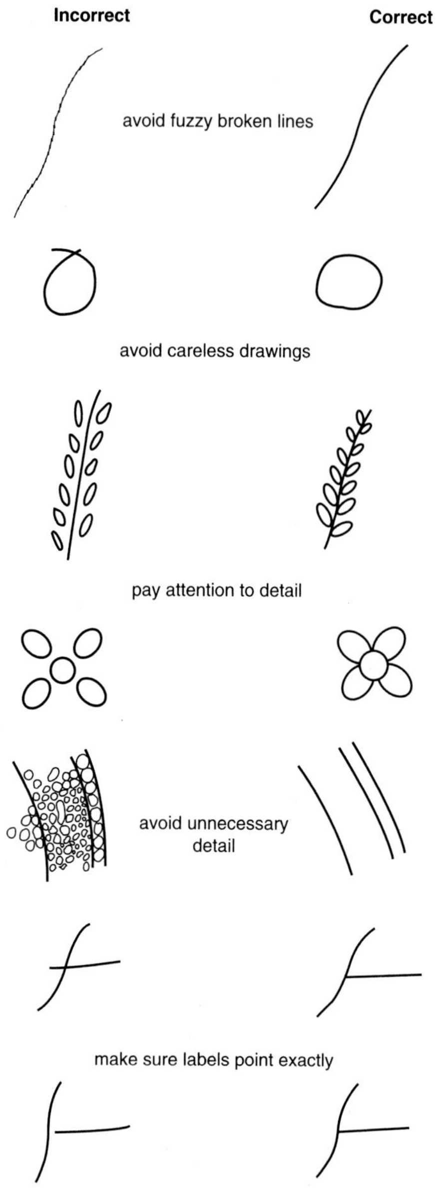

Fig. 1.7 Common Errors in Biological Drawings

Make sure that junctions between lines are properly drawn; for example, if you are drawing a plant, observe carefully exactly how the leaves are attached to the main stem. Is there a little stalk joining the main leaf blade to the stem or does the blade join directly on to the stem? Look at the exact arrangements of the leaves. Are the two leaves arranged exactly opposite each other or are they alternating? And so forth....

9. Draw exactly what you see and not what you expect to see and **definitely do not copy from a textbook.**
10. Shading or use of coloured pencils is not normally allowed. Indicate different areas by using stippling, hatching or cross-hatching. Once you are satisfied with your effort go over with firm darker lines, rubbing out any mistakes and fuzzy, broken lines.
11. Any drawing, no matter how beautifully executed is absolutely useless unless it is **labelled** clearly. Always keep all labels well away from the drawing. Print using a sharp pencil on either side of the drawing, with lines drawn with a ruler, pointing **precisely** to the structure. Labels should never cross each other and should be written clearly. Annotations are strongly recommended.
12. Work out the magnification and write it down neatly at the side.

Microscopic drawing

Drawing what you see under the microscope can be quite daunting, but it can be learnt.

1. Initially draw the **main plan** at low power, making sure to keep all major structures in proportion. Avoid fuzzy or broken lines. Be **precise** about detail.
2. Later you can draw certain parts or structures at a higher power as a separate drawing. If the whole slide shows similar cells it is pointless to draw the whole thing in great detail. It is quite sufficient to draw a small part. It is useful to indicate on the initial drawing the portion you have drawn in detail.

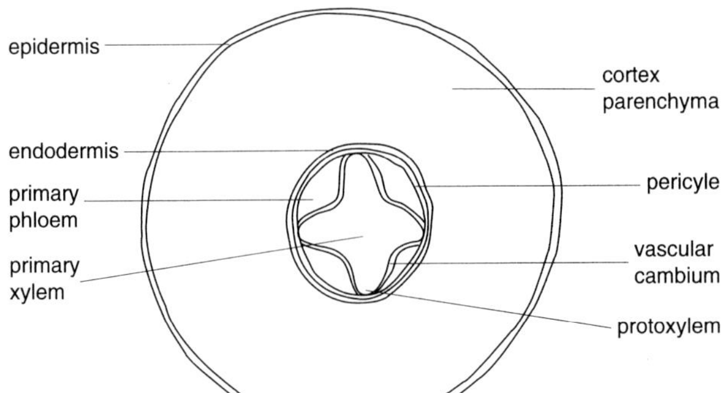

Fig. 1.8 Plan diagram of a Dicotyledon Root TS

3. Give the drawing its main label, (usually what is written on the slide e.g. T.S. of a dicotyledon stem) and make a habit of always indicating at what magnification (see chapter on microscope) the observations were made.
4. A plan **diagram** or a **map** is a special form of recording where only the boundaries between tissue are marked and no cellular details are included **Fig. 1.8**.

Basic safety rules for laboratory work

Science laboratory is potentially a hazardous place. Although any potential dangers are pointed out in each investigation remember it is your responsibility to be constantly vigilant about any hazards not only to yourself but to others, in the laboratory.

1. Observe, understand and follow **all warning** labels for specific hazards **Fig. 1.9**.

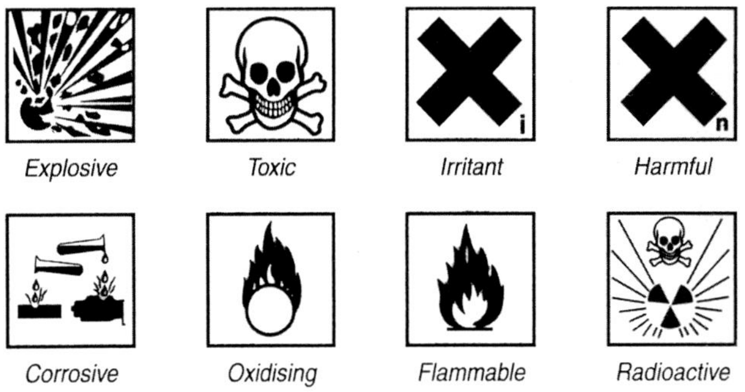

Fig. 1.9 Signs for Hazardous Substances

2. Make sure you know what to do in case of fire, including how to raise the fire alarm, and the location of the fire extinguisher. Remember that the most important consideration at all times is human life.
3. Wear a lab coat at all times.
4. Know the location of the **FIRST AID** kit.
5. Report all accidents and dangers to the staff.
6. Never eat, drink, or smoke in the laboratory.
7. Do not allow electrical equipment to come into contact with water.
8. Be particularly careful with glassware.
9. Treat ALL chemicals as hazardous.
10. Know what you are doing before you start to work.
11. Work in a logical, tidy manner and clean up afterwards.
12. Heating anything with a Bunsen burner has its risks. Make sure to hold test tubes so that they point away from you and everyone else.
13. Always wash your hands before leaving the laboratory.

Measurements used in biology

The international conventions for measurements are governed by the **Systeme International d'Unitéd**, usually referred to as **SI units**. This is an internationally recognised form of measurement and represents the accepted scientific convention for measurement of physical quantities.
Units and symbols that you are likely to encounter in this course are listed below.
Most measurements consist of a number and a unit. The number expresses the ratio of the fixed quantity to a fixed standard and the unit is the name for the measure or the dimension **Fig. 1.10**.
Certain measurements can be expressed as dimensionless ratios or logarithms (e.g. pH) and thus do not require a qualifying unit.

Measured quantity	Name of SI unit	Symbol
Length	Meter	m
Mass	Kilogram	kg
Volumes (solids)	Meter	m^3
Volumes (fluids)	Litre	dm^3
Time	Second	S
Frequency	Hertz	Hz
Energy	Joule	J
Pressure	Pascal	Pa
Force	Newton	N
Enzyme activity	Katal	kat
Temperature	Kelvin Celsius	K ºC
Luminous intensity	Candela	cd

Fig. 1.10 The base and supplementary SI units

The units of length likely to arise in your biological study are: meter (m), millimetre (mm), micrometer (µm), nanometer (nm) and Ångstrom (Å) (an older unit of measurement 10^{-10}m) **Fig. 1.11**.

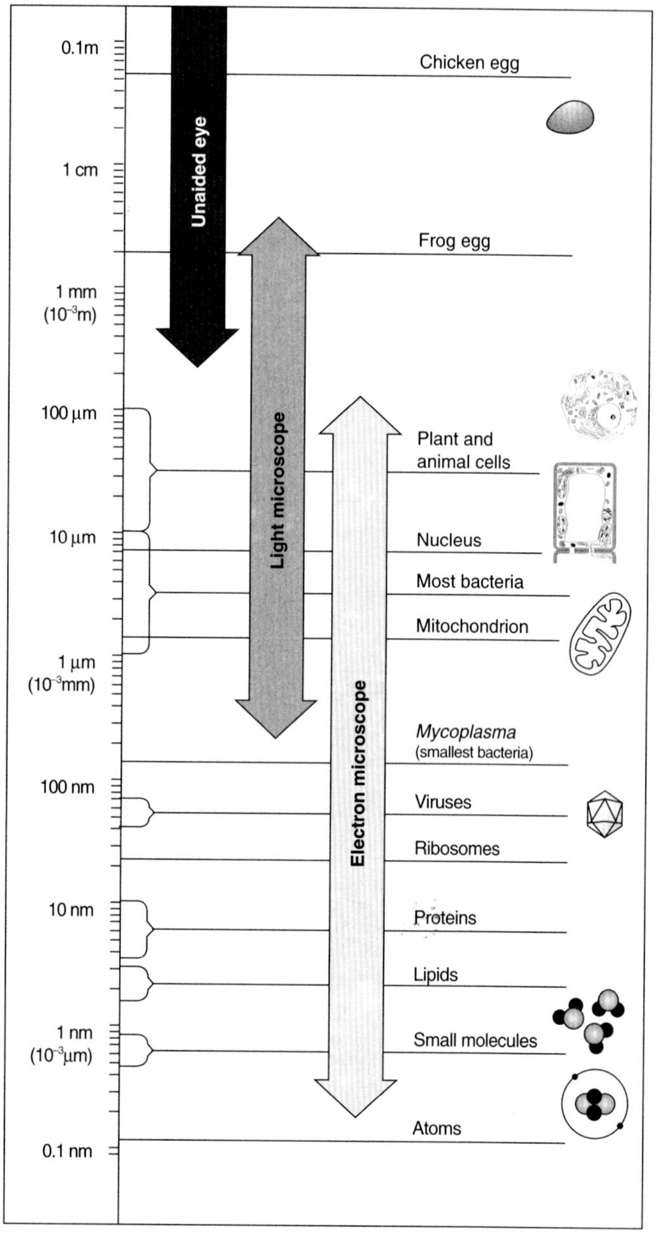

Fig. 1.11 Size Scale
The scale is logrithmic. Each division marks a tenfold change in size.

Using glassware

Choose the right glassware to measure liquids, keeping in mind the accuracy required, the volumes being dispensed and the number of times the job must be done.

Care with glassware:

1. Don't use chipped or cracked glassware – it may break on heating or under the slightest strain.
2. If possible use Pyrex glassware, especially if heating and cooling is involved.
3. Don't force stoppers in glassware, they are very hard to take out and you may cause breakage and injury. **(If you do cut yourself report to staff.)**
4. Dispose of broken glass with care, so that the cleaning staff does not get injured.
5. Wear safety glasses.

Certain liquids may cause problems:

1. Viscous liquids such as glycerol, may be difficult to dispense: allow time for all the liquid to transfer.
2. Organic solvents evaporate quickly, making measurements inaccurate and difficult: work rapidly and seal containers quickly. Work in a fume cupboard or in well ventilated room.
3. Certain solutions such as proteins and detergents are prone to frothing: try to avoid forming bubbles by dispensing gently.
4. Suspensions such as cell cultures, soil samples etc. tend to sediment. Mix thoroughly before dispensing.

Measuring accurately:

1. Stand the measuring cylinder or volumetric flask on a level surface.

2. Fill to just **below** the required volume, with the eye in level with the meniscus, (take the measurement from the bottom level of the meniscus).
3. Fill carefully to final mark using a Pasture pipette until the meniscus is in level with the final mark.
4. Allow time for the solution to run down the wall of the cylinder or flask.

Graduated pipettes

1. These come in various sizes. Choose the right size for the volume to be dispensed (i.e. do not use 10 cm^3 pipette to dispense $0.1cm^3$, use 1.0 cm^3 pipette).
2. Take care and **check the volume scale** before use. Some scales empty from full volume to zero, others from zero to full and some refer to the shoulder of the tip, others to the tip by gravity or by blowing out.
3. **Never** mouth-pipette hazardous chemicals such as acids or poisonous solutions. Use a syringe or a pipette pump.

Check with staff if uncertain. That is why they are here.

Bulb pipettes

1. These are of fixed volume, for example 5, 10, 50 cm^3, and are very accurate.
2. Touch the tip of the pipette to the side of the glassware to allow the last drop to trickle out.
3. Do not blow out the last drop.

Syringes

1. Syringes are often used instead of pipettes these days. If the needle is not required remove it with care.
2. Place the tip into the solution and gently pull the plunger to a little more than the required volume on the scale.
3. Expel any air bubbles by inverting and gently tap the syringe, and expel the air and the excess.

Balances

1. Balances can also be used to weigh out accurately the liquid you have dispensed.
2. Convert mass to volume using the following equation:

   Mass/density = volume

3. Density of most liquids is written on the bottle, or can be looked up in textbooks.

   Remember density is temperature dependent and hence you will need to know the temperature of the liquid.

Solutions

A solution is a homogenous liquid formed by the addition of solute to a solvent (usually water in most biological systems). Most experiments require solutions of a particular concentration. Before preparing any such solutions make sure you understand exactly what is required for the particular task.

What is a concentration?

In SI units the concentration of a solute is expressed in **mol m^{-3}** which is convenient for most biological purposes. The concentration of a solute is represented by square brackets, e.g. [KCl]. However, there are a number of alternate ways of expressing concentration and you may come across them in your practical work, or in textbooks.

A 1.0 molar (1.0 mol l^{-1}) KCl solution would contain 74.55g in a litre of solution. (The molecular mass is usually written on the side of the container; K = 39.10, Cl = 35.45 = 74.55g) **Fig. 1.12.**

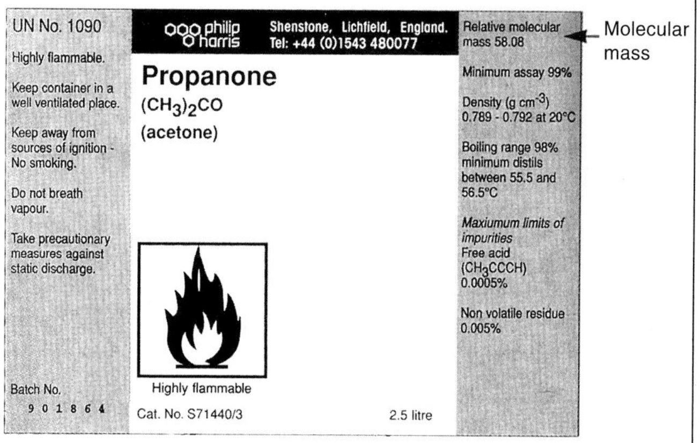

Fig. 1.12 Label on a Chemical Container has lots of useful Information

Detail of how such a solution is prepared is given below.

Molarity

This is the term used to denote concentration **C**, expressed as moles of solute per litre volume of solution (mol dm^{-3} = molar). The symbols in common use for molar (M) and millimolar (mM) solutions are at odds with SI system and now mol dm^{-3} and mmol dm^{-3} are preferred.

A 1.0 molar (1.0 mol dm^{-3}) NaCl solution would contain 58.44g (the molecular mass, usually written on the side of the container, Na = 23, Cl = 35.45; 23 + 35.45 = 58.45), in a litre (dm^{-3}) of solution.

Molality

This is the term used to express the concentration of a solute relative to the **mass** of solvent, i.e. mol kg^{-1}. **Molality** is a means of expressing solute concentration; it is **temperature independent** and is rarely used except when the osmotic properties of solution are of interest.

Example

A 0.1 **molal** solution of NaCI would contain 58.44 x 0.1 = 5.84g NaCI per kg of water.

Percent composition (% w/w)

This contains the solute mass (in g) per 100g solution. This is a very convenient way of preparing solution, and is frequently used.

Example

A 10% w/w sucrose solution contains **10g** sucrose and **90g** water.

Similarly parts per thousand ($^0/_{00}$), i.e. mg g^{-1} and parts per million (p.p.m.), i.e. µg g^{-1}, are used.

Percent concentration (%w/v and v/v)

For solute added in solid form, this is the number of grams of solute per $100cm^3$ solution. This is more commonly used than percent composition, as solution can be accurately prepared by weighing out the required amount of solute and then making this up to a known volume using a volumetric flask or a measuring cylinder.

Example

A 10% w/v sucrose solution contains 10g sucrose made up to $100cm^3$ with water.

Note:

When water is the solvent this is not usually specified e.g. a 80% v/v ethanol solution would contain 80% ethanol and 20% water.

Practical 1 – MAKING AQUEOUS SOLUTIONS OF KNOWN CONCENTRATION

In most cases, solutions are made for you by technicians and laboratory staff but you should know how to prepare one should the need arise. Follow this simple procedure.

1. Work out and decide on the concentration of the chemical required for your investigation.
2. Work out the total volume of solution required (always make a little extra as you may spill some or make a mistake in dispensing).
3. Find the **molecular mass** of the chemical. (This is the sum of the atomic elements and can usually be found on the side of the container) **Fig. 1.12**.
4. Work out the mass of the chemical required that would give the desired concentration in the required volume, which can be calculated using the following equation:

$$C = \frac{\text{mass of solute/molecular mass}}{\text{volume of solution}}$$

Suppose you need to make 200 cm^3 (0.2 dm^3) of 0.5 mol dm^{-3} NaCl solution,

$$\text{Using the above equation } 0.5 = \frac{\text{mass of solute/58.44}}{0.2}$$

$$\text{Therefore mass of solute} = 0.5 \times 0.2 \times 58.44$$
$$\text{which is} = 5.844\text{g}$$

Weighing

1. Make sure you know how to use the balance accurately.
2. Never weigh anything directly onto a balance pan: you may contaminate from previous users.
3. Use a clean spatula and new piece of aluminium foil or filter paper. Otherwise, weigh directly into the vessel in which you are mixing the solution.

Making the solution

1. Add the weighed chemical to a clean beaker.
2. Then add distilled water, a little less than the final volume required.
3. Stir until all the chemical is dissolved (you may need to heat gently to dissolve some chemicals. Make sure the chemicals do not alter with heating).
4. Check and adjust the pH, if required.
5. Adjust the volume accurately using a measuring cylinder.

Now prepare 100 cm^3 of 0.1 mol dm^{-3} NaCl solution.
Molecular mass of NaCl is 58.45.
To make 1.0 dm^3 (litre) of 1.0 mol dm^{-3} solution you would need 58.45 g of NaCl.
You are only making 100 cm^3 of 0.1 mol dm^{-3}

$$\text{therefore } \frac{58.45}{100} = 0.5845$$

You require 0.5845g of NaCl in 100 cm^3 of water.

Proceed as follows:

1. Label a 100 cm^3 beaker 0.1 mol dm^{-3} NaCl.
2. Weigh out 0.59g of NaCl either straight into the beaker or on a piece of filter paper depending on the balance available to you.
3. Mix the NaCl with distilled water in the beaker until all the salt dissolves.
4. Transfer the solution to a volumetric flask or a $100cm^3$ measuring cylinder and adjust the final volume, adding the last few cm^3 with a Pasture pipette, and holding the measuring cylinder up to your eye level. The bottom of the meniscus should touch the final volume mark.
5. Transfer the solution to a labelled reagent bottle.

Useful Tips

If the mass required is too small to be weighed accurately consider the following:

1. Make up a greater volume of solution.
2. Make up a stock solution, which can be diluted further.
3. Use the right glassware for the job; e.g. do not use a litre measuring cylinder to measure 50 cm^3, use a $50cm^3$ or a 100 cm^3 measuring cylinder.

4. Do not pipette 0.1 cm^3 using a 10cm^3 pipette, use a 1 cm^3 pipette.
5. Make sure the glassware is clean (sterilised if required).
6. Always use distilled deionised water to make solutions.
7. Always make sure all the solute is dissolved prior to adjusting the final volume.
8. Adjust the pH, if required, **before** adjusting the final volume.
9. Use a funnel when pouring the solution to avoid spillage.
10. Make up the volume using the meniscus at eye level.
11. Transfer the solution to a **labelled** reagent bottle.

Labeling and storing solutions

1. Label all stored solutions/chemicals carefully with the following information: the chemical name, the concentration, pH if measured, and the date when made.
2. Make sure solutions are stored appropriately, in either the refrigerator or a freezer and allow time for them to come to room temperature before use.

Dilutions

Now suppose you need to dilute 200cm^3 of your 0.5 mol dm^{-3} NaCl solution to a final concentration of 0.1 mol dm^{-3}, the following relationship is very useful:

$$C_1 V_1 = C_2 V_2$$

Where:
C_1 and C_2 are initial and final concentrations, and
V_1 and V_2 are their respective volumes.

Therefore $0.5 \times 200 = 0.1 \times V_2$

$$V_2 = \frac{0.5 \times 200}{0.1} = 1000$$

$$V_2 = 1000$$

that is 200 cm^3 of 0.5 mol dm^{-3} NaCl made up to a litre will give the final concentration of 0.1 mol dm^{-3}.

Stock solutions and serial dilutions

Stock solutions are very useful if you are making a range of solutions of various concentrations or for serial dilutions. Stock solution is always made more concentrated than the final requirement, and is diluted as required.

Make up 100cm^3 of each of the following sucrose solutions: 10%, 5%, 2.5%, 1.25%, pH 7.
Prepare 200cm^3 of 10% stock solution as follows:

1. Weigh out 20g of sucrose in a beaker.
2. Add about 150cm^3 distilled water and dissolve the sucrose.
3. Adjust the pH if required using dilute hydrochloric acid or sodium hydroxide solution as required.
4. Transfer the solution to a 250cm^3 measuring cylinder. Adjust the final volume using a Pasteur pipette to add the last few cm^3.
5. Transfer to a labelled reagent bottle.

Useful tips

- Clearly label the vessel containing each dilution, it is easy to get confused!
- Solutions must be thoroughly mixed before measuring out volumes for the next dilution.
- When deciding on the final volume required, allow for the volume removed when making up the next dilution in the series.
- Remember to discard the excess from the last vessel in the series, if volumes are critical.

Dilution of stock solution

Now dilute this to 100 cm^3 of each of the 5%, 2.5%, and 1.25% solutions:

1. Label 3 beakers 5%, 2.5% and 1.25%.
2. 50cm^3 of 10% made up to 100cm^3 with distilled water will give you 100cm^3 of 0.5% solution.
3. 50cm^3 of the 0.5% solution made up to 100cm^3 will give you 100cm^3 0.25% and so forth....

Use the 10% stock solution to prepare the following dilutions: 1%, 0.1%, 0.01% and 0.001%.

1. Label four test tubes: 1, 0.1, 0.01 and 0.001
2. Add 9cm^3 of distilled water into each of the four test tubes.
3. Add 1 cm^3 of 10% solution to test tube 1, mix well.
4. Transfer 1 cm^3 from this test tube to test tube labelled 0.1, mix and transfer 1 cm^3 from this test tube to test tube labelled 0.01 and so forth....
5. Discard 1 cm^3 from the last dilution if final volume is critical.

pH and Buffer solutions

pH is a measure of the amount of hydrogen ions [H^+] in a solution, a measure of the solution's acidity. The term is taken from French *pouvoir hydrogène,* "hydrogen power". This affects the solubility of many substances and the activity of most biological systems. Slight changes in the pH of the body's internal environment can adversely effect the physiology. The rate of chemical reactions alter with slight changes in the pH because of the shape of protein molecules and thus the functioning of enzymes is profoundly affected by pH changes.
The pH scale runs from 0 to 14. The concentration of ions in pure water is chosen as the midpoint (7) on the scale of acidity and alkalinity known as the pH scale.
At pH 7 the concentration of hydrogen ions [H^+] is equal to the concentration of hydroxyl ions [OH^-], and the solution is considered as neutral at 22°C, room temperature.
The lower values of pH (<7.0) refer to acid conditions, with more hydrogen ions in solution. The higher values (>7.0) refer to alkaline or basic conditions, with fewer

hydrogen ions than hydroxide ions in solution.
Many compounds act as acids, bases or alkalis: those which are almost completely ionised in solution are usually called strong acids or strong bases, while weak acids or bases ionise only slightly in solution **Fig. 1.13**.

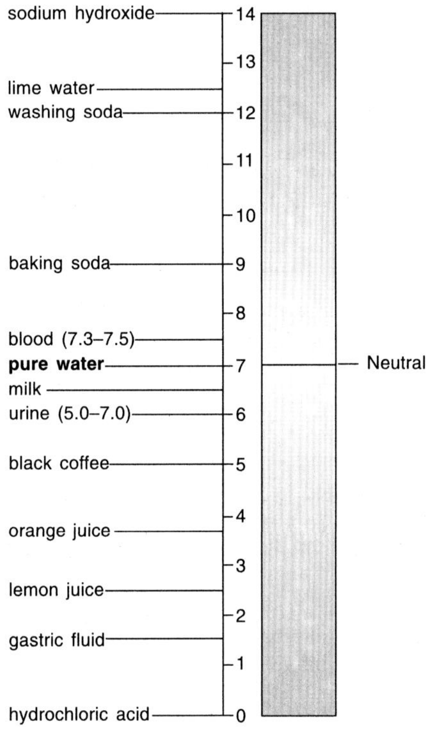

Fig. 1.13 pH of some Common Solutions

pH is strictly the negative logarithmic (base 10) of H^+ activity, although in practice H^+ concentration (in kmol m^{-3}, equivalent to mol l^{-1}) is mostly used. ***The pH scale is not SI*** **nevertheless; it is still widely used in biological science.**

$$pH = -\log_{10} [H^+]$$

pH is determined experimentally using either coloured indicators or an electronic pH meter, which is equipped with a probe sensitive to hydrogen ions **Fig. 1.14.**

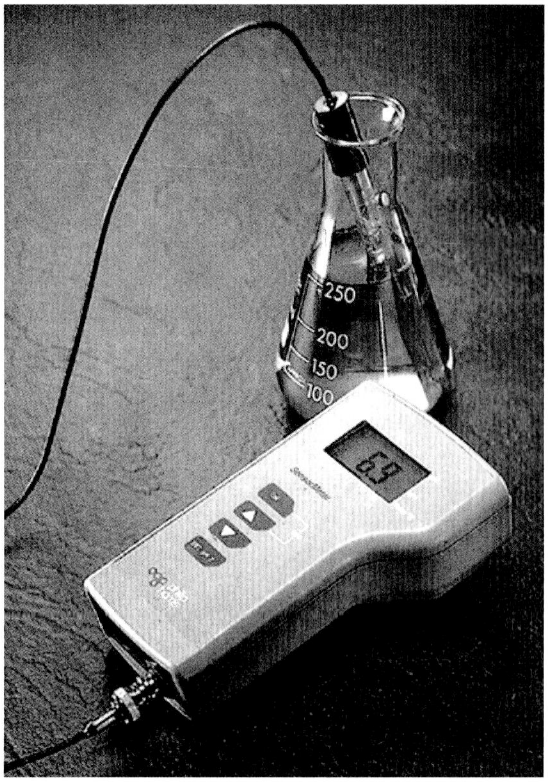

Fig. 1.14 Portable Combined pH Meter

Remember

Acid is a compound that acts as a proton donor.
Base is a compound that acts as a proton acceptor.
Alkali is a compound that liberates hydroxyl ions when it dissociates. Since hydroxyl ions are strongly basic, this will reduce the proton concentration.
Ampholyte is a compound that can act both as an acid or a base. Water is an ampholyte since it can dissociate to give a proton and a hydroxyl ion.
Conjugate pair is an acid together with its corresponding base.

Buffer Solutions

A solution that resists change in its pH when small amounts of acid or alkaline are added is called a buffer solution. Buffers are usually made by mixing week acid and the soluble salt of the same acid. A buffer of any pH can be made by selecting a suitable acid and the appropriate acid to salt ratio.
Buffers are common in biological systems, because the complex biological reactions in living organisms are very sensitive to pH. Even a very slight change in pH can result in death e.g. the pH of human blood is 7.35, a change of more than 0.3 of pH unit could be fatal.

2 Microscopy

Microscopy

The human eye can distinguish two objects apart, unaided, at best if the distance between them is 0.2mm (200μm). The resolving power of the human eye therefore is 200μm. Many features of interest to biologists are far too small to be observed without the use of microscopes; for example most cells have a diameter of about 10μm and therefore can not be seen without a microscope.

The resolving power of a light microscope is about 0.0002mm-(0.2μm). With the light microscope a trained observer can not only observe cells but also their internal content, cytoplasmic streaming and even cell division.

All microscopes consist of a co-ordinated system of lenses arranged so that a magnified image of the specimen can be seen. The main difference is the wavelength of the light source (electromagnetic radiation) used to produce the image. Microscopes allow an image to be viewed **magnified** (enlarged) with increased **resolution** and **contrast**.

Resolution is the ability to distinguish clearly between two points on the specimen – the better the resolution the better the image. The resolution is dependent on the lens and the wavelength of radiation used.

Contrast is the difference in intensity perceived between different parts of an image. This can be improved with use of suitable stains and microscope adjustments, usually at the expense of resolution.

There are three main forms of microscopy used in biology: **light microscopy, transmission electron microscopy (TEM)**, and **scanning electron microscopy (SEM)**.

Practical 2 – THE COMPOUND MICROSCOPE

The compound microscope is a precision instrument in which the magnifying powers of two convex lenses, the eyepiece and objective lens are used to produce a magnified image of very small objects. Light rays are focused on to a transparent specimen by a condenser lens. The rays pass through the specimen and are focused again by two more lenses – the objective lens and the eyepiece lens. The total magnification of the microscope is determined by the focal lengths of the two lens systems. These two lenses can produce a magnified image up to x 2000 or more.

As specimens are often colourless and transparent, stains are used frequently to make different parts stand out. These stains usually colour specific parts of a cell and are extremely useful. So long as the specimen is thin and transparent there is no limit as to what you can view under the light microscope. Living, moving cells and 'fixed' stained sections can be examined and present no problems.

Precautions when using a microscope

(a) **The compound microscope is an expensive precision instrument,** ***handle it with care*** and protect it from dust by storing it under cover or in a box.

(b) When carrying the instrument always use two hands, holding it by the limb and under the base and put it down on the bench workstation without jarring. (**Never carry a microscope by the microscope tube or stage.)**

(c) Keep the lenses and working surface (the stage) clean and dry, uncontaminated by reagents, stains and fixatives. Take special care to avoid touching the lenses and make sure any of the solvents, stains and mounting fluids do not come into contact with the lenses either.

(d) Lenses and the mirror should be wiped only with the lens tissue or a lint-free soft duster, kept solely for this purpose.

(e) Do not use direct sunlight to illuminate the mirror or condenser lens of the microscope, as sunlight when focused on to the retina may damage the light-sensitive cells there.

Setting up a microscope at low power

Caution: *follow these instructions carefully. Failure to do so would result in breaking the slide and may damage the microscope.*

Before using the microscope, familiarise yourself with its components. Time spent now in learning to set your instrument to give the best possible image will pay dividends later. The microscope will be your companion in many investigations throughout your course. If possible, try and use the same microscope each time, so that you can familiarise yourself with it.

Note: If you wear glasses, remove them, as the microscope adjustment will accommodate most eyesight deficiencies (except astigmatism).

With reference to **Fig. 2.1** proceed as follows:

1. Place the microscope on the bench in front of you, so that you can sit comfortably and look down the **eyepiece lens** without straining yourself.
2. Plug in and adjust the **lamp setting** to the minimum and switch on. Adjust the lamp setting to about (two-thirds) of the maximum.

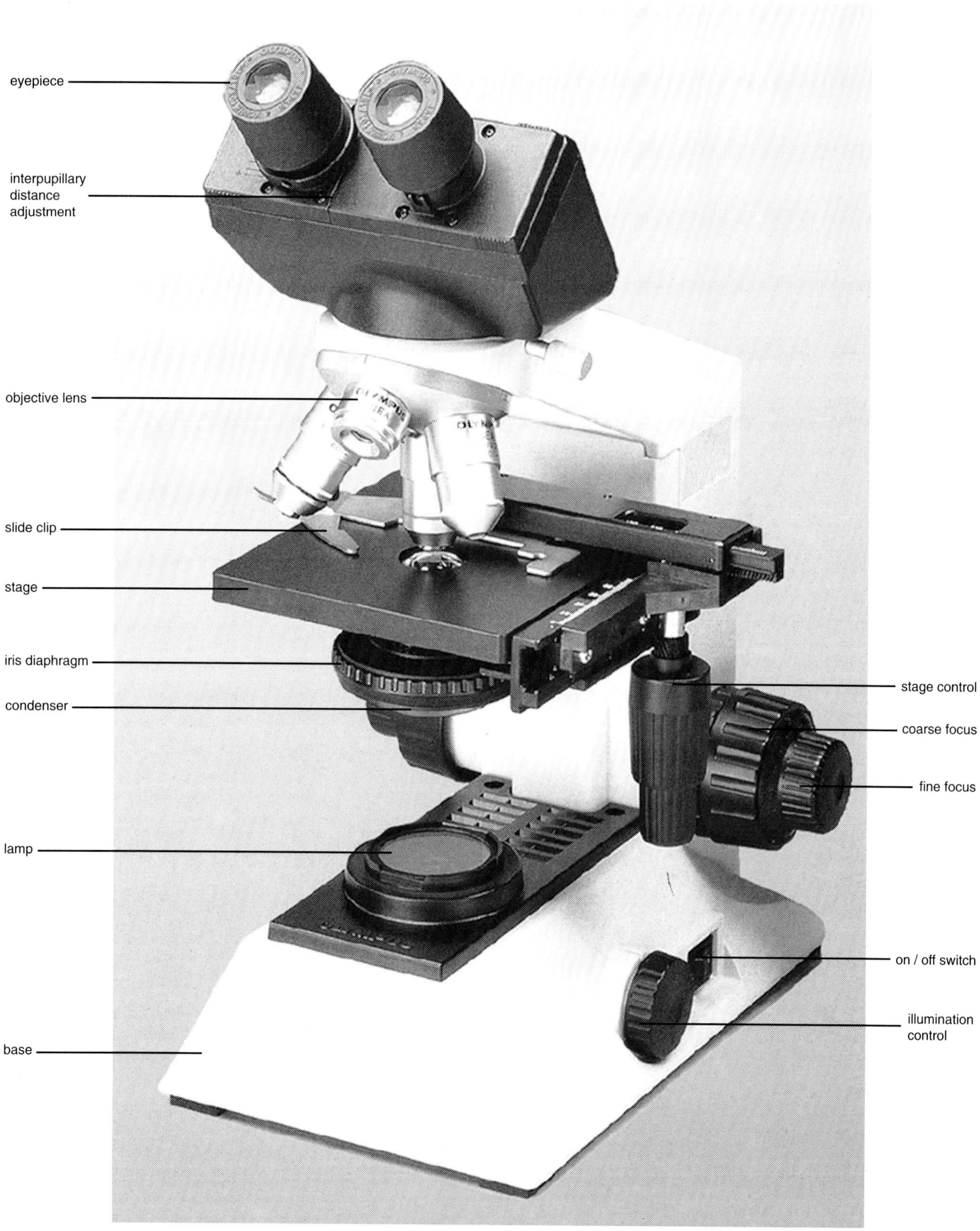

Fig. 2.1 The Compound Light Microscope

3. Familiarise yourself with the various **objective lenses** (x4, x10, x40, and x100) mounted on a rotating turret called the **nosepiece**, which clicks into position. Rotate the turret to click low power (x4 or x10) objective into position.
4. Now find the **coarse and fine adjustment knobs**, movement of which usually moves the microscope tube (in some microscopes the stage moves) and focuses the image.
5. Below the **stage**, examine the movement (focusing) of the **condenser**, and the control lever of the **iris diaphragm**. (There is often a filter ring or tray at the base of the condenser too, with its own handle.)
6. When you are fully familiar with these controls, find a suitable stained slide, place it on the stage with the coverslip (thin glass covering the section) uppermost, and clip it into position so that the specimen is illuminated from the **lamp** beam below.
7. Check that the iris diaphragm of the condenser lens (operated by the iris **diaphragm lever** below the condenser) is about half open.
8. Now focus the image of the specimen first with the **coarse adjustment knob then with the fine adjustment knob** until the image is in sharp focus.
9. If both eyepiece lenses are adjustable set your **interpupillary distance** (distance between the two eyes) on the scale for each lens. Close your left eye, look through the eyepiece with your right eye and focus the image using the coarse and fine focus knobs. Repeat this with your right eye but focus the image by rotating the eyepiece holder. Note these settings for future reference.

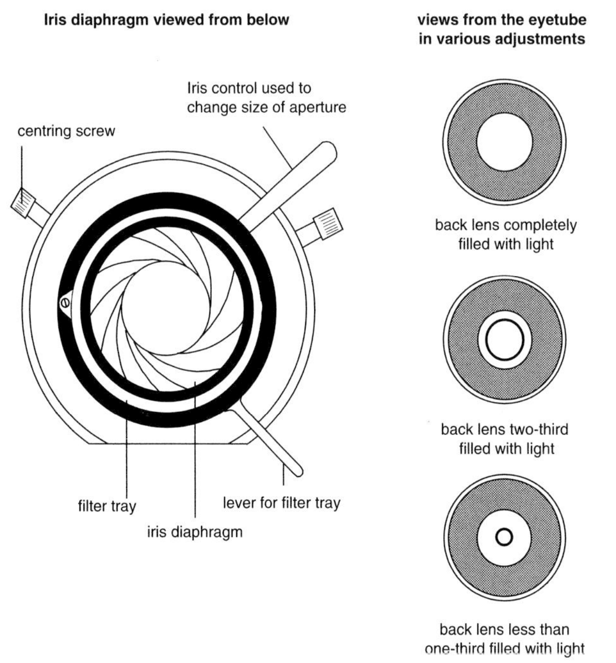

Fig. 2.2 Fine Adjustment of the Iris Diaphragm

10. Close the iris diaphragm **Fig. 2.2**, then open it slowly to a position such that further opening has no effect on the brightness of the image. The edge of the diaphragm should not be in view. Reduce the illumination if too bright.
11. Now the condenser must be focused. Place the tip of a sharp pencil or a pointer on the light source, adjust the **condenser setting** until the pointed tip and the specimen are in sharp focus. The condenser and iris diaphragm should be just outside the field of view.
12. Your microscope is now set to give you the best possible image.
13. You do not have to adjust the condenser every time you use the microscope, but you should know how to adjust it.
14. Observe prepared slides of *ameoba, paramesium, algae, blood and other suitable tissues.*

Setting up a microscope at high power

1. For high power magnification, first focus the microscope using the specimen to be examined as described above using the **coarse adjustment knob** only.
2. Then carefully turn the objective nosepiece round till the relevant high power objective (x40 or x100) is clicked into place (if the microscope was in focus at low/medium power, then the high power objective lens will be close to the prepared slide but not touching it).
3. Look down the microscope and fine-focus the image by **slowly** racking up with the **fine adjustment knob only**. ***Using the coarse focus knob will break the slide and may damage the microscope.***
4. With some specimens it is possible to see a sharp image with the x100 objective but in most cases immersion oil is required (see practical 3) with this objective.
5. Do not remove the slide with the high power objective lens in position. First turn back to low power objective, then lower the stage and remove the slide.
6. Examine prepared slides at low and high magnification, until you are sure you can do so with ease.
7. When you have finished your observations, re-set the microscope objectives to medium power.
8. Remove the prepared slide and store it in the correct slide tray, see that the microscope is clean and dry before you put it away.

Note:

- ***Do not remove eyepieces, objectives etc. without permission of staff and unless you know exactly what you are doing.***
- ***If there is dust inside your instrument ask the staff to help you as unnecessarily opening these parts introduces more dust into the instrument.***

Practical 3 – OBSERVING TRANSPARENT MICROSCOPIC SPECIMENS

Transparent preparations that have not been stained are difficult to see when the microscope is set as described above. By closing down the condenser-iris diaphragm contrast can be improved but in doing so diffraction haloes appear around the edges of the specimen which may result in loss of resolution. Nevertheless the image is easier to interpret.

Oil-immersion microscopy

Oil-immersion microscopy, though a little difficult, provides the best resolution possible with the light microscope, especially when bacterial preparations are examined.

A drop of special immersion oil, which has the same refractive index as the lens is introduced between the specimen slide and the objective lens. This reduces the loss of light by reflection, and refraction at the glass/air interface, resulting in an increased resolution, brightness and clarity of the image.

1. Set up your microscope so the slide is focused for high power examination (x40 objective).
2. Swing away the x 40 objective, but do not engage the oil-immersion objective (x100) immediately. Lower the stage.
3. Apply a single drop of immersion oil to the slide, over the object being viewed **Fig. 2.3**.
4. Now click the oil-immersion lens into place. **Look from the side**, and very slowly lower the objective using the fine focussing knob until the oil **just** touches the objective. Now, using the fine focussing knob, very carefully continue lowering the objective until it **just** touches the coverslip on the slide ***(continuing to turn the knob any further will break the slide and may damage the objective)***. Look down the microscope and gently focus, using the fine focus adjustment knob, until the specimen comes into focus.
5. Observe prepared slides, especially of bacteria.
6. After completing your observations, wipe all immersion oil from the objective lens and the slide, using lens tissues.

Magnification of a microscopic image

The magnification of a microscopic image is calculated by multiplying the objective magnification by the eyepiece magnification. This however bears no relationship to the magnification of your drawing; you may choose to draw the same image 10mm or 10cm. For this reason it is essential to work out and record the magnification on all your drawings.

A rough estimate of the magnification can be made by comparing the size of the image to the diameter of the field of view. The field of view can be roughly estimated by focussing on a millimetre transparent ruler under low power.

For example, if the field of view at an overall magnification of x40 is 4mm, at an overall magnification of x100 it will be: 40/100 x4mm = 1.6mm (1 600μm).

A better method is to use an **eyepiece graticule**, **(see pages 20–22)** which is a piece of glass with a fine scale etched on it, that fits inside the eyepiece lens. The scale on the graticule is calibrated using a **stage micrometer** (a slide with a scale on it). The procedure is described in practical 4.

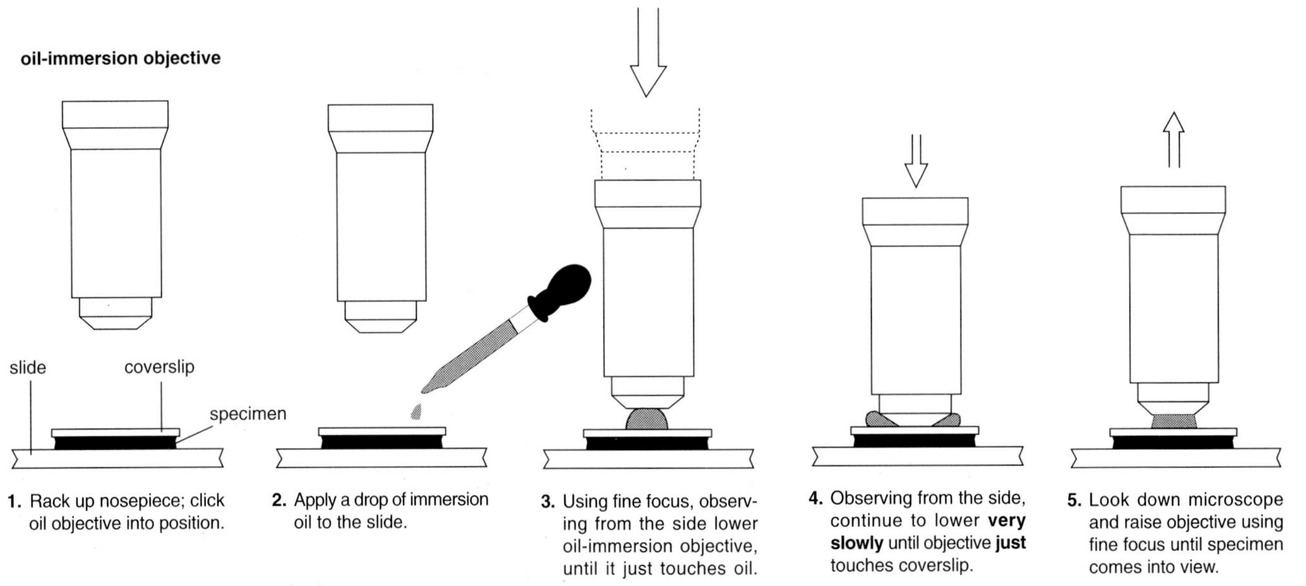

Fig. 2.3 Setting up Oil-Immersion Microscopy

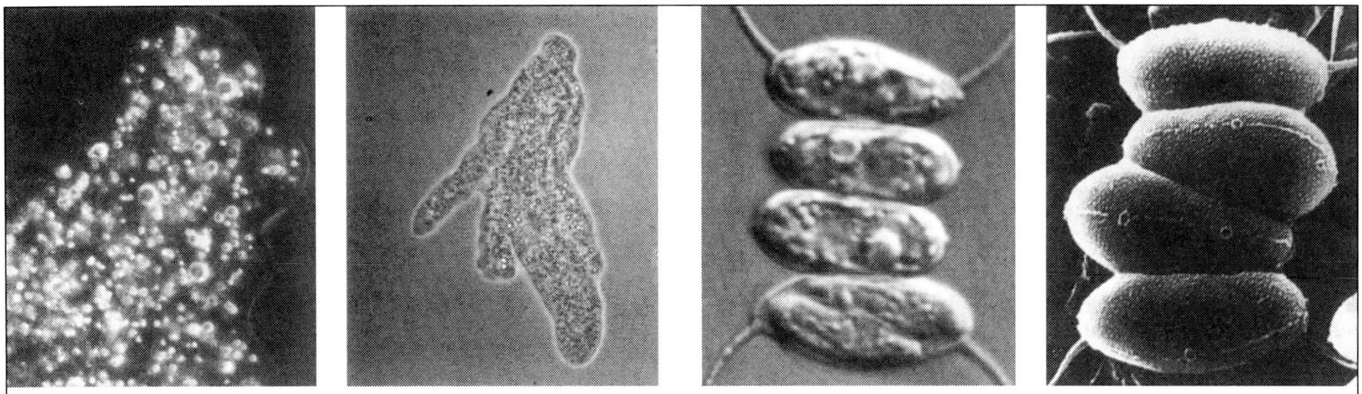

Fig. 2.4 Images with Different Microscopic Techniques

Other Microscopic Techniques

Dark ground microscopy

In dark ground microscopy **Fig. 2.4 (a)** a special condenser allows only rays of light scattered by structures within the specimen to enter the objective lens and form the image. The result is an image that appears bright against a dark background, with a high degree of contrast. Resolution is usually not as good as that obtained using normal (bright field) transmitted light, but the technique does make it possible to view living, unstained cells.

Phase contrast microscopy

The phase contrast microscope **Fig. 2.4 (b)** has a special fitments (**phase plates**) added to the objective lens and an **annulus** is fitted to the sub-stage condenser. As a result, structure within living things such as unstained cells becomes visible in high contrast and with exceptional resolution of very fine detail. Phase contrast microscopy avoids the need to kill cells or to add dyes to a specimen before it is observed microscopically.

Electron microscopy

The magnification of an optical microscope is limited by the wavelength of visible light. The electron microscopy (EM) offers magnification and resolution that is far greater (about x250) than that of an optical (light) microscope. This is because radiation of shorter wavelengths in the form of an electron beam is used. The wavelength of visible light is about 500nm, whereas that of an electron beam is 0.005nm.The shorter the wavelength the better the resolution. At best the light microscope can distinguish between two points which are 200nm (0.2μm) apart, whereas the transmission electron microscope can resolve points 0.5–1.0nm apart when used on biological specimens. **Magnification of up to x250 000 can be obtained with an electron microscope.** In principle, an electron microscope operates on the same basis as a light microscope. An electron beam replaces light rays.

In electron microscopy electrons are produced by tungsten filament operating in a vacuum. The resulting beam is focused by electromagnets and is projected on to a fluorescent screen for direct viewing, or on to a photographic plate for permanent recording. The resulting photographs are referred to as **electron micrographs** (EM) or simply micrographs.

There are two basic types of electron microscopes: **transmission electron microscope** (TEM) and **scanning electron microscope** (SEM). They differ in the way in which the electrons interact with the specimen: in TEM **Fig. 2.4 (c)** the beam passes through the specimen while in SEM **Fig. 2.4 (d)** it is scanned across the specimen and is reflected from the surface. In both cases it must fall on a fluorescent screen before the image can be seen. SEMS have a most impressive depth of field.

In SEM the resolution of the microscope is limited by the size of the electron beam, and is rarely better than 0.01μm, which is much poorer than the transmission electron microscope, but greatly superior to that of a light microscope.

Preparation of biological materials for SEM

Specimens are usually fixed or freeze dried to preserve their shape, and are then showered with heavy metal, prior to exposure to the SE microscope. Because of the vacuum, specimens must be completely dehydrated, and living material cannot be examined; only ultra-thin sections or very small objects can be used. Cell membranes and other fine structures must first be made electron opaque by the use of special stains.

Preparation of biological materials for TEM

The specimen is killed, chemically 'fixed' and dehydrated in a life like condition. It is embedded in a resin medium and sectioned on an **ultramicrotome** to less than 2μm thickness. Fragile specimens are floated of the knifepoint on to a supporting fine copper grid. Sections are then stained with electron dense materials such as solutions of lead salts (for lipid containing membranes) or uranyl salts (for proteins and nucleic acids). The dried grids with the stained sections are transferred to the EM.

Preparation of Biological Material for Optical Microscopy

Preparation techniques are crucial to successful microscopic investigations. Although biological specimen, living or preserved, can both be observed with the compound microscope, usually killed, fixed and stained specimens are used.
'Contrast' is the highlighting of tiny differences in the structure of the specimen. In biological material, which is too transparent, contrast is normally achieved by staining the material.

Staining

Much of what is known about the structure of cells was first learnt by observation of thin sections of tissues which had been preserved, sectioned, stained and permanently mounted on microscope slides. In light microscopy staining is used to add contrast to the image as well as to highlight components of interest and to locate particular cells, tissues or organs.
In ultraviolet (UV) microscopy, contrast is obtained using florescent stains. Physico-chemical properties of the stain cause it to attach to certain structures preferentially or be taken up across cell membranes. Living cells take up some dyes, known as vital dyes or stains. These dyes colour particular structures within the cells. For example, if yeast cells are treated with dilute neutral red dye or Congo Red dye solutions (these dyes are also acid/base indicators, like litmus) and then fed to *Paramecium*, the stages of digestion of the yeast cells in the *Paramecium* cytoplasm can be observed.

Preserved and stained tissues

The steps in this process are as follows:

1. **Fixation:** The main purpose of fixation is to preserve material in as life-like a manner as possible. This is usually achieved by immersion in chemicals such as formalin. This hardens and preserves the tissue with minimum of shrinkage, allowing sections to be cut easily.
2. **Sectioning:** The tissue is mounted in pith, wax or plastic and then sectioned. The sections have to be extremely thin, thin enough to allow light to pass through. This is usually done by a microtome, an automatic micro-thin section cutter.
3. **Staining:** The development of the German dye industry in the nineteenth century led to the use of many stains in microscopy. The section is stained by immersion in a suitable dye. Stains are selectively absorbed by important structures inside the cell, such as nuclei and chromosomes, which can therefore be seen more clearly. The use of Gram's stain allows bacteria to be divided into two main classes (**Gram-positive** and **Gram-negative**), which differ in the chemical composition of their cell walls see below. The technique of staining is highly well documented for every possible preparation in microbiology textbooks.
4. **Dehydration:** Immersion of stained sections in ethanol to remove water is called dehydration. This helps make the tissue transparent and prevents it from becoming opaque. Dehydration is carried out gradually, using a series of increasing concentrations of ethanol in water until 'absolute' (nearly pure) alcohol is reached.
5. **Clearing:** A liquid such as xylol replaces alcohol in the specimens, which is miscible with the mounting medium. This also completes the process of making the material transparent.
6. **Mounting:** Sections are mounted on a microscope slide in a medium (e.g. Canada Balsam) which excludes air and protects it indefinitely. A cover slip is added, and the mounting medium hardens.

Other techniques used for observation of biological material

Cell fractionation

Cell fractionation is the technique by which the tiny structures within the cells, known as organelles, are isolated so that structure and function can be investigated outside the organisms. The steps in cell fractionation are summarised in **Fig. 2.5**.

Practical 4 – MEASURING MICROSCOPIC OBJECTS

It is important to measure the dimensions of biological material. The size of an object observed under the microscope can be measured by using **an eyepiece graticule** and a **stage micrometer slide**.

Procedure

1. You are provided with a stage micrometer slide and an eyepiece graticule, which is a tiny printed grid etched on a circular piece of glass. Familiarise yourself with both and observe the grid on them by holding up to the light and by means of a hand lens **Fig. 2.6**.
2. Get your teacher to demonstrate how to install the graticule into the microscope before you attempt it yourself.
3. Clean them both with lens tissue or a fine soft cloth, and avoid getting fingerprints on them as you install them in the microscope.
4. Carefully remove the eyepiece from the microscope and then unscrew the top lens **Fig. 2.6**.
5. Place the graticule on the 'shelf' halfway down, *correct side up* (you will have to practice doing this).
6. Replace the upper eye piece lens and return the eyepiece to the microscope. Carry out these steps

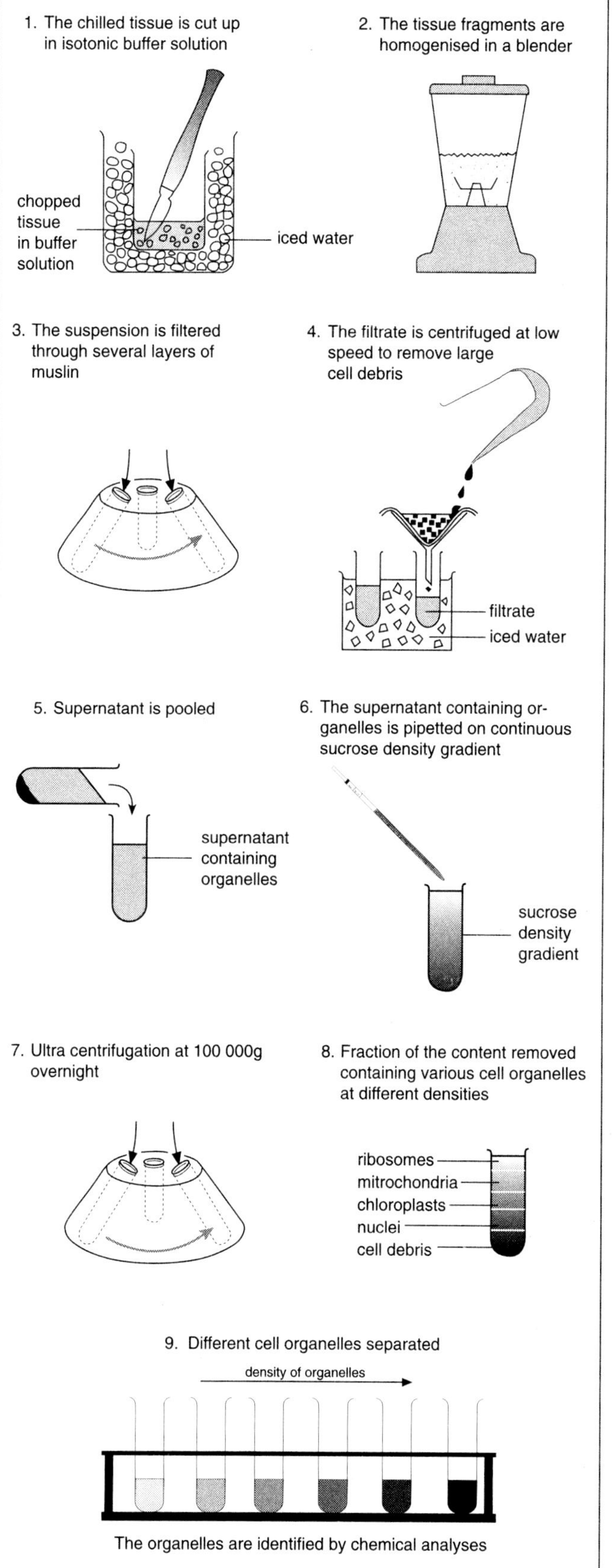

Fig. 2.5 Cell Fractionation to Isolate Cell Organelles
All steps are carried out at 0°C to minimise self-digestoin of cell organelles by the enzymes released from cell vesiceles in cell disruption.

quickly to avoid dust entering the microscope tube.

7. Replace the upper eyepiece lens, and return the eyepiece to the microscope. The eyepiece graticule is held in the plane of the primary image and therefore, is always in focus, whatever the magnification.
8. Using a prepared stained slide of unicellular animals such as *amoeba,* or *paramesium* measure the organism by mounting the slide on the microscope stage and focusing on the relevant part of the specimen. You may need to rotate the eyepiece so that the scale lies across the object.
9. Record the dimension of the organism in **arbitrary** units (a graticule has numbered divisions). Note the magnification.
10. Repeat this technique by taking measurements of the following:
    (a) the diameter of a parenchyma cell from the central pith of the stem;
    (b) the diameter of a nucleus (stained preparation);
    (c) the width of a capillary;
    (d) the length of an *amoeba* (stained preparation);
    (e) the diameter of the largest xylem vessel in the stem (TS);
    (f) the diameter of a red blood cell.

Calibration of the eyepiece graticule

1. Now the eyepiece graticule has to be calibrated. Hold up the stage micrometer slide in the light and observe the scale by means of a hand lens.
2. Most micrometer slides have a scale printed on them, e.g. 1cm with either 10 or 100 divisions. Each division is therefore equal to 10μm or 100μm (1μm = 0.001mm). Remember the scale on the micrometer slide can vary. *Check on the micrometer slide.*
3. Focus on the calibration scale and examine the micrometer slide under the microscope. Rotate the eyepiece until the graticule scale lies superimposed **Fig. 2.6.** Observe how many eyepiece divisions are equivalent to how many slide divisions. Do this at both medium and high-power magnification, for as the magnification is increased the eyepiece scale will cover a smaller area of the object, and each division measures a smaller length. Record the size of the divisions at each magnification.
4. List the eyepiece measurements (arbitrary units) of the objects you measured above, recording whether at medium or high power magnification. Multiply these measurements by the length calculated for the divisions at the magnification used.
   For example at low power, 60 eyepiece divisions are equivalent to 30-micrometer divisions.
   Therefore 60 eyepiece divisions = 3000μm

   $$1 \text{ eyepiece division} = \frac{3\,000}{60} = 50 \ \mu\text{m}$$

5. Record the size of various unicellular organisms and cells.

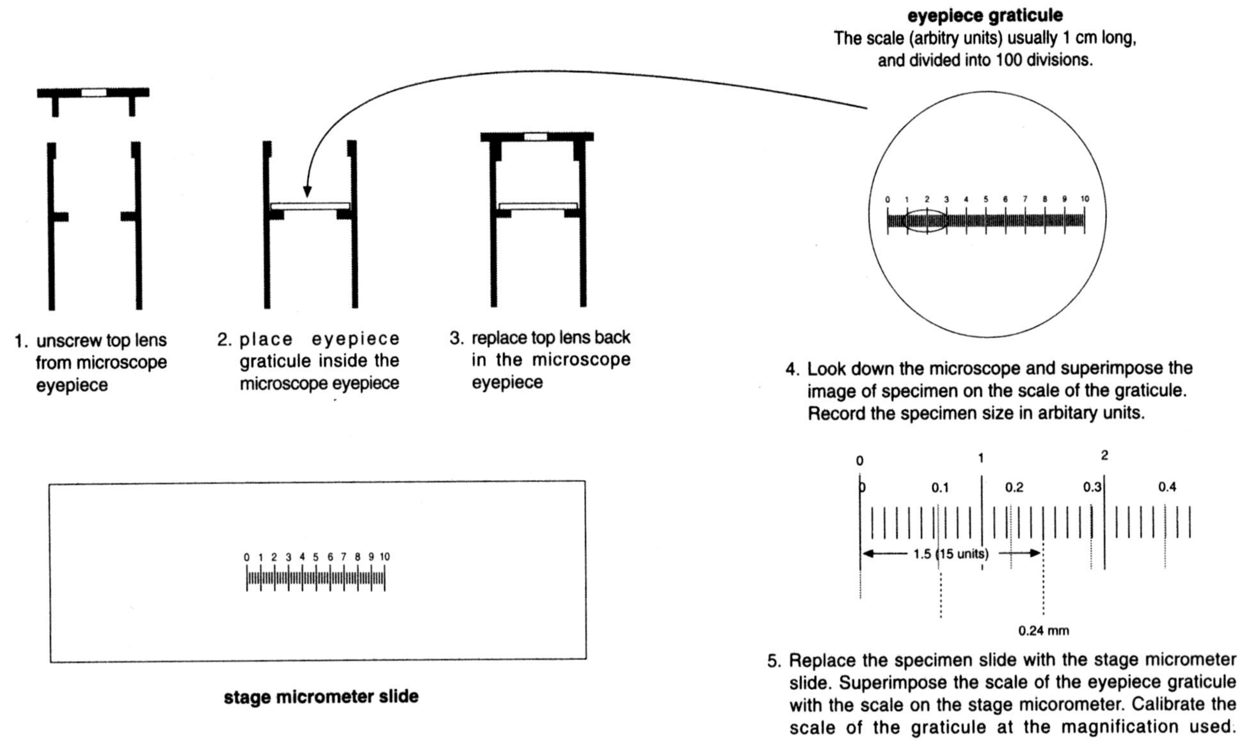

Fig. 2.6 Micrometer Slide and Eyepiece Graticule

For consideration

(a) Compare and contrast plant cells with animal cells in respect to size and structural organisation. Tabulate your observations.

(b) When preparing permanent slides, 'fixing' attempts to minimise the shrinking (due to dehydration) that occurs when biological materials are sectioned and stained for microscope examination. How could this be taken into account when investigating the actual size of the specimen?

3 The Cell

The Cell

Background Summary

A common characteristic shown by nearly all living things is that they all consist of cells. Cells were first described by Robert Hook in 1665 and are now known to be of universal occurrence in living organisms.

The **cell** is the functional unit of all tissues. It has the capacity to perform independently all life functions. Within the various tissues of the body, cells exhibit a wide range of specialisation, which are, merely amplifications of one or more of the cellular processes. Reflecting their particular functional specialization, mammalian cells have an extraordinary range of morphological forms, **Fig. 3.1** varying in size and shape, yet all cells conform to a basic model of cell structure. As viewed by the light microscope, all cells are seen to consist of **cytoplasm surrounded**

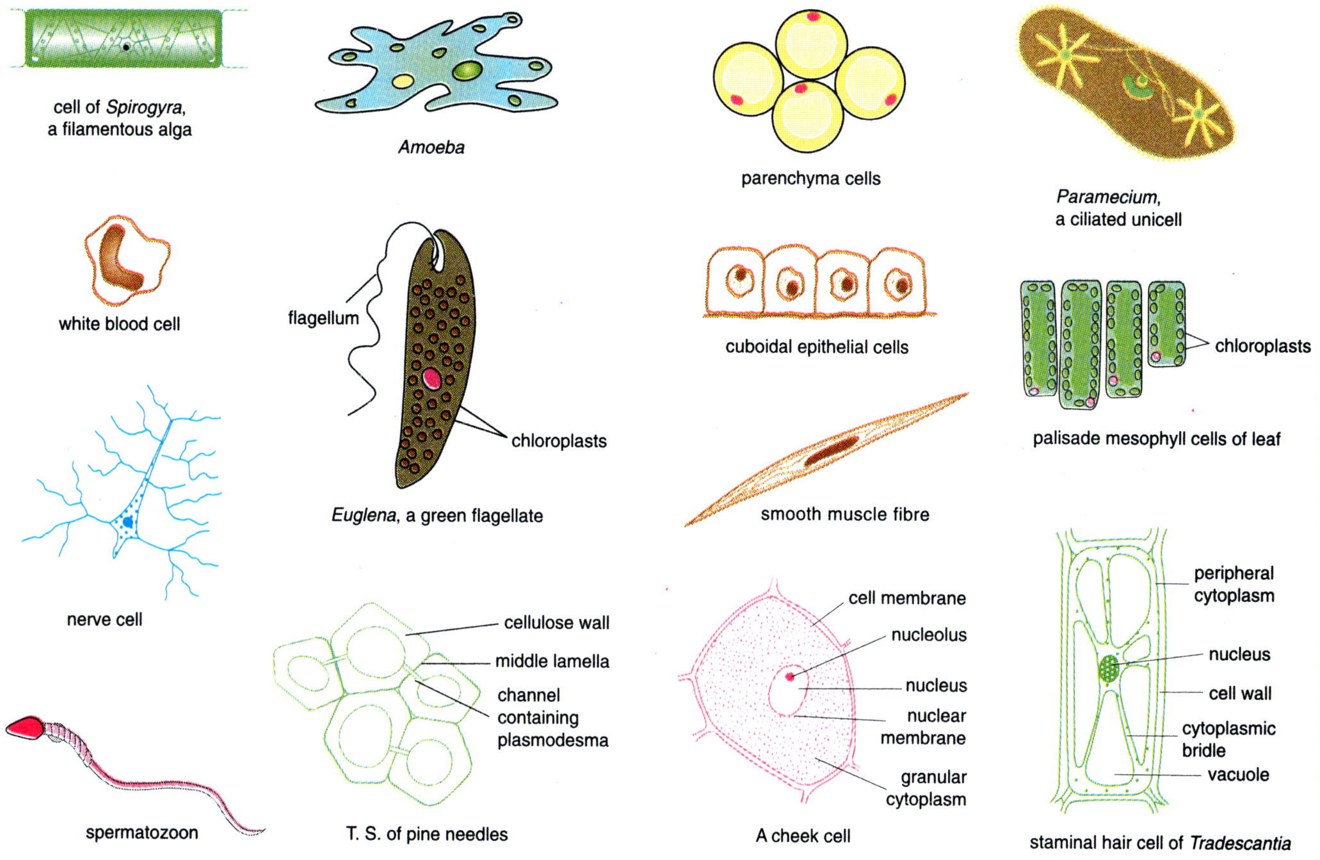

Fig. 3.1 A Variety of Different Cells (not to scale)
All cells are fundamentally similar, possessing a nucleus and cytoplasm with an array of organelles, enclosed within a membrane.

by a plasma membrane, and to contain a nucleus. As and when microscopic techniques advanced it became increasingly obvious that both the nucleus and the cytoplasm contain a number of subcellular elements, which are, called **organelles**. Typical plant cells differ from animal cells in lacking cillia or flagella and in possessing cellulose wall, chloroplasts, starch grains and permanent sap vacuole.

Most structures within cells are far too small to be resolved by light microscopy but can be observed with an electron microscope, see **Figs. 3.2–3.5.** The resolving power of the light microscope is limited to about 0.20μm (200 nm) and the study of the ultrastructure of the cell had to await the advent of the electron microscope, which at present permits the resolution of structures as small as 3.0nm (30 angstrom units).

Electron microscopy, together with the technique of **cell fractionation** i.e. disruption of cells to isolate the internal structures, **Fig. 2.5** has established a range of organelles. These cell organelles can be separated by **differentiation centrifugation** and are studied individually to ascertain their functions. The roles of the different organelles in the growth, behaviour and metabolism of cells are understood, at least in part.

Some organisms are unicellular whilst others are multicellular. Multicellular organisms show a great range of

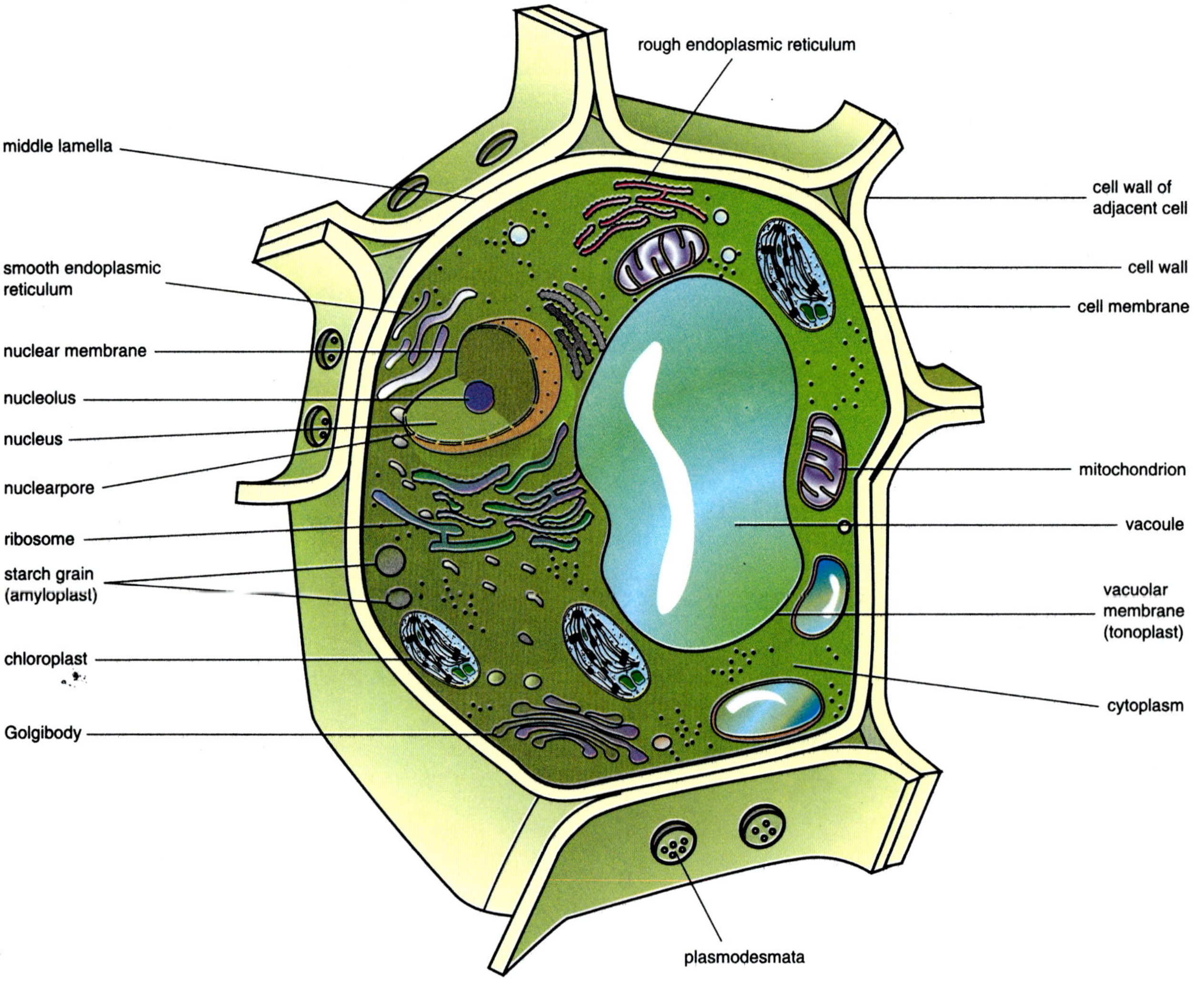

Fig. 3.2 Diagram of a Generalised Plant Cell as seen in the Electron Micoroscope

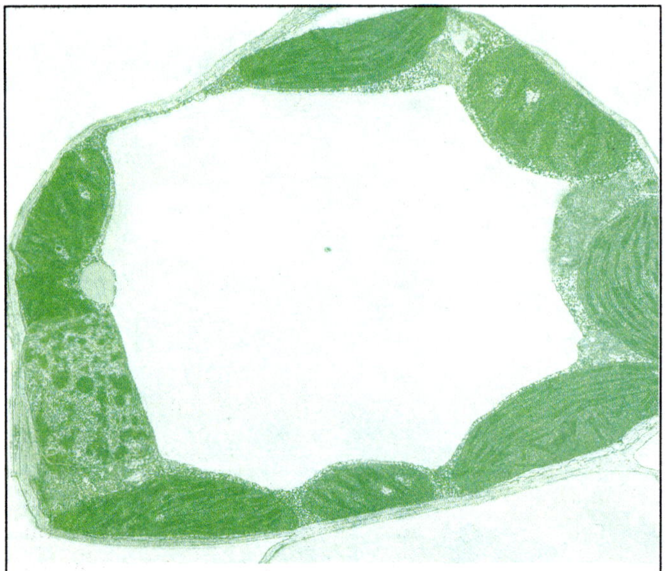

Fig. 3.3 TEM of a Plant Cell

complexity, from multicellular colonies with little or no co-ordination of component cells to multicellular organisms consisting of a vast number of cells showing marked division of labour. The specialised cells of multicellular organisms make up **tissues** (cells of similar structure that perform particular function), **organs** (collection of tissues) which combine together to form systems e.g. nervous system.

The structure of the **prokaryotic** cells is fundamentally different from that of **eukaryotes**. The prokaryotes are smaller (0.5-5μm) do not have an organised nucleus or the range of organelles that can be seen in eukaryotic cells. The eukaryotes are much larger (up to 40μm) and have a well defined nucleus and many cell organelles. The structure of the cell wall is also different **(see page 50)**.

Viruses are non-cellular. They consist of nucleic acid and protein. Within a specific host cell they bring about their own replication and subsequent release, leading to the possibility of fresh invasions of other host cells.

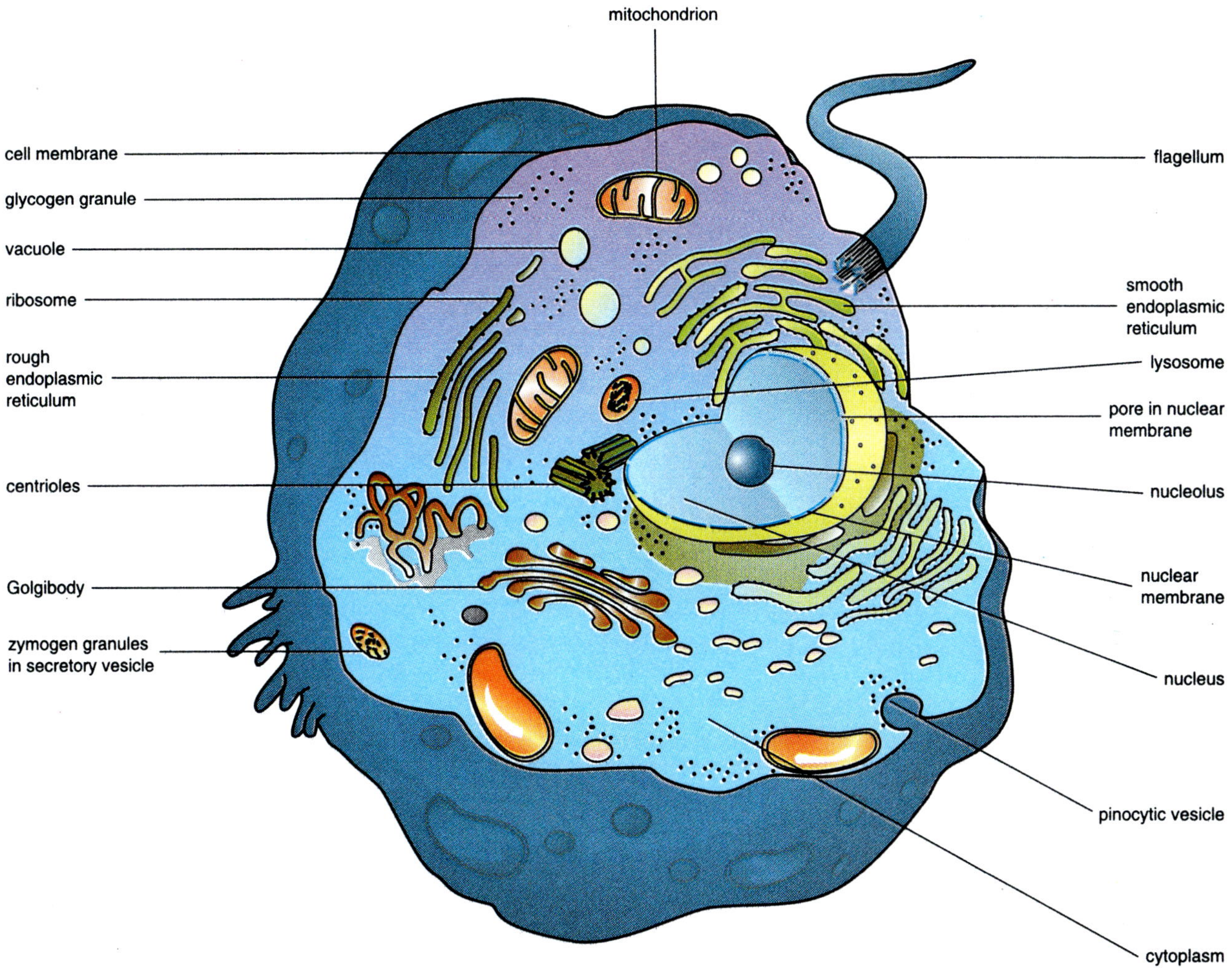

Fig. 3.4 Diagram of a Generalised Animal Cell as seen in the Electron Micoroscope

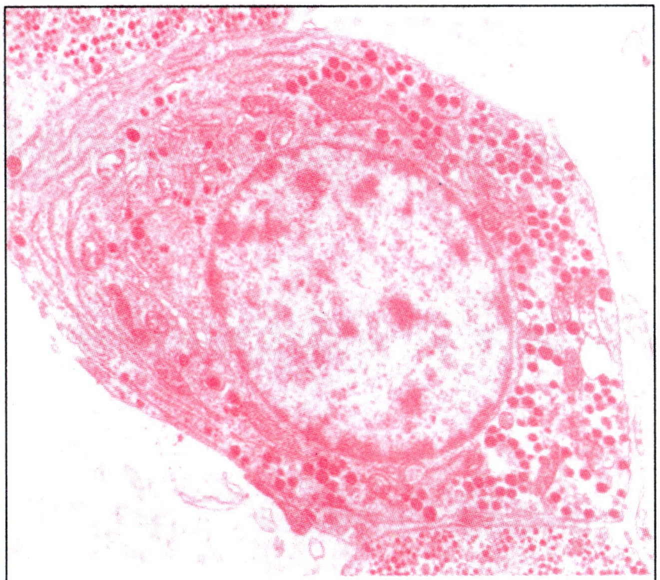

Fig. 3.5 TEM of an Aminal Cell

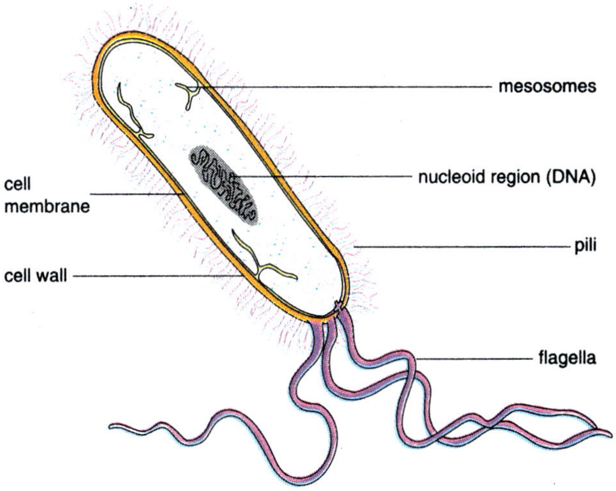

Fig. 3.6 A Prokaryotic Cell

Practical 5 – OBSERVING CELL STRUCTURE

Individual cells are extremely small and almost transparent, and are therefore difficult to observe unless treated with special stains. The various structures that are crammed into a theoretical diagram of a generalised cell are not all visible in any one cell. So to piece together the structure of a typical cell it is necessary to look at more than one type of cell. In light microscopy, it is common practice to add dyes or stains **(see page 20)** to introduce sufficient contrast, and observe different structures. Dyes and stains that are taken up by living cells are especially useful in this. The choice of stain is important since certain stains are specific to certain structures; for example actinocarmine stain is picked up by the nucleus and its contents, whereas iodine stains starch grains.

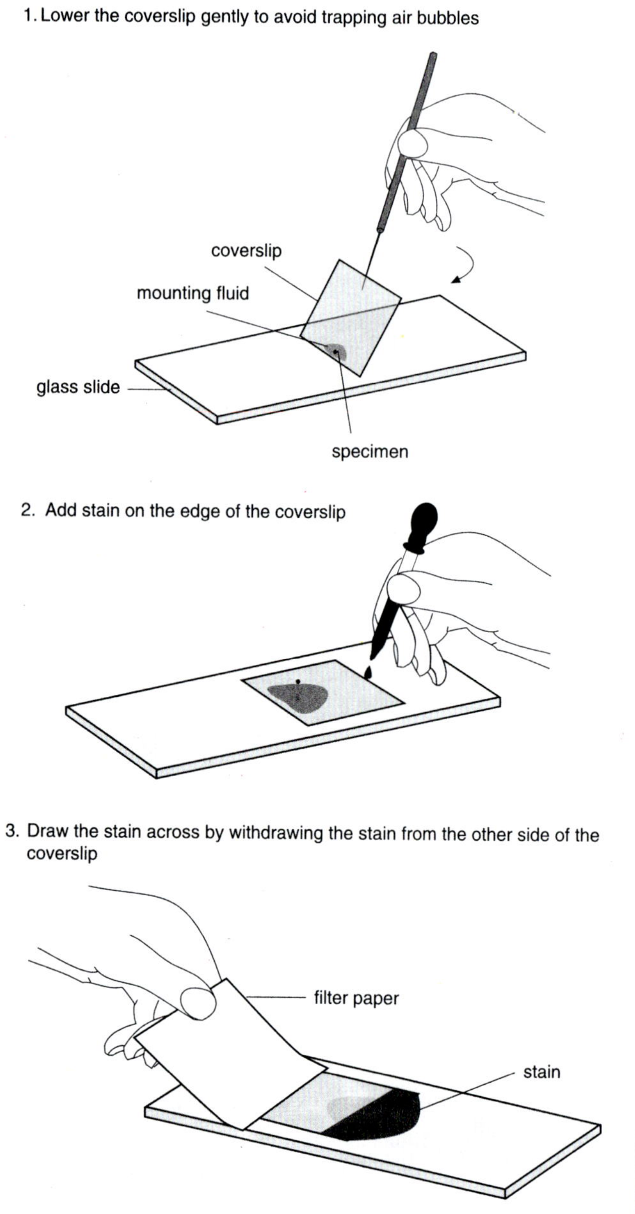

Fig. 3.7 Preparation of a Temporary Slide

Caution:

- *When working with dyes and stains, avoid contact with skin or clothing.*
- *Take care when using sharp dissection equipment.*

Observing human cheek cells

Caution:

Wash hands before you begin, and dispose of the slide in a beaker of disinfectant or absolute ethanol.

1. Gently wipe the inside lining of a your own cheek using a **fresh, clean** cotton bud or **sterilised** spatula.
2. Mount the scrapings in a drop of water on a clean microscope slide. Add a coverslip.
3. Observe first under low power, then under high power. Some of the cells will appear crumpled and irregular in outline because the cell membrane is extremely delicate and thin **Fig. 3.8.**

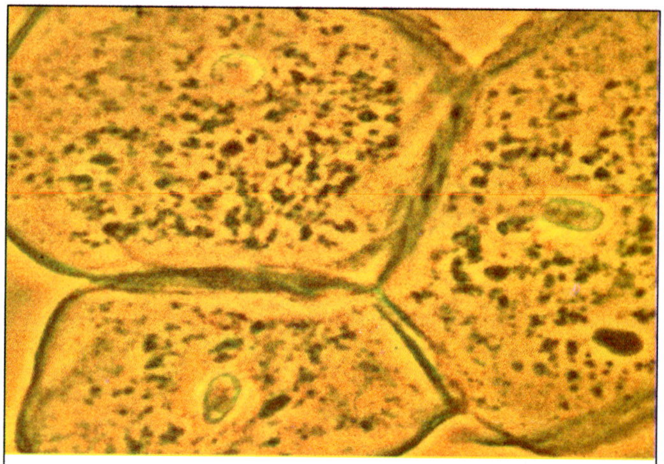

Fig. 3.8 Cells from Lining of Cheek Epithelium

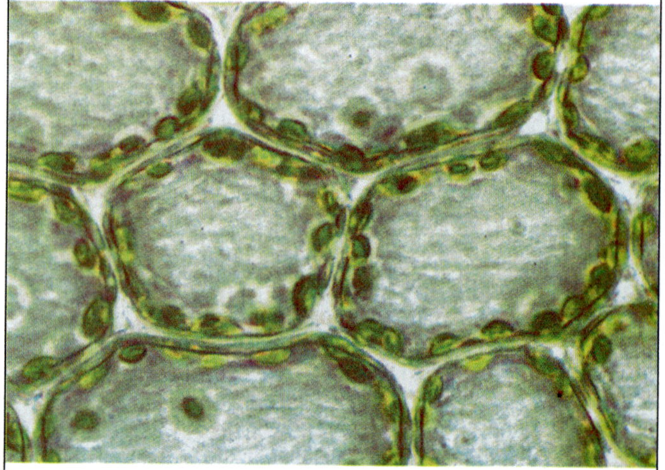

Fig. 3.9 Cells in a Moss Leaf

4. Find a single intact cell and draw your observations. Label nucleus, nuclear membrane, nucleoplasm, chromatin granules, nucleolus, granular cytoplasm and cell membrane.
5. Prepare another cheek cell slide as before.
6. Add a drop of methylene blue dye to the edge of the coverslip and remove the bulk of the dye, by withdrawing it with a piece of filter paper from the other edge **Fig. 3.7.** Examine some of the individual cells present under medium and high power magnification.
7. Observe and record your observations with annotated drawings. When drawing cells remember that each cell has its own separate cell wall, connecting to the adjacent cell with the middle lamella **Fig. 3.10**. Look for nucleus, cell membrane, and the granular cytoplasm. Pay special consideration to how the cells join with adjacent cells and the shape of cells.
8. Work out the total magnification of your drawings.
9. Now using prepared slides examine as many different plant and animal cell types as possible.

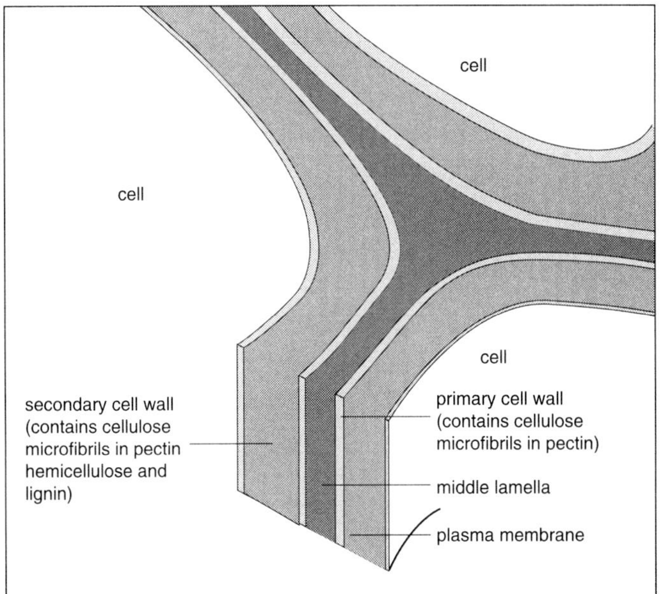

Fig. 3.10 Diagram of Cell Walls of three Connected Plant Cells

Observing chloroplasts

1. The leaf of the moss plant *(Mnium sp.)* is typically one cell thick. Place a single leaf from a moss plant, mount it on a microscope slide in a drop of glycerol, and carefully add a coverslip. Avoid trapping air bubbles.
2. Then examine individual cells under low and high power of your microscope **Fig. 3.9**.
3. Make labelled drawings of your observations.

For consideration

(a) What is the green colour of the chloroplasts caused by?

(b) What other structures (if any) of these plant cells are visible?

(c) When cells were first observed why do you think it was easier to observe plant cells than animal cells?

Observing onion (Alluim cepa) epidermis cells

1. Slice an onion bulb into half, and cut into pieces about 0.5 cm long. With a fine forceps peel off the epidermis from the inner, curved surface of one of these pieces.
2. Place this film of tissue on a microscope slide in a drop of iodine solution (I_2/KI) and carefully place a coverslip on top, making sure the tissue layer is flat and not folded. Avoid trapping air bubbles **Fig. 3.7.**
3. Leave this **temporary mount** for one or two minutes whilst the iodine penetrates the cell membrane.
4. Examine and make a labelled drawing of the cells under medium and high power magnification.
5. Notice that the iodine solution stains the living contents a light yellow colour, but the nucleus takes up the stain more strongly than the cytoplasm. The bulk of these cells are filled by a vacuole which remains unstained.
6. Observe the nucleus, nucleoli, and chromatin granules inside the nucleus, the distribution of granular cytoplasm surrounding the vacuole and the cellulose cell wall.
7. Record your observations by drawing.

For consideration

(a) Why do you think onion tissue was chosen for this exercise?

(b) What can you say about the 3-dimensional shape of the cells?

(c) The onion is a plant organ but why does it not contain chloroplasts?

(d) The leaf bases of the onion bulb are concerned with food storage, but the onion does not store carbohydrate as starch. Why do you think this is fortunate for this investigation?

(e) Make a table of the cell structures observed and relate them to their functions. Also record how each responded to the stains used.

(f) What value, if any, is there in the concept of 'the generalised plant or animal cell'?

(g) Examine some electron micrographs of plant and animal cells, identifying as many structures as possible with reference to **Figs. 3.3, 3.5.**

(h) Work out and record the size of the cell and of each organelle you have observed from the scale given on the electron micrograph.

(i) Compare the structure of plant and animal cells observed.

Observing cytoplasmic streaming

Take a few **staminal hairs** from the flower of *Tradescantia*. Mount in water and observe under high power. Notice the nucleus is suspended in the centre of the cell by thin strands of cytoplasm, attached to the peripheral layer of the cytoplasm **Fig. 3.11.**

Observe steaming of the cytoplasm by the movement of cytoplasmic granules. (You will need to focus up and down under high power to observe this. ***Make sure you only use the fine focus knob***).

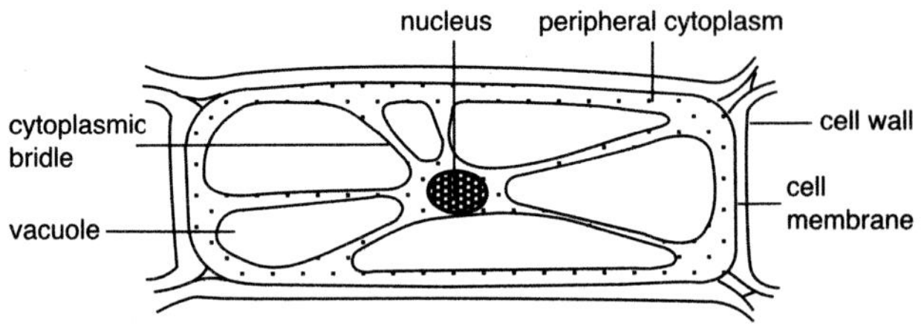

Fig. 3.11 Staminal Hair Cell of *Tradescantia*

Practical 6 – USING THE HAEMOCYTOMETER TO COUNT CELLS

Haemocytometer **Fig. 3.12** is a special microscope slide used to count the number of cells in a known volume. It can be used to count the number of red blood cells, white blood cells, yeast cells or any other kind of cells. The total number in a population of non-motile, unicellular organisms may be estimated by counting the number of cells in a representative sample.

Caution:

The haemocytometer (and its special coverslip) is an expensive piece of equipment. Treat it with care.

1. Observe the grid on the slide by holding it up against the light and/or by using a hand lens.
2. Using a Pasture pipette, place a drop of yeast cell suspension to fill the well over the grid at the centre of the slide. Carefully place the special (thickened) coverslip over the slide, without trapping any air bubbles. Move the coverslip backwards and forwards with some pressure, until you can see a coloured interference ring (Newton's rings) at the sides. The slide and coverslip are now very close together, and the depth in the central chamber is uniform. You can now count a known volume of cell suspension.
3. Examine the grid microscopically, using a x10 eyepiece with a x10 objective lens (low power) for initial focus. The central squared area (**A**) of the slide fills a field of view at this magnification. You will observe that the central squared area is subdivided into 5 x 5 = 25 smaller squares (**B**).
4. Now switch to x40 objective (high power). Note that the 25 smaller squares are each subdivided into 4 x 4 = 16 of the smaller squares (**C**).
5. Focus onto the cells present in one of the smallest squares (**C**). Count the number of cells in several of the smallest squares. **Include the cells that touch or are situated across the upper and right-hand boundary, but ignore those that cross the bottom and the left-hand boundaries**. [**Note:** for dilute suspensions count the larger squares (**B**), but for dense culture, count the smaller ones (**C**). If the culture is very dense you may need to make known dilutions of the culture before counting. Consult staff if you are uncertain.]
6. Once you are comfortable with the procedure, standardise your technique. Make known dilution of the cell suspension, make sure to stir well before you take a sample and repeat this procedure several times, taking a fresh sample every time. The approach is time-consuming, and it is sometimes difficult to differentiate between single cells and a small clump, so careful observation is essential.
7. Clean and dry the haemocytometer between counts of different samples, and also when all counts are finished. Clean it by rinsing with a jet of distilled water and dry by washing in ethanol and allowing it to evaporate. Wipe the haemocytometer with a lens tissue or a fine, soft cloth.
8. Place the haemocytometer and the coverslip in its box.

Calculation of cell numbers

The counting chamber is 0.1 mm deep. The central squared area is a 1mm square, divided into 25 main squares, each of which is subdivided into 16 smaller squares. The volume of suspension above the smallest square is **0.00025 mm^3**. Thus the number of cells in the culture suspension given is:

$$\frac{D \times N}{S \times C}$$

Where D = dilution of the original culture (if necessary)
N = total number of cells counted
S = number of squares counted
C = the volume of one 'square'.

If you have difficulty in working this out, try to work it out step by step:
Area of a small square is 0.05 x 0.05 mm^2.
Volume of small 'square' is 0.05 x 0.05 x 0.1mm^3.
Since there are 10 mm^3 in 1 cm^3, the volume of a small 'square' is : 0.05 x 0.05 x 0.1 x 10^{-3}= 2.5 x 10^{-7}cm^3.
There are 1/(2.5 x 10^{-7}) or 4 x 10^6 small squares in 1 cm^3.
If each one contains an average of three cells, the approximate number of cells per cm^3 is 1.2 x 10^7.

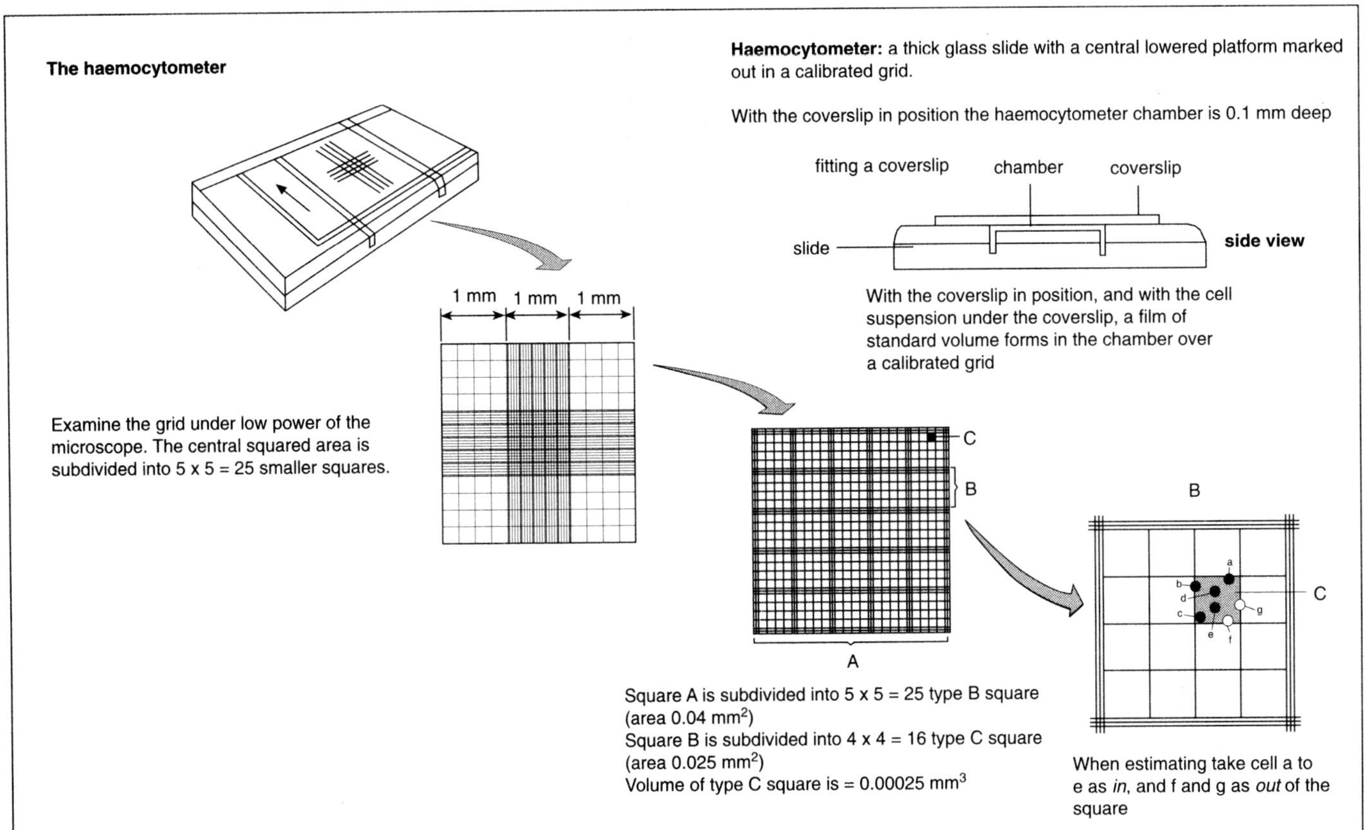

Fig. 3.12 Using a Haemocytometer

For consideration

(a) Calculate the total number of cells present. Remember that a very large number of cells need to be counted for the results to be significant. Why is this so?
(b) The count does not discriminate between living and dead cells. How would you distinguish between the two?
(c) Would this observation be significant if you were counting the cells to estimate cell population?
(d) Consider in which other circumstances the haemocytometer can be used.
(e) How are blood cells counted in modern clinical tests?
(f) Pool class data or group data to work out cell density.
(g) Do you think your estimations would remain constant over the time you took to make your observations? Explain.

Practical 7 – OBSERVING BACTERIAL CELLS

Bacteria are prokaryotes, and as such are extremely small cells; many bacteria are little larger than certain of the organelles in eukaryotic cells. Bacteria require to be stained to make them visible for viewing by high-power/oil-immersion microscopy.

Caution:

1. *Bacteria can multiply by growth and cell division in a matter of minutes rather than hours in favourable conditions and some bacteria are dangerous pathogens. Great care must therefore, be taken in all bacteriological work as a matter of essential routine.*
2. *Do not put your fingers near your mouth, nose or eyes during the experimental work.*
3. *Have a working area marked out with a sheet of lining paper and keep the apparatus you use within this zone.*
4. *At the end of the experiment, place the lining paper and all disposables in a plastic bag to be incinerated and swab down the bench with disinfectant.*
5. *Submerge tools and equipment that have come into contact with bacterial preparations in sterilising fluid immediately after use; sterilise wire loops in a hot Bunsen flame.*
6. *Wash your hands with soap and water after all practical work with bacteria.*

Bacteria in Yoghurt

1. Pass a glass slide through the blue flame of a Bunsen burner using a pair of forceps, to remove grease.
2. Transfer a drop of sterilised distilled water on to the slide using a heat sterilised inoculating loop. Dip the sterilised cooled inoculating loop in the yoghurt. Mix about half a loopful of the yoghurt with the water on the slide.
3. Smear the resultant mixture in the centre of the slide **Fig. 3.13** using another glass slide.
4. Allow the **smear** to air dry. Then **heat-fix** the smear by quickly passing the slide through the blue flame of the Bunsen burner. The slide should not become too hot for comfort when touched against the back of your hand.
5. Using a dropper, flood the slide with crystal violet stain and leave for one minute.
6. Wash clear with a gentle flow of distilled water. Blot and allow to air dry.
7. Examine the stained smear directly (without a coverslip) first under high power, and then under immersion oil (**see page 18**). Bacteria are coloured red-violet.
8. Record your observations by drawing what you see.

Bacteria in Plaque (tooth scrapings)

1. Using a sterilised inoculating loop add two drops of sterilised distilled water to a clean microscope slid.
2. Using a sterile toothpick, scrape the surface and the crevices between your teeth and mix the scrapings with the distilled water on the slide.
3. Transfer a loopful of the mixture to another clean glass slide, add a drop of nigrosin, mix and prepare a smear using the end of another glass slide.
4. Air-dry the smear and dispose of other used slides in the sterilising fluid.
5. Observe and record your observations with annotated drawings under high power/oil-immersion without a coverslip. The bacteria appear colourless with an intense blue/black background (negative staining).
6. If time permits, use an eyepiece graticule and a stage micrometer slide to estimate the size and range of bacteria present (**see page 20**).

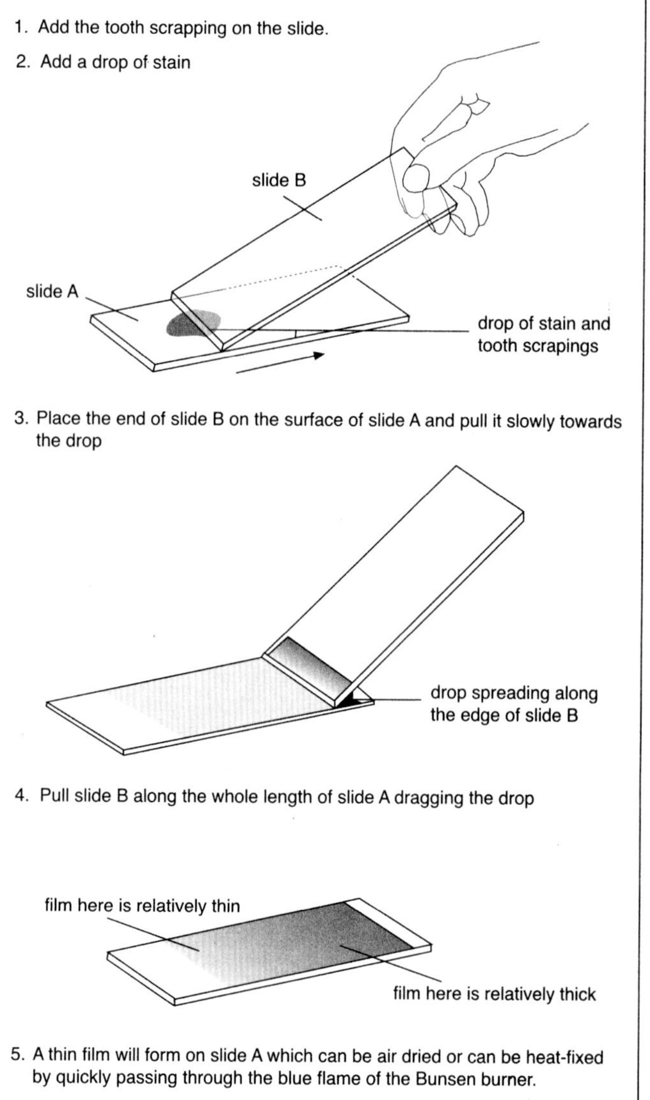

Fig. 3.13 Preparation of a Smear

For consideration

(a) Compare and contrast bacterial cells with other cells you have observed in previous investigations.

(b) What are the sources of danger from bacteria when you are working with materials such as yoghurt and tooth scrapings?

4 Transfer of Substances through the Cell

Transfer of Substances through the Cell

Cells and Osmosis

Red Blood Cells

Plant Epidermis

Filamentous Algae

Effect of Temperature on Cell Membrane

Movement of Ions through the Cell Membrane

The Water Potential of Cells of an Inflorescence Stalk

Osmotic Fragility of Red Blood Cells

Water Potential of Plant Cells

Transfer of Substances through the Cell

Background Summary

Substances move in and out of cells by crossing the cell membrane by **diffusion**, **osmosis**, **active transport**, **endocytosis** and **exocytosis**. The cell membrane actively controls transport in and out of the cell.

Diffusion is the net movement of particles from a region of high concentration to a region of lower concentration. Diffusion satisfies the metabolic needs of small organisms whose **surface-volume ratio** is large and where the diffusion distance is small. Large organisms, whose surface-volume ratio is small, and where the diffusion distance is great, have special ways of acquiring essential materials and transporting them within the body.

Facilitated diffusion–protein carriers in the cell membrane help to move the molecules or ions down concentration gradients **Fig. 4.1**.

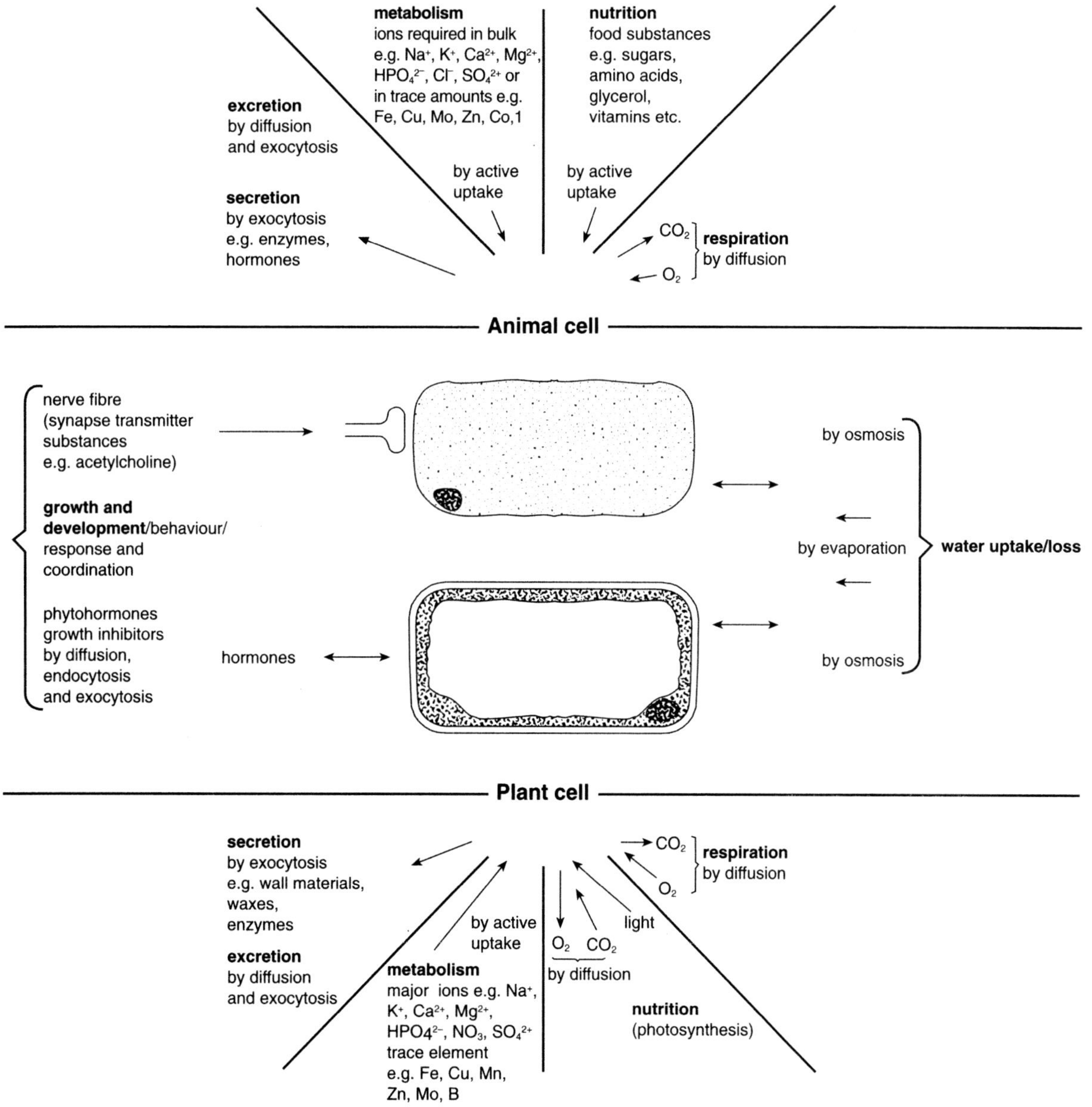

Fig. 4.1 Summary of Movement of Substances in and out of Cells

Osmosis

Osmosis is the one-way net diffusion of solvent (particularly water) across a **selectively permeable membrane.** It plays a vital role in cell homeostasis. Cell water relations are determined by osmotic concentration of the cell sap (**solute potential**) and the **pressure potential** of the cell (pressure due to the cell wall or the turgidity of the cell).

The osmotic movement of water can be expressed in terms of **osmotic pressure**. This is the tendency of a solution to take in water across a selectively permeable membrane.

An animal cell immersed in a **hypotonic** (external solution more dilute than the cell) solution swells and may burst unless it has means of disposing of the water that enters by osmosis. In a **hypertonic** solution the cell shrinks and the cell membrane crinkles. Whereas a plant cell immersed in water or a hypotonic solution becomes **turgid**. If immersed in a hypertonic solution the protoplast shrinks and **plasmolysis** occurs. (The protoplast membrane is selectively permeable but the cellulose wall is fully permeable.)

As a way of expressing water movement, osmotic pressure is increasingly being replaced by the **water potential** concept. For practical purposes, water potential is the capacity of a system to give out water, and it is given a negative sign. The component of the water potential, which is caused by the presence of solutes, is called the **osmotic potential**. The symbol for water potential and related energy potentials is the Greek letter psi (ψ).

The water relations of a plant cell can be summarised as follows:

$$\psi_{cell} = \psi_s + \psi_p$$

Where:

ψ_{cell} is the water potential of the cell (usually negative),

ψ_s is the osmotic potential of the sap (negative),

ψ_p is the **pressure potential** – that is the inward pressure exerted by the cell wall against the protoplast (zero or positive).

The water potential of a plant tissue can be determined by balancing it with an external solution, which produces no mass or volume change in the tissue. The osmotic potential can be determined by balancing it with an external solution that produces incipient plasmolysis.

Active transport is a highly selective process in which the movement of particles is against a concentration gradient. It is an energy requiring process involving the use of protein carriers in the cell membrane.

Bulk transport of substances in the cells takes place by invagination of the cell membrane to form vesicles, generally referred to as **endocytosis.** There are three types of endocytosis, **phagocytosis** ('cellular eating'), **pinocytosis** ('cellular drinking') and **receptor-mediated endocytosis**. The reverse process is known as **exocytosis** (expulsion out of cells). Basically the cell wraps pseudopodia around the substance to be engulfed, forming a membrane-enclosed vacuole. The package is digested after the vacuole is fused with a lysosome containing hydrolytic enzyme. The receptor-mediated endocytosis is very specific. The extracellular substance binds to the receptor (called **ligand**) located in the cell membrane, forming a pit and the substance is transferred inside this pit. Endocytosis and exocytosis provides a means by which liquids and macromolecules may be brought in and out of cells.

Practical 8 – CELLS AND OSMOSIS

All cells are enclosed in a selectively permeable membrane. If an animal cell is placed in hypotonic solution water enters the cell by osmosis and the cell swells. In extreme cases the cell bursts. If, however, the external solution is hypertonic, water leaves the cell and the cell shrinks.

In plant cells the cellulose wall, though fairly rigid, is fully permeable to both water and solutes. In hypertonic solutions the plant cell displays plasmolysis but the cell shape does not alter. In hypotonic solution the cell is seen to become turgid **Fig. 4.2.**

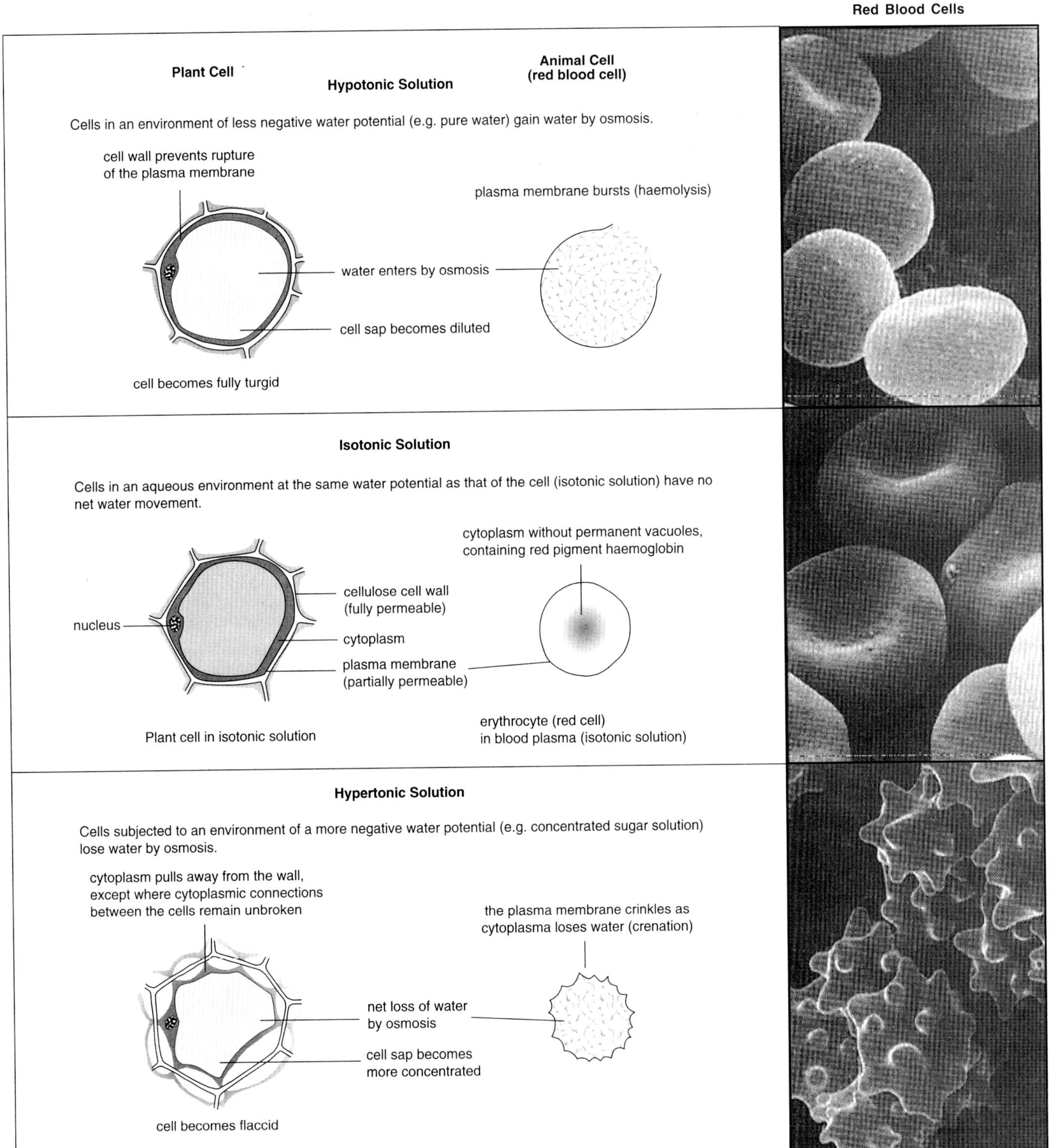

Fig. 4.2 Cells and Osmosis

Procedure

Red blood cells

1. Place a drop of blood on a slide.
2. Add a drop of 0.5% NaCl solution to the drop of blood. Mix.
3. Observe under high power of the microscope for the next five minutes.
4. Record your observations with labelled drawings.
5. Repeat steps 1–4 using 0.9% NaCl solution and then 3.0% NaCl solution on a clean glass slide each time.
6. Interpret your observations as fully as you can.

Plant epidermis

1. Strip off small pieces of epidermis from a plant stem or leaf. (The outer epidermis from the surface of red onion scale or the red pigmented epidermis from a leaf of *Tradescantia virginiana* is recommended.)
2. Mount one piece in water and the other in a solution of sucrose (1.0 mol dm^{-3}).

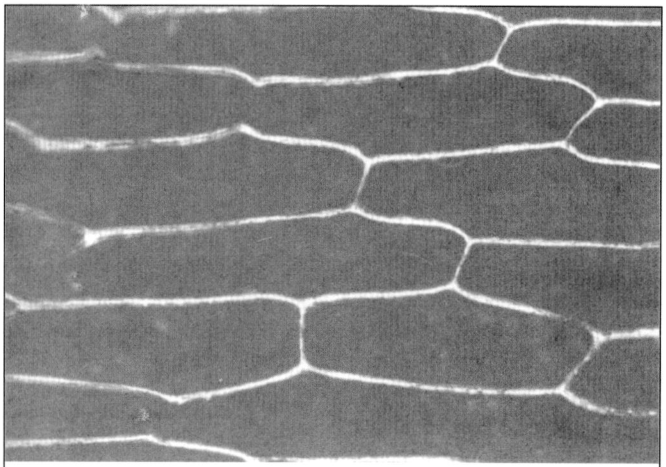

Fig. 4.3 Turgid Cells of Onion Epidermis

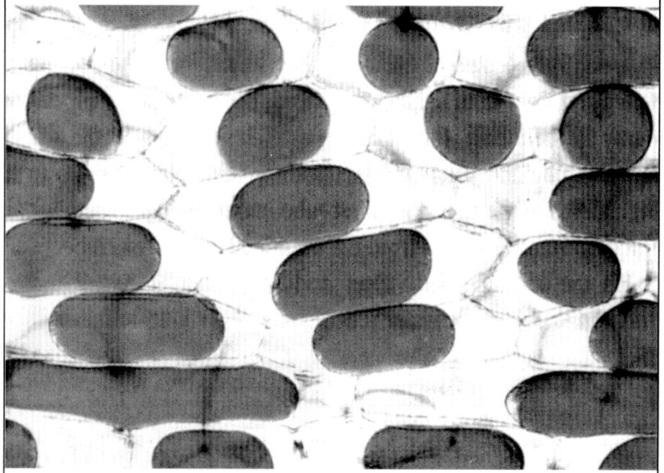

Fig. 4.4 Plasmolysed Cells of Onion Epidermis

3. Observe and record your observations by drawing what you see at once and then after 5 minutes **Fig. 4.3** and **Fig. 4.4.**
4. Prepare another slide in a solution of potassium nitrate (1.0 mol dm^{-3}), and observe at once and then after 5 minutes. Compare with the slide mounted in sucrose solution.
5. Observe exactly where the red pigment is located within the cell.
6. Irrigate the piece of epidermis, which you mounted in sucrose, with distilled water. Use filter paper to draw the water beneath the coverslip **Fig. 3.5** and look down the microscope as you do so. Observe what happens and interpret your result.

Reference: UCLES, Question 2, 26th May, 1993.

Reference: UCLES, Question 2, 9th Nov. 1994.

Reference: UCLES, Question 2, 3rd Nov. 1997.

Filamentous algae

1. Mount one small piece of the filamentous algae *Cladophora* in water, and a second piece in a strong sucrose solution (1.0 mol dm^{-3}).
2. Compare the two slides and interpret your observations.
3. Mount one piece of *Cladophora* in a 1.0 mol dm^{-3} solution of sucrose, and a second piece in a 1.0 mol dm^{-3} solution of sodium chloride.
4. Compare:
   (i) how long it takes for plasmolysis to occur in each solution?
   (ii) Which one works faster?
   (iii) Can you suggest a reason?
   (iv) What does this tell you about the nature of osmosis?
   (v) Why is it better to do this experiment using *Cladophora* rather than plant epidermal tissue?

For consideration

(a) What can you infer from your observations about the molecular mass of the pigment?

(b) Both the sucrose and the potassium nitrate are equimolar. Explain any differences in your observations (think about the size/molecular mass of the ions in the solutions).

(c) What is the relevance of your observations on the osmotic properties of cells to the organisms concerned?

(d) Did you find it easier to observe plasmolysis in the algae cells than in the plant epidermal cells, and if so why?

Practical 9 – EFFECT OF TEMPERATURE ON CELL MEMBRANE

Beetroot contains a water-soluble red pigment called anthocyanin, which occurs in the cell vacuoles. The vacuole is surrounded by a **tonoplast membrane**, outside which is the cytoplasm surrounded by the plasma membrane. It is not possible to observe the structure of the membranes under the light microscope but we can observe the effect of temperature on it and the rate at which anthocyanin leaves the cell through these membranes.

Procedure

1. In a $250cm^3$ beaker heat distilled water to 100˚C.
2. Label twelve test tubes and twelve $100cm^3$ beakers as 85, 80, 75, 70, 65, 60, 55, 50, 45, 40, 35 and 30.
3. Add 10 cm^3 of distilled water (at room temperature) into each of the labelled test tubes.
4. Carefully pour small amount of hot distilled water labelled 85 (enough to cover a beetroot cylinder) into the beaker and adjust the temperature to 85˚C **Fig. 4.5.**
5. Place a beetroot cylinder, into the beaker of water at 85˚C for exactly one minute.
6. After one minute transfer the cylinder to the test tube of cold water marked 85 using forceps. Note the time.
7. Repeat steps 4–6, using a fresh cylinder each time, at the following temperatures: 80˚C, 75˚C, 70˚C, 65˚C, 60˚C, 55˚C, 50˚C, 45˚C, 40˚C, 35˚C, and 30˚C.
8. Leave each cylinder in the test tube of distilled water for **exactly** 30 minutes.
9. After 30 minutes shake the test tubes and remove and discard the beetroot cylinders. By now you should have twelve test tubes containing red coloured water.
10. Using a colorimeter (for a red solution a blue filter is required) compare the amount of red pigment, which has diffused out of the beetroot cylinder. (If you do not have access to a colorimeter, grade the colours visually, denoting zero to distilled water and 12 to the darkest solution.)
11. Tabulate your data, and plot a graph of optical density against temperature.

For consideration

(a) According to the current theory of the structure of the cell membrane explain what prevents the pigment anthocyanin from diffusing out of the cells at room temperature?

(b) What implications do these results have for bacteria living in hot springs at 80˚C?

(c) Why is it useful for the beetroot to have the anthocyanin pigment in the vacuole of their cells?

(d) How can you take your investigations further, given more time?

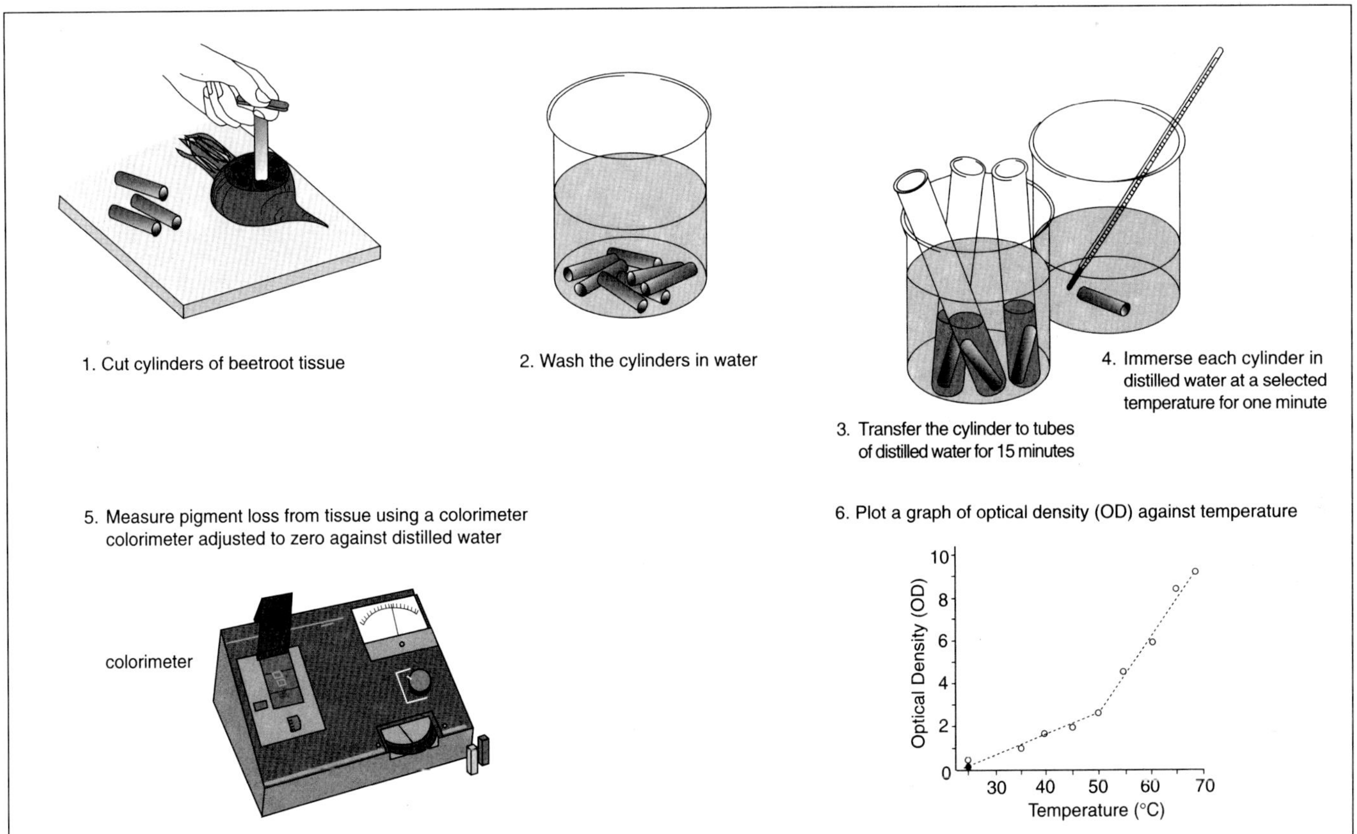

Fig. 4.5 Effect of Temperature on Cell Membrane

Practical 10 (a) – MOVEMENT OF IONS THROUGH THE CELL MEMBRANE

Ions move across the cell membrane at different rates, depending on the cell membrane, solubility in lipids and the availability of protein-carrier molecule present to recognise the ion and to take it across the membrane by facilitated diffusion or active transport.
The red pigment anthocyanin, found in red cabbage and beetroot, is confined within the vacuole of the cells. It is pH sensitive and is *red* at neutral and acidic pH but turns *blue* in alkaline conditions. Ammonium chloride is a weakly acidic compound, which dissociates completely in solution into ammonium and chloride ions. These ions can move across the membrane independently. In this investigation a change in the colour of the anthocyanin pigment is used as indication of the movement of these ions.

Procedure

1. Tear a piece of cabbage leaf, twisting it whilst tearing it to enable you to peel off the thin transparent upper or lower epidermis away from the underlying tissue.
2. Mount a small piece of the epidermal layer in distilled water. Carefully place a coverslip on top and observe under high power.
3. Prepare two more slides; mount one in distilled water, the other in 1.0 mol dm^{-3} ammonium chloride solution. Label them appropriately and examine them under high power **after** five minutes.
4. Record your observations with annotated drawings. Note the colour and shape of the cell content.

Reference: UCLES, Question 2, 7th Nov. 1994.

For consideration

(a) What can you say about the water potential of the ammonium chloride solution?
(b) What evidence suggests that the ammonium and the chloride ions do not migrate together?
(c) Which of the two ions migrate faster across cell membranes? (The radius of the ammonium ion is 0.143nm and that of the chloride ion is 0.198nm).
(d) Which of the two ions is likely to be more useful to the plant cell and why?

Practical 10 (b) – THE WATER POTENTIAL OF CELLS OF AN INFLORESCENCE STALK

Procedure

1. Cut narrow strips of tissue about 2mm wide, from a length of a hollow stalk of dandelion (*Taraxacum officinate)* inflorescence, each 2.0cm in length. It is advisable to try and cut the strips from the same region of the stalk.
2. Prepare solutions of varying concentrations from 0-0.5 mol dm^{-3} in labelled covered Petri dishes using a 1.0 mol dm^{-3} stock solution of sucrose and distilled water.
3. Immerse at least two strips in each solution.
4. Observe and record by drawing, the change in shape of the strips after 5 and 10 minutes of immersion.

Reference: UCLES, Question 2, 21st May, 1991
Reference: UCLES, Question 2, 19th May, 1998.

For consideration

(a) Write a full report giving details of your experimental procedure, results, conclusion and any further suggestions.
(b) Why was it necessary to cut the strips from the same region of stalk?
(c) Exactly how much sucrose ($C_{12}H_{22}O_{11,}$ M.Wt = 342) should be weighed out to prepare one litre of 1.0 mol dm^{-3} solution?
(d) Why are the Petri dishes kept covered?
(e) What type of cells form the outer margins of the stalk, and how do they differ in structure from the cells of the outer cortex (the remaining cells of the tissue strips)?
(f) What changes have occurred in the cells of the tissue strips immersed in 0.5 mol dm^{-3} sucrose solution to cause the change in their shape?
(g) What is the approximate water potential of the stalk cells? Explain your reasoning.
(h) If the experiment was repeated with a dandelion plant growing on a high exposed wall after a period of low rainfall, what difference in results would you anticipate?
(i) What results would you expect if the tissue were immersed in ethanol prior to immersion in sucrose solution?

Practical 11 – OSMOTIC FRAGILITY OF RED BLOOD CELLS

Red blood cells like all eukaryotic cells are enclosed in a selectively permeable membrane (plasma membrane). The plasma membrane is not a rigid array of molecules. The phospholipids flip-flop freely within their own half of the bi-layer structure and hence the membrane is fairly fragile. If a red blood cell is placed in hypotonic solution, water enters by osmosis and the cell swells, and eventually bursts, releasing the enclosed haemoglobin (haemolysis). In hypertonic solutions the reverse takes place and the cell 'crinkles' (crenation) see **Fig. 4.2.** Red blood cells, which are more prone to haemolysis, help in diagnosing blood diseases such as haemolytic anaemia. In this investigation you will examine the effect of hypotonic and hypertonic solutions on mammalian red blood cells and investigate the mechanical properties of the plasma membrane.

Procedure

1. Label seven centrifuge tubes: 0, 0.1, 0.3, 0.5, 0.7, 0.9 and 1.0.
2. Using distilled water and 1.0% NaCl solution as stock, make up 10 ml of each of the following NaCl solutions: 0, 0.1, 0.3, 0.5, 0.7, 0.9 and 1.0% in the centrifuge tubes.
3. Mix the defibrinated blood thoroughly to insure an even distribution of the red blood cells.
4. Add 0.1 cm^3 of defibrinated blood to the first centrifuge tube, mix well and examine a drop of the solution under the microscope at once and at 2-minute intervals for ten minutes.
5. Repeat steps 3 and 4 with each of the other remaining tubes.
6. Using the diluted blood in 0.9% solution and a haemocytometer, estimate the number of red blood cells per cm^3 of blood (use of haemocytometer **(see page 30).**
7. Centrifuge the remaining solutions for 3 minutes at full speed (about 5000 rpm) in a bench centrifuge.
8. If a colorimeter is available measure the absorbance of the supernatant in each tube against distilled water.
9. If you do not have access to a colorimeter use the haemocytometer to count the intact red blood cells in each tube.
10. Calculate the percentage haemolysis for each solution assuming that all the cells are haemolysed in distilled water.
11. Compare and comment on the amount of sediment in each tube.
12. Plot an osmotic fragility curve from your results (% haemolysed against NaCl concentration %): No haemolysis should occur in 0.9% solution as the cells are in an **isotonic solution**, (external environment is similar to the internal environment), so this tube should give normal blood count.

To calculate the number of haemolysed cells per mm^3 of blood in the other tubes subtract the number of intact cells present in each sample from the number in the 0.9% NaCl.

Calculate the percentage of cells haemolysed:

$$\text{Percentage haemolysis} = \frac{a}{b}$$

Where:
a = number of haemolysed cells per mm^3
b = number of intact cells per mm^3 in 0.9 % NaCl
Plot percentage haemolysis (y-axis) against the concentration of the NaCl solutions (x-*axis*).

For consideration

(a) Explain your observations in step 4 for each dilution.
(b) Comment on the shape of the curve?
(c) Did all red blood cells haemolyse at the same NaCl concentration? If not, explain why.
(d) Comment on the mechanical properties of the plasma membranes.

Practical 12 – WATER POTENTIAL OF PLANT CELLS

Plant cells are surrounded by a cellulose cell wall. Though it is porous and permeable to aqueous solution, it is fairly tough and elastic. The protoplast is enclosed within the cell membrane, which is more permeable to water than to many other kinds of solutes. Most of the sap is localised in one or more large vacuoles bounded by a tonoplast membrane.

If a plant cell is immersed in an isotonic solution there is no net loss or gain of water; the water potential of the external solution will be equal to the water potential of the cell.

This can be demonstrated by using plant tissue such as a potato tuber. Samples of tissue are immersed in a range of external solutions of different concentrations. The solution that induces neither an increase nor a decrease in the volume or mass of the tissue has the same water potential as that of the cells in the tissue.

Procedure

1. Label the base of six Petri dishes: 0, 0.1, 0.2, 0.3, 0.4, and 0.5.
2. Using the 0.5 mol dm^{-3} sucrose solution and distilled water, prepare 20 cm^3 of sucrose solutions of 0.1–0.5 mol dm^{-3} in the appropriate Petri dishes.
3. Place 20 cm^3 of distilled water in the Petri dish labelled 0.
4. Carefully cut 12 potato cylinders, each 2cm in length.
5. If an accurate balance is available, weigh and record the weight and the exact length of a pair of 2cm-potato cylinder after wiping them dry with a tissue. (In each case weigh them on the piece of filter paper, then weigh the filter paper alone, and subtract one from the other to get the mass of the cylinder.) Record the mass and length of each cylinder in the table. (If you do not have access to a balance, record the length only.)

Conc.	IL (mm)	FL (mm)	Diff. L (mm)	Avg. L (mm)	IM (mg)	FM (mg)	Diff. M (mg)	Avg. M (mg)	KPa
0									
0									
0.1									
0.1									
0.2									
0.2									
0.3									
0.3									
0.4									
0.4									
0.4									
0.5									
0.5									

IL = initial length (mm), FL = final length (mm), IM = initial mass (mg), FM = final mass (mg),
Diff. L = difference in length, Diff. M = difference in mass, Avg. L = average length, Avg. M = average mass

6. Place two cylinders of known mass and length in the first Petri dish. Cover with a lid and leave overnight.
7. Place pairs of potato cylinders of known mass and length in each of the other Petri dishes.
8. After about 24 hours remove a cylinder from a Petri dish, wipe away any surplus fluid with tissue or filter paper. Then re-weigh, re-measure and record the new mass and length in the table for each cylinder.
9. Plot a graph of percentage change in mass (change in mass multiplied by 100 divided by original mass) against the concentration (molarity) of the sucrose solutions. The latter, being the independent variable should be on the horizontal axis, the former on the vertical axis on the left-hand side. Plot on the same graph, change in length against the concentration of sucrose solution, showing the length on the right hand vertical axis.
10. Calculate the water potential of the potato cells as follows:
Find the point on your graph corresponding to a percentage mass/length of zero. The concentration of sucrose corresponding to this zero mass/length change can now be read from the horizontal axis. In the table below find the water potential of a sucrose solution of that concentration. That is the water potential of your sample of potato cells. Express your result in kPa.

Relationship between concentration and osmotic potential of sucrose solutions

Molarity (mol dm^{-3})	Osmotic potential (kPa)
0.05	-130
0.10	-260
0.15	-410
0.20	-540
0.25	-680
0.30	-860
0.35	-970
0.40	-1120
0.45	-1280
0.50	-1450
0.55	-1620
0.60	-1620
0.65	-1980
0.70	-2180
0.75	-2370
0.80	-2580
0.85	-2790
0.95	-3250
0.90	-3000
1.00	-3500

For consideration

(a) Criticise this method of finding the water potential of plant cells. Suggest how it could be improved?
(b) With what kind of plant tissue might it be possible to use a change in volume rather than mass or length for estimating the water potential?
(c) Explain the change observed in your potato cylinders.
(d) Why is turgidity of cells important to plants?
(e) How does the value of the water potential differ from the osmotic potential of the solution in the vacuole?
(f) Could this technique be used with animal tissue? Explain.
(g) What was the reason for using a pair of cylinders and why was it necessary to standardise the procedure for drying the cylinders?
(h) In constructing your graph did you join the points with straight lines or a smooth curve? Justify whichever techique you used.

Reference: UCLES, Question 2, 21st May, 1991.

5 Bacteriology

Bateriology

Background Summary

Bacteria are unicellular, prokaryotic organisms that occur in vast numbers, practically everywhere. They are extremely small colourless cells (average diameter about 1μm) and although they can be seen with phase contrast microscopy without staining to be viewed under the light microscope (high powered/oil-immersion) they have to be killed and stained. Whilst some bacteria are parasitic and cause disease, most are **saprotrophic** (feed on dead organic material) and harmless (in fact many are very useful and essential for life!)
Although most species of bacteria are harmless to humans we should handle all cultures as if they were pathogenic. If even a small number of harmless bacteria happen to enter our body by accident via ingestion or a cut they could have ill effects, since in favourable conditions bacteria can multiply within minutes. Contamination by pathogenic species could be lethal.
Consequently, pathogens should only be handled by experienced bacteriologists, and even non-pathogenic species should be handled with extreme care under aseptic (sterile) conditions.

Essential Precautions

Aseptic techniques are an essential part of safety procedures and must be followed carefully whenever cell cultures are handled.

The following are essential precautions to take in all microbiological work:

(a) Wash your hands thoroughly with soap and water before and after all practical work.
(b) Never eat or drink in the laboratory.
(c) Do not put your fingers in your mouth, nose and eyes whilst working with bacterial cultures.
(d) Never 'mouth pipette' bacterial cultures. Instead use a pipette pump.
(e) Cover the worktop with a sheet of lining paper, and keep all apparatus within this zone.
(f) Keep containers such as Petri dishes and flasks covered, except when opening them for inoculation.
(g) Tape Petri dish lids to the dish bases immediately after they are inoculated (but not all the way round since this might exclude air and encourage growth of anaerobic bacteria, if present). Do not open these Petri dishes unless they have been sterilised.
(h) Do not incubate cultures above 30°C or near human body temperature.
(i) Used plates must be sterilised (in a pressure cooker or autoclave) before the contents are disposed of and the dishes washed.
(j) At the end of the experiment, incinerate the lining paper, and swab down the bench with disinfectant.

Aseptic Techniques

Bacteria and fungal spores are abundant in our environment; hence aseptic (sterile) techniques are applied to prevent contamination of cultures. All equipment, distilled water etc. has to be sterilised, usually by heat treatment or in some cases by radiation. Usually sterilised covered glass or plastic plates called Petri dishes are used to grow bacteria cultures either on solid media (agar) or in an appropriate liquid medium.

Setting up sterile nutrient agar plates

Bacteria are normally grown over agar plates in Petri dishes. Agar is a long chain polysaccharide obtained commercially from red algae. A 1-2% aqueous solution of agar is usually prepared which melts at about 95-100°C and sets to give a firm transparent gel which remains solid below 44°C. Micro-organisms do not normally digest agar and hence can be grown on the solid agar gel surface or added to the liquid, if they are not damaged around 44°C. Appropriate nutrients for the growth of particular micro-organisms are added to the agar. Nutrient agar is a formulation commercially available, containing peptone, meat extract and water.

Practical 13 – EXAMINING BACTERIA IN MILK

Note: this investigation may take over 24 hours.

During milking, bacteria inevitably enter the milk even under the most hygienic conditions. This is why milk should be **Pasteurised** (a process of rapidly heating and then cooling and again heating, first attempted by Louis Pasteur) before consumption. Although most pathogenic bacteria are killed during pasteurisation many non-pathogenic bacteria survive. The most commonly found bacteria present in milk are *Streptococcus lactis* (spherical in shape, often in chains) and *Lactobacillus* (rod shaped, stuck together to form chains) **Fig. 5.1.**
These cause the milk to sour by producing lactic acid, as the lactose in milk ferments anaerobically. There may also be other bacteria present as well.
For this investigation you are provided with fresh unboiled milk, boiled milk, (kept in an ordinary refrigerator) stale milk (left at room temperature overnight), sterile nutrient agar, peptone agar and Petri dishes. Plan your own investigation, and investigate the number of bacteria in the different milk samples over a period of 24 hours.
After inoculation, the plates should be kept at 30°C in an incubator, if available or at room temperature.
Carefully plan your investigation on paper, with the following points in mind:

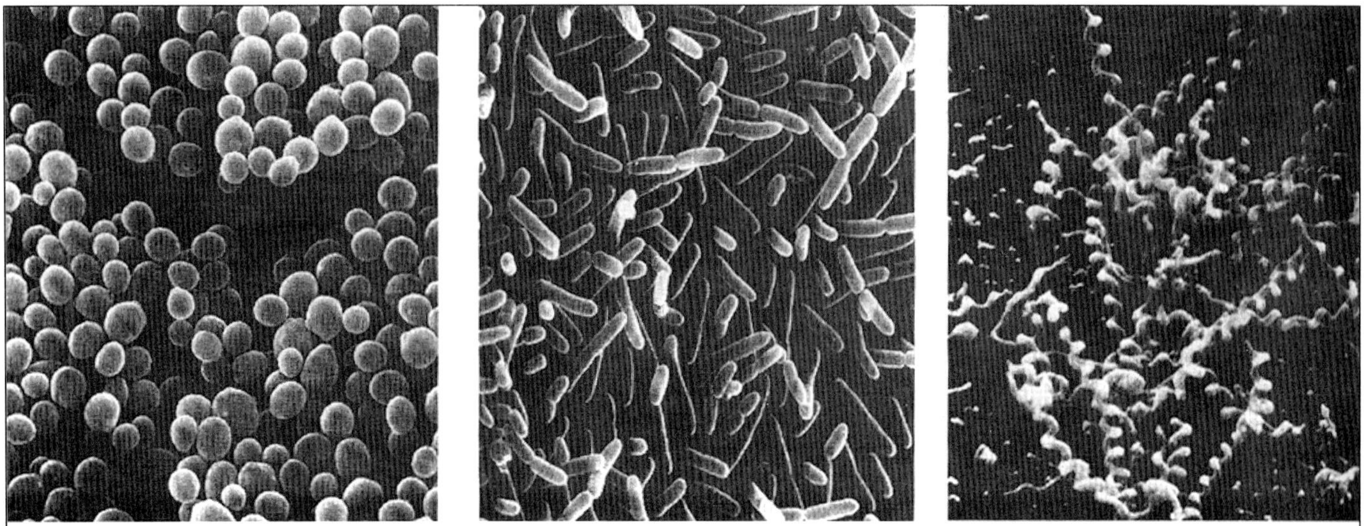

Fig. 5.1 SEM of Common Shapes of Prokeryotes

(i) Decide on how many plates you would require, remembering to add some kind of control in your investigations, (pour a few extra plates).

(ii) Make sure you know exactly what to do before you begin, ask for help if unsure.

(iii) Read the precautions given on **page 31**.

(iv) Begin by pouring out the plates, making sure to follow aseptic techniques to avoid contamination.

(v) The numbers of bacteria in milk are very high. If undiluted milk is poured on a plate and incubated overnight, so many colonies of bacteria will grow that it will be impossible to distinguish them for counting. Prepare serial dilutions **Fig. 5.2** of your sample using sterilised pipettes, test tubes and sterilised distilled water. (To 1 cm^3 of milk or milk dilution add 9 cm^3 of sterilised distilled water each time, and mix thoroughly before sampling further.)

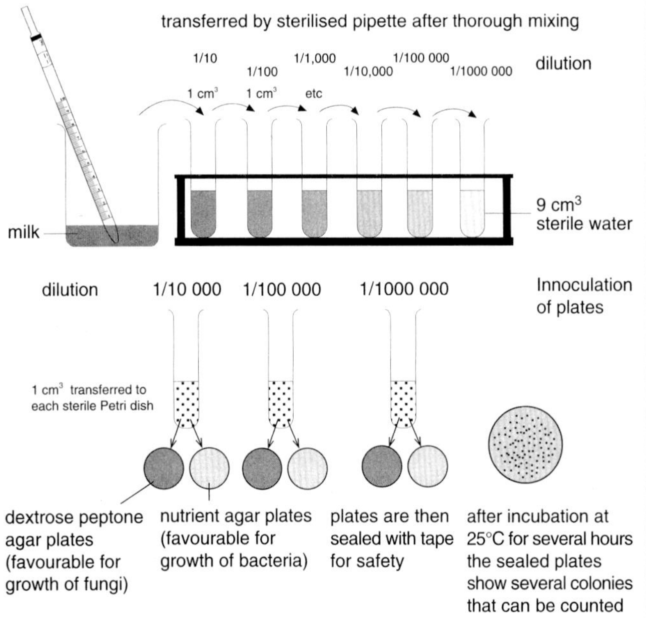

Fig. 5.2 Serial Dilutions

(vi) It is suggested that you make the following dilutions: 1/10, 1/100, and 1/1000 and then estimate the number of bacteria present in the original sample.

Pouring agar plates Fig. 5.3

1. Place the flask of agar in a beaker of boiling water, to melt the agar. When the agar is completely molten, remove the flask and leave it to cool to a temperate just comfortable to handle (about 50°C, but no cooler, for agar sets at 44°C).
2. Now pour the agar into the sterilised Petri dishes as follows: hold the flask in one hand, remove the cotton plug and flame the mouth of the flask for two to three seconds in the Bunsen flame.
3. Lift the lid of the Petri dish just enough to allow the neck of the flask to enter. Pour the molten agar into the dish very carefully.
4. Replace the lid and swirl the dish gently, so that the agar is evenly distributed without any air bubbles.
5. Leave the agar plate to cool and set solid.
6. When set place the plate upside down, resting on its lid, to stop condensation from dripping on the agar. The plate is now ready for use.
7. Label the outer edges of the base of the plate with the following information: your initials, date, and dilution.

Inoculating and incubating plates

Introduction of a small number of micro-organisms on or into the medium is called **inoculation**. This is usually carried out using a sterilised wire loop (inoculation loop), **Fig. 5.4** but in this investigation, a known volume of **inoculum** is introduced by a pipette.

1. Transfer 0.1 cm^3 of each dilution of milk over the surface of a labelled sterile nutrient agar plate, using a clean sterilised pipette.
2. Secure the lid of the Petri dish to the base with clear adhesive tape, without excluding the entry of air (anaerobic species are more likely to be dangerous).

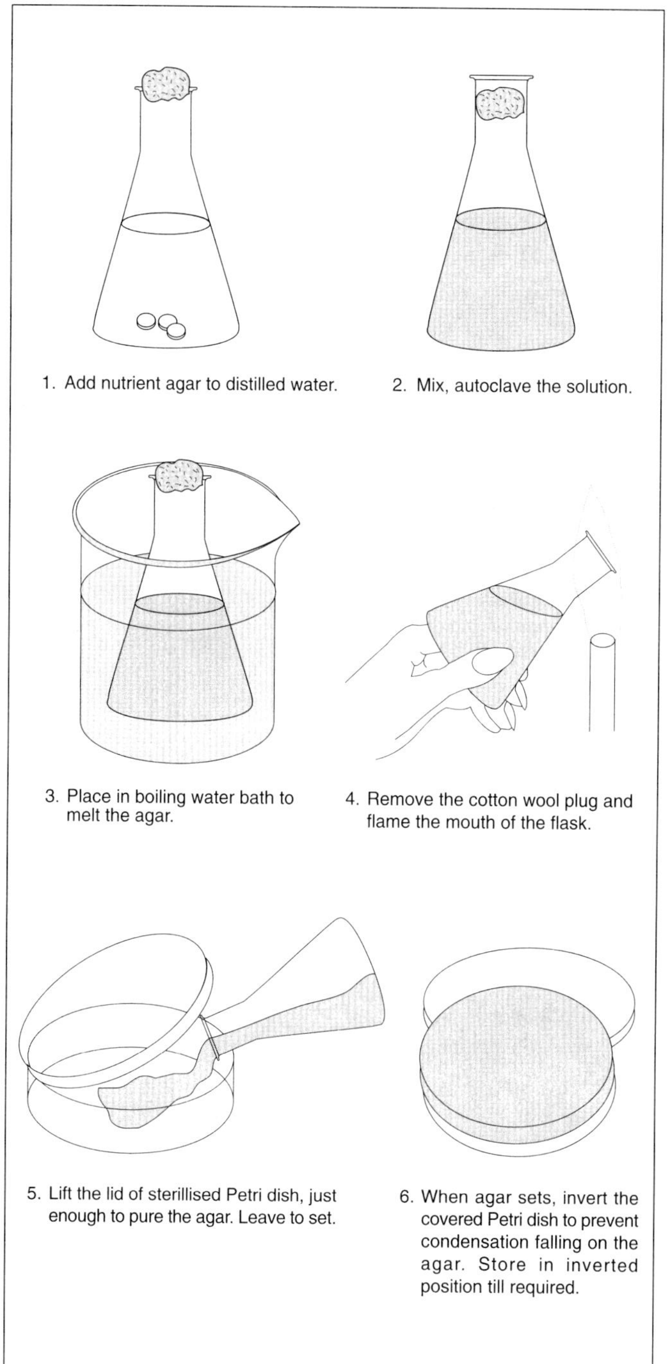

Fig. 5.3 Preparing Agar Plates

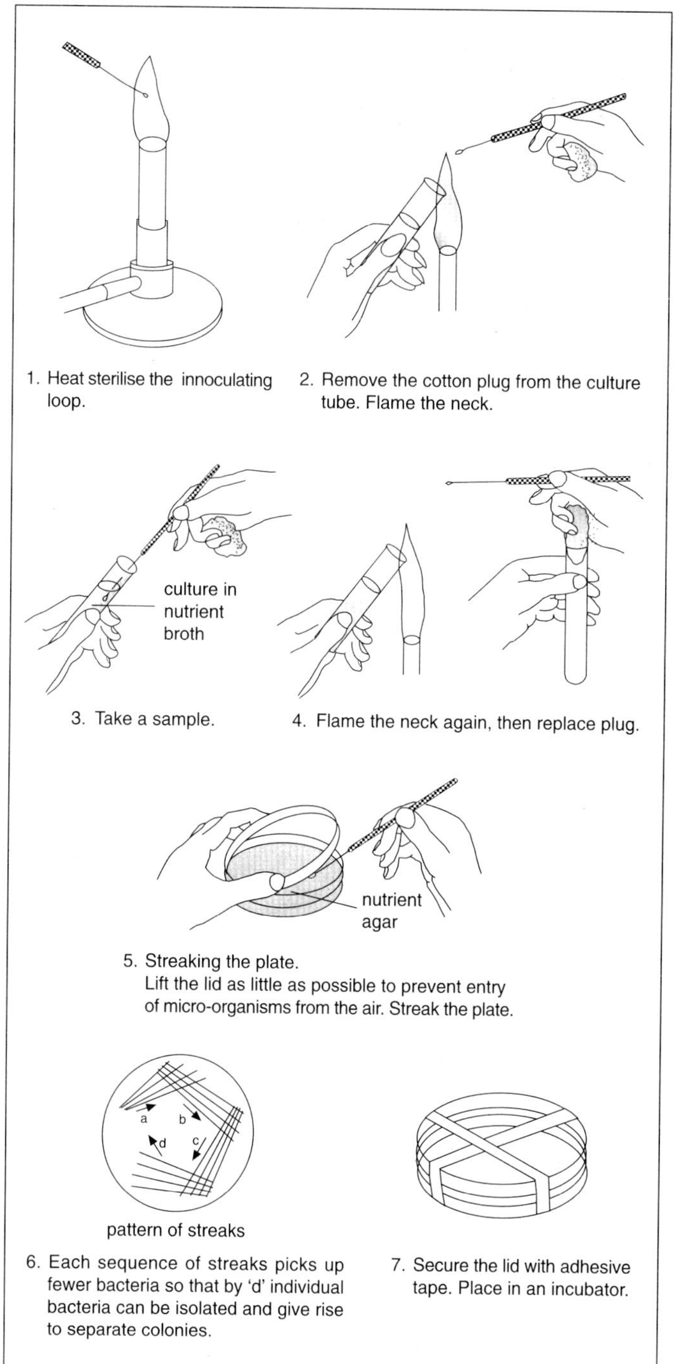

Fig. 5.4 Inoculation and Incubation of Agar Plates

3. Place the Petri dishes in an incubator at 30°C, for 24 hours or more. (Incubation at 10°C will promote the growth of *Streptococcus lactis*.)

Examining growing cultures

Do not open your Petri dish. Examine it with the adhesive tape intact.

1. If possible examine your plate daily. Once the colonies have appeared, illuminate the plate from the back and record your observations by means of annotated drawings **Fig. 5.7.**
2. Record the following: time of appearance (growth time) and the number of colonies, colony characteristics such as shape, size, colour, margin's edge and surface texture and elevation (flat or raised), apparent interactions between particular colonies.
3. Count the number of individual colonies that appear, and then multiply this count by the dilution employed. This gives you an estimate of the number of bacteria in 1 cm^3 of the milk sample.
4. Record in a table your estimates of the change in the number along with time, of bacteria in 1 cm^3 of milk.
5. Plot a graph of your results.

For consideration

(a) Comment on the effect of pasteurisation and ageing on 'fresh' milk.

(b) What might be the likely source of bacteria in your sample?

(c) How can you show that the bacterial colonies observed, actually grow from the 'inoculum', and not from contamination?

(These plates could also be used for the following investigation).

Practical 14 – MICROSCOPIC EXAMINATION OF BACTERIA

Procedure

1. Prepare a smear on a clean microscope slide as follows:
   i. Using a flamed loop, place a drop of sterilised distilled water in the centre of the slide.
   ii. Gently scrape a single colony from the surface of the agar plate using the sterilised loop, mix gently with the water and spread the bacteria with the loop. (A thick layer will not do; a very thin transparent coating is required).
2. Heat sterilise the loop.
3. Allow the smear to air dry. (Don't wave it around).
4. Observe and record your observations with labelled drawings under high power/oil-immersion using oil immersion objectives at a total magnification of x1000. Look for the following: Motility (true motility due to presence of flagella) and **cell shape**. Bacteria normally dart around the field of view, changing direction in zigzag, tumbling movements.

Cell shape **Fig. 5.1**

Bacteria are divided into the following groups:

Cocci (singular coccus): spherical, and almost spherical, sometimes growing in pairs (diplococci), chains and clumps e.g. *Staphylococus aureus* (lives in nasal passage), *Streptococcus thremophilus* (gives creamy flavour to yoghurt).

Bacilli (singular bacillus): rods, straight, cylindrical cells with flattened ends. May form chains, *Staphylobacillus e.g. Lactobacillus* (causes souring of milk), *Bacillus anthracis* (causes anthrax).

Vibrio: comma shaped e.g. *Vibrio cholerae,* (causes Cholera).

Filamentous: with flagella e.g. *Treponema pallidium* (causes syphilis).

Many bacteria are **pleomorphic**, varying in shape according to growth conditions/culture age; thus other characteristics are required for identification which are well documented in microbiology textbooks.

(a) Compare bacterial cells (prokaryotic) with eukaryotic cells.

Staining Bacteria for microscopic examination

Although bacteria can be seen under the light microscope without staining and appear colourless, it is common practice to kill and stain them before examination. Most commonly used method is **Gram-staining** which relies on the difference in structure of the cell wall of the bacteria.

Gram-staining

This is the most important differential staining technique in bacteriology, invented by Danish scientist **Hans Christian Gram.** It enables us to divide bacteria into two distinct groups, **Gram-positive** and **Gram-negative**, according to a particular staining procedure dependent on difference in the structure of the cell walls.

Both Gram-negative (e.g. *Salmonella* and *E.Coli*) and Gram-positive (e.g. *Staphylococcus, Bacillus* and *Lactobacillus*) bacteria have a cell wall containing **peptidoglycans** (mureins). Gram-positive bacteria have a thick cell wall made up of a single layer of peptidoglycans right next to the cell surface membrane **Fig. 5.5.**

Gram-negative bacteria however, have two membranes. There is a standard cell surface membrane, with a thin peptidoglycan layer lying just outside it. Outside this thin layer is a layer of **lipoprotein**, and then a second, outer, membrane, made up of **lipopoly saccharides**, which protects them from lysozyme (an antibacterial enzyme), and penicillin.

Absence of this second outer membrane allows lysozyme to digest the peptidoglycan backbone of Gram-positive bacteria, causing lysis of the cell. Action of penicillin interferes with the structure of the peptidoglycan backbone, making them prone to lysis.

Lipopolysaccharides are peculiar to bacteria and as yet have not been found in any other living organisms.

Spores are often visible as unstained areas in older vegetative cells of *Bacillus* and *Clostridium.* Other stains can be used to demonstrate spores, capsules or flagella. Additional tests are needed to characterise the organisms further.

Preparation of a heat-fixed smear

1. Take a clean glass slide and pass it through a Bunsen flame to ensure it is free of grease. Allow it to cool.
2. Using a sterilised inoculating loop, place a single

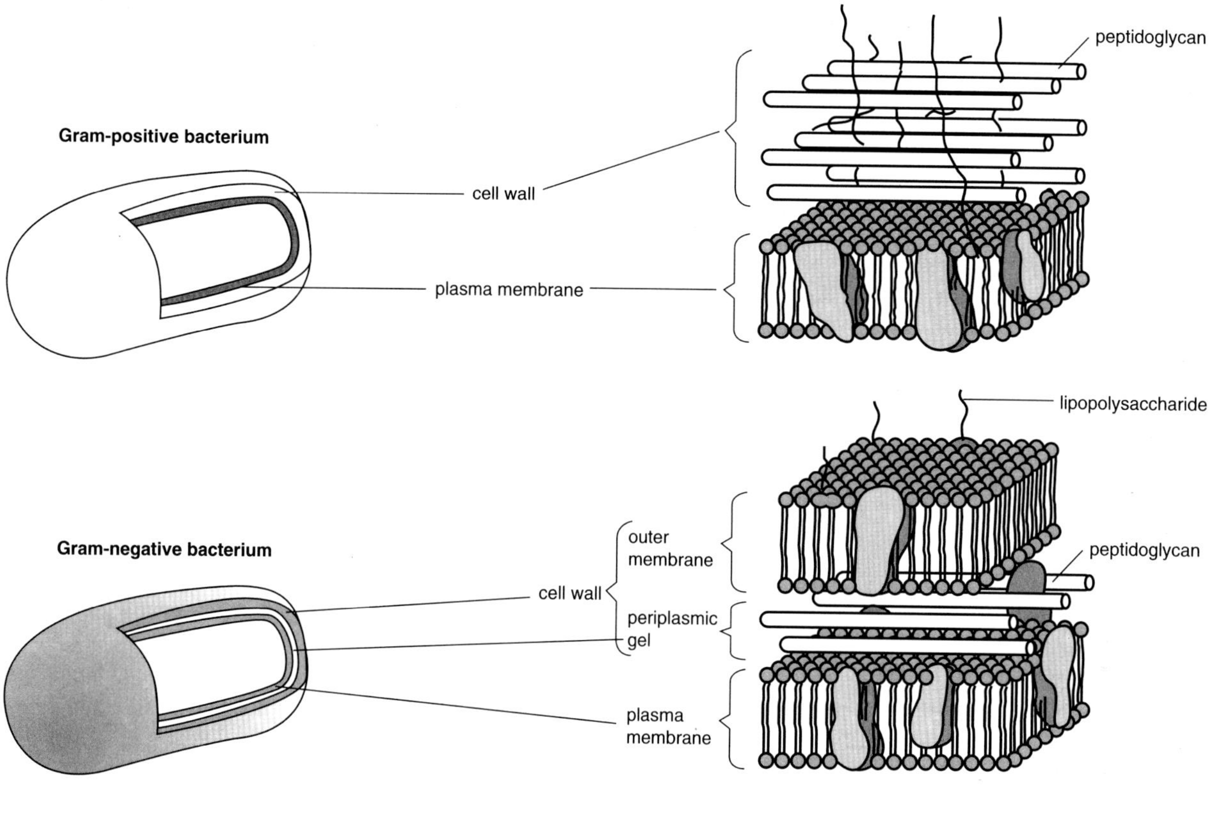

Fig. 5.5 The Gram Stain

drop of water in the centre of the slide then mix a small amount of sample from a single colony. Prepare a smear **Fig. 3.13**.

3. Allow to air-dry, or dry keeping the slide high above a Bunsen flame.
4. Fix, by passing the slide quickly through a blue Bunsen flame. The temperature of the slide should not be too hot to touch the back of your hand. Allow it to cool.

Gram-staining procedure *(Hucker's method)*

Caution: ***acetone is flammable. Turn OFF the Bunsen burners.***

1. Flood a heat fixed smear with a 0.5% w/v crystal violet in 20% v/v ethanol: water. Leave for 1 minute.
2. Wash with tap water. Flood with Gram's iodine for 1 min.
3. Decolourise by adding acetone. Add acetone drop by drop to the slide until the colour appears in the effluent. This step is critical since acetone is a powerful decolourising solvent and must not be left on the slide for too long, 2-3 seconds is all it takes.
4. Immediately immerse the slide in tap water and counter-stain using 1% aqueous safranin.
5. Pour off safranin, rinse briefly with tap water and blot dry gently.
6. Observe under oil-immersion without a coverslip. Record your results by means of annotated drawings and photographs. Gram-positive bacteria retain the crystal violet (primary stain) and appear purple.
7. Gram-negative bacteria are decolourised by acetone and are stained pink or red with safranin.

For further identification

Identification kits are commercially available and various biochemical tests such as oxidase and catalase tests can be performed and are well documented in micro biology textbooks.

Important Note:

Sterilisation and disposal of old plates/cultures

Place all swabs, lining paper from work surfaces and all disposable material in plastic bags to be incinerated. All used slides and glassware should be placed in a bucket of fresh disinfectant.

Place old cultures that are no longer required in their (unopened) Petri dishes, together in an autoclavable bag or other containers, and put them into the autoclave or pressure cooker to be sterilised. After sterilisation, dispose of the plastic equipment in the dustbin, and wash the glass equipment for re-use.

Practical 15 – BACTERIAL GROWTH IN THE PRESENCE OF ANTIBIOTICS

It is advised that students give a list of requirements to the staff prior to the day of the practical.

Micro-organisms are present virtually everywhere and multiply rapidly under suitable conditions. However, bacterial growth can be inhibited with many antibiotics. You are required to plan your own investigation, exposing agar plates to various environmental conditions to introduce micro-organisms and to observe inhibition of growth in the presence of antibiotics.

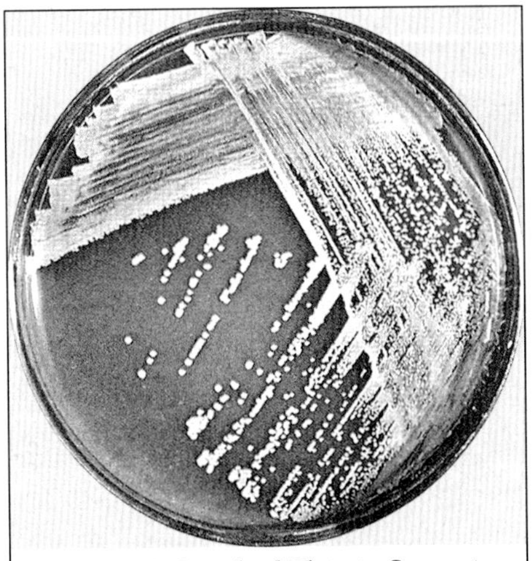

Fig. 5.7 A Streaked Plate to Separate Individual Bacterial Colonies

Procedure

1. Place the nutrient agar flask in a boiling water bath to melt.
2. Plan your investigation on paper before you begin.
3. Decide exactly how you are going to introduce micro-organisms on to your sterilised plates. You may try coughing on a plate or leaving them exposed to air in the laboratory or outside, or inoculating with a swab from the door handle, or touching the surface of the gel with your fingers etc. You need to prepare an identical plate as a control.
4. Decide how many plates you will require altogether. It is suggested you try 2-3 different conditions. (Remember to include controls, and then add a couple extras.)
5. Pour your own plates, as described on **pages 48, 49** observing all the rules of aseptic techniques.
6. On the underside of the Petri dish write the date, your initials, and indicate the type of exposure. Do the same on another plate, and mark it as control.
7. Introduce the micro-organisms on both the experimental and the control plates. Seal the control plate with adhesive tape.
8. Using a separate sterilised forceps for each (**do not contaminate**), place 3-4 discs impregnated with different antibiotic on the surface of your plate as indicated in **Fig. 5.6.** Make sure the disc lies flat on the agar.
9. Mark on the underside of the Petri dish the initials of the antibiotic of each disc. Seal with adhesive.
10. Incubate all plates at 30°C for 24 hours.
11. After 24 hours examine the cultures without opening them **Fig. 5.7** and **Fig. 5.8.**
12. Compare the plate with your control.
13. Record your observations by means of annotated drawings and photographs.

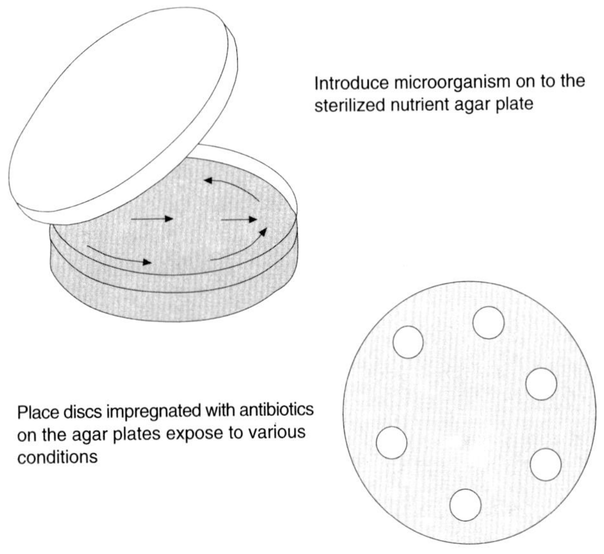

Fig. 5.6 Bacterial Growth in the Presence of Antibiotics

For consideration

(a) Which antibiotics are most effective? Can you explain why?
(b) From where are the antibiotics extracted?
(c) Can you try and explain their role in nature?
(d) How have the antibiotics reached the cells of the bacteria to inhibit growth?
(e) Why is it necessary to keep the plates sealed even in presence of antibiotics?
(f) How can you modify this procedure to take your investigations further?

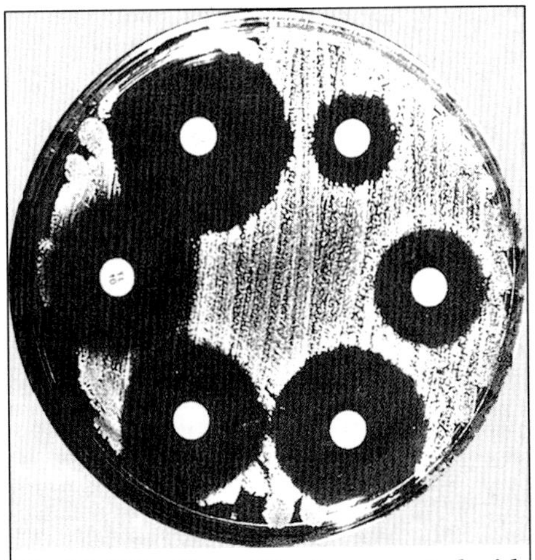

Fig. 5.8 Filter Paper Disc Impregnated with Antibiotics placed on Nutrient Agar

6 Biological Molecules

Biological Molecules

Background Summary

Living organisms are made up of a limited number of elements, namely hydrogen, carbon, nitrogen, oxygen, phosphorous and sulphur. These elements combine together to form organic molecules of life, such as **carbohydrates, lipids, proteins, nucleic acids and vitamins**. Inorganic constituents include **water, bases, salts** and **acids**. All of which should be part of a balanced diet. Absence or shortage of any one of these leads to deficiency diseases, such as rickets, scurvy and pellagra.

Water, the most abundant constituent of organisms, (between 60-95% of fresh mass) is a fundamental requirement for life. The importance of water as a medium for all chemical reactions is due to its unique solvent properties, heat capacity, surface tension, evaporation and freezing properties.

Acids and bases are also important in that they determine the pH of an organism's body fluids. The correct functioning of cells depend on the pH being kept constant, maintenance of salts or their ion concentration within a specific limit, imbalance of which could be devastating to the cell or to the organism as a whole.

Carbohydrates are divided into three main groups: **monosaccharides, disaccharides** and **polysaccharides**. Monosaccharides and disaccharides are water-soluble reducing sugars, (except for sucrose) **see page 57**. Polysaccharides are insoluble non-reducing sugars such as starch, cellulose and glycogen. Carbohydrates are vital as energy sources and are important structurally. These large molecules being insoluble in water exert no chemical or osmotic influence on the cell. They fold into compact shapes and are easily converted to sugars by hydrolysis whenever energy is required

Starch, a polysaccharide, is a major fuel source for plants. It is found in chloroplasts in leaves or in storage organs such as potato tubers. It is a mixture of two polysaccharides, **amylose** and **amylopectin**. **Glycogen**, the animal equivalent of starch, is found notably in liver and muscle cells. Its structure is similar to amylopectin, but shows more branching **Fig. 6.1**.

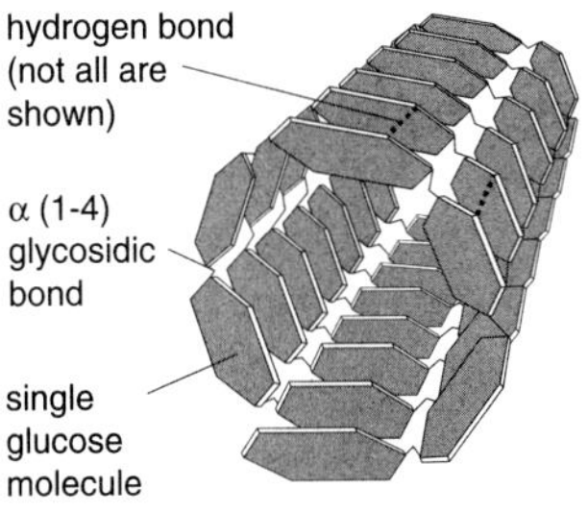

Structure of starch molecule

Starch is a mixture of polysaccharides, amylose and amylopectin. Both are polymers of α – glucose. The long molecule consists of 1–4 linked α – glucose units, coiled into a helix forming a cylinder.

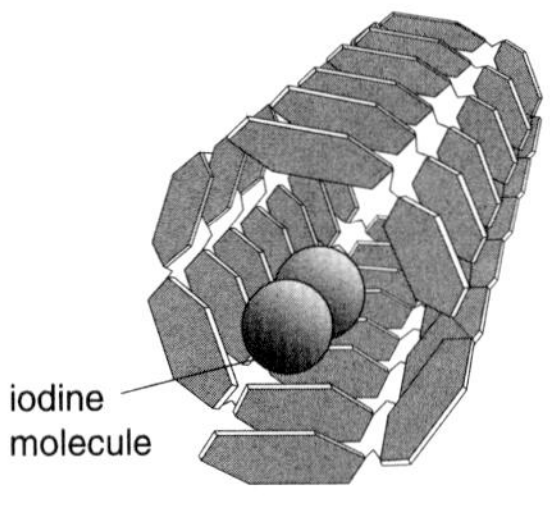

Starch-iodine mixture

The iodine molecule fits neatly into the cylindrical starch structure and produces the blue/black colour of starch-iodine mixture.

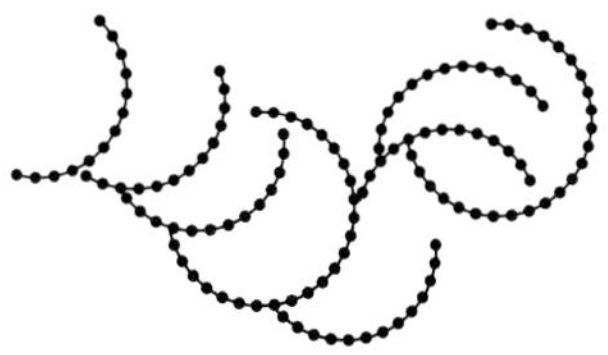

Part of a Glycogen Molecule

Glycogen and amylopectin are both branched molecules. Branching reduces the tendency to spiral.

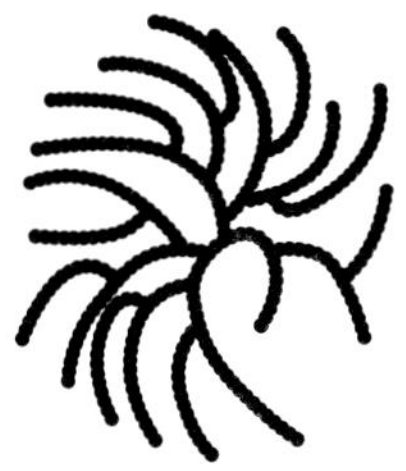

Part of an Amylopectin Molecule

Amylopectin is a branched polysacchiride found in starch.

Fig. 6.1 Biological Molecules

Cellulose, the most abundant of all polysaccharides is a material of great commercial importance, for it becomes impregnated with **lignin** to form wood.

Some sugars contain nitrogen and are therefore called **amino sugars**. Polysaccharides that contain amino sugars are called **mucopolysaccharides.** Mucopolysaccharides are found in the basement membrane of epithelia, the matrix of connective tissue, as well as in the bacterial cell wall (**murein**) and in **chitin**, a carbohydrate found in exoskeleton of arthropods and fungal cell walls.

Proteins are the most abundant organic molecules found within the cells. They are very large molecules, which can be converted to both fat and carbohydrates by the cell and play a vital structural and metabolic role in organisms. Proteins are required for the body's own protein building program. They are made up of numerous amino acids, which can be combined by condensation to form polypeptide chains and ultimately an unlimited variety of proteins. The sequence of amino acids is specific to a particular protein and is genetically controlled by the DNA of that particular cell. Of the twenty common types of amino acids, eight are **essential amino acids**, which our bodies cannot synthesize, so we must obtain them from our diet. The rest, the body synthesizes by **transamination.**

The sequence of amino acids make up the **primary structure** of the protein. The chain of amino acids may be coiled into an α **helix**, which constitutes the **secondary structure** of the protein. Further coiling or folding gives the protein its **tertiary structure**. Finally, several polypeptide chains may be combined in the finished protein molecule, giving it its **quaternary structure.** The quaternary structure may also combine further with other compounds, called **prosthetic groups** to form a **conjugate protein.** In haemoglobin, four **porphyrin (haem)** groups combine with the protein and in mucous it combines with a carbohydrate as **glycoprotein**.

The exact shape of the protein molecule is extremely important and is directly related to its function. Proteins are classified as **globular** or **fibrous**. The **globular** proteins are usually metabolically active, soluble and perform regulatory functions in the body (e.g. enzymes). An important function of globular protein is **buffering**. This is due to the presence of both positively and negatively charged groups in the polypeptide chain. The grouping together of globular protein molecules forms certain structures, e.g. microfilaments and microtubules. Fibrous proteins perform structural functions (e.g. myosin, keratin, collagen and silk).

Lipids include fats and oils, which are water insoluble organic substances. They are important sources of energy and also carry out structural roles, as they provide insulation beneath the skin. Lipids also form the waxy cuticle of plants and insects thus rendering them waterproof. The three most important groups of lipids found in living organisms are **triglycerides, phospholipids** and **steroids**. The phospholipid **lecithin** is an important component of cell membranes in addition to glycerol and fatty acids. Many membranes also contain **cholesterol**.

The body can synthesise most of its own fats, including cholesterol from protein and carbohydrates. The fats it cannot produce are called **essential fatty acids**, but whole foods etc. provide plenty of them.

Steroids are a group of lipid-like compounds with important biological functions e.g. in the formation of hormones.

Nucleic acids, like proteins are very large molecules essential for life. They constitute the genetic material for all living organisms including viral particles. They are formed from building blocks called **nucleotides**. These combine together to form very long molecules called **polynucleotides**.

Vitamins, a mixed assortment of organic compounds, are required by organisms for various metabolic purposes. Some of them function as co-enzymes. They cannot be synthesized by the body, so must be present in the diet. Vitamin A, D, and K are fat-soluble and all others are water-soluble.

Practical 16 – TESTING FOR THE PRESENCE OF CARBOHYDRATES

The chemical composition of any substance can be investigated in two main ways. One is to homogenise the tissue, and extract the juices from it, either by filtration or by centrifugation and perform chemical tests on the extract. (It may be necessary to decolourise the extract as pigments interfere with some colour tests.) Alternatively, microscopically examine a thin section of the tissue, stained with a reagent specific to its chemical constituent. This method has the advantage that the distribution of individual compounds within the cells can be studied in detail.

Carbohydrates

If a carbohydrate is suspected it can be tested by using one of the following tests:

- Starch test
- reducing sugar test
- non-reducing sugar test

Starch Test

The starch test is simple and quick and should be carried out first when testing for an unknown carbohydrate.
A solution of iodine and potassium iodide (iodine solution) will react with starch grains giving a blue/black colour **Fig. 6.1**. The iodine forms complex with the starch molecule and prevents the amylase from reacting with the starch molecule. Therefore if you intend to use mylase as part of the investigation do not test the carbohydrate with iodine solution first.

Starch Test

Carry out the following procedure on a white tile. Add a few drops of iodine/potassium iodide (iodine solution) to a crushed sample, or add the crushed sample to a test tube and add approximately 4 cm^3 (quarter of a test tube) of distilled water, centrifuge if necessary and then add two drops of iodine solution. A blue-black colour indicates the presence of starch.

Procedure

1. Irrigate a thin section of potato tuber on a slide with iodine solution. Watch the starch grains turning blue as the iodine reaches them.
2. Now examine the distribution of starch in a potato tuber by cutting thin sections and mounting them in iodine solution. Starch grains stain blue and can be located within the cells.
3. Next take a 1cm^3 of potato tuber and crush it. Transfer it to a test tube, and add 4 cm^3 distilled water and 2 drops of iodine solution. Observe the resulting solution on a microscope slide under the microscope or with the aid of a hand lens.
4. Starch grains of different carbohydrates differ in shape and structure. Observe carefully their size, shape and other similarities and differences under the microscope.
5. Test other food substances for the presence of starch.
6. Record your observations in a table and with annotated drawings.
7. Tabulate your results as follows:

Sample	Test	Observations	Conclusion
Potato	Starch	turns black	Starch present/+ive

8. Observe using a hand lens or under microscope the individual grains stained with iodine in a starch solution.
9. Also observe the structure of the iodine stained grains after heating the starch solution.

For consideration

(a) Explain your observations with reference to the structure of starch molecules.
(b) Can this test be used to detect if a true solution is formed with starch prior to heating?
(c) What changes take place when a starch solution is heated?
(d) Is it possible to identify a substance by observing its starch grains?

Practical 17 – TESTING FOR THE PRESENCE OF SUGARS

All monosaccharides and certain disaccharides, including maltose and lactose are reducing sugars, because these sugars reduce an alkaline solution of copper (II) sulphate to a brick red precipitate of copper (I) oxide. Hence, such sugars are called **reducing sugars**, but you cannot distinguish one from the other with this test. Sucrose is a non-reducing sugar. The chemistry of the reduction is related to the aldehyde group of aldo sugars and the combined ketone and primary alcohol groups of keto sugars. In non-reducing sugars these groups do not participate in the reaction because they are linked together in the glycosidic bond. Two common tests for reducing sugars, Benedict's and Fehling's make use of the ability of these sugars to reduce copper from a valency of II to a valency of I. Both tests involve use of an alkaline solution of copper (II) sulphate ($CuSO_4$) which is reduced to insoluble copper (I) oxide (Cu_2O).

$$Cu^{2+} + e^- \rightarrow Cu^+$$

blue solution   brick red solution

Reducing sugar test (Benedict's Test)

To approximately 2 cm^3 of glucose solution in a test tube add an equal quantity of Benedict's reagent. Shake and bring to the boil by heating the test tube in a water bath. A precipitate indicates reducing sugar. The colour and density of the precipitate gives a rough indication of the amount of sugar present. A green precipitate means relatively little sugar, a brown or brick red precipitate means progressively more sugar.

Boiling Water Baths

Although it takes time to set up and reach boiling point the use of water bath is highly recommended in this investigation since:

(i) it is safer and prevents liquids from spurting out from test tubes on heating;
(ii) a controlled temperature is easier to achieve;
(iii) if more than one sample is being tested it is quicker and the results are more comparable.

T. Tube →	1	2	3	4	5	6	7
Conc. →	0%	1%	0.5%	0.25%	0.12%	0.06%	0.03%
D. Water	2	0	2	2	2	2	2
Glucose 1%	0	2	2	0	0	0	0
Transfer			-2 →	-2 →	-2 →	-2 →	-2
Benedict's	2	2	2	2	2	2	2

Procedure

1. To familiarise yourself with the test, dissolve a small spatula full of glucose in about $2cm^3$ of water, carry out the Benedict's test on it.
2. Using a 1% solution of glucose make up serial dilutions in seven test tubes:
3. Label seven test tubes 1–7. Add $2cm^3$ of distilled water in test tubes 1, 3, 4, 5, 6, and 7.
4. Add $2cm^3$ of 1% glucose solution to test tubes 2 and 3. Mix well.
5. Transfer $2cm^3$ of glucose solution from test tube 3 to 4. Mix well. Transfer $2cm^3$ from test tube 4 to 5 and so on. Mix thoroughly before transferring the solution at each step. After mixing thoroughly discard $2cm^3$ from the last test tube, numbered 7.
6. Add $2cm^3$ of Benedict's to each of the 7 test tubes.
7. Heat in a boiling water bath for 5 minutes.
8. If you have a colorimeter, record optical density of each tube, using test tube 1 to adjust the instrument to zero. If a colorimeter is not available observe colour visually using the following criteria:

   clear blue solution – no trace of sugar;

   turbid green – 0.25%

   yellow – 0.5%

   brick red – 2% and above.
9. Record colour against concentration in a table.
10. Plot a graph of your results.

Testing food for the presence of reducing sugars

1. Cut a cube of apple of about 1 cm^3. Grind it up in a mortar or crush it very fine on a clean white tile.
2. Transfer the material to a test tube, add $2cm^3$ water.
3. Add an equal volume of Benedict's reagent and heat to boiling in a water bath.
4. Examine other food substances such as potatoes, peas, starch powder etc. for the presence of reducing sugars.
5. Record your results and conclusions in a table.
6. Use the graph to quantify your results.
   (a) Why is it necessary to crush the solid sample to be tested?
   (b) Suggest how you could improve your procedure.
7. The main reducing sugar in apple tissue is fructose. Investigate its distribution within the cell as follows: cut thin sections with a razor blade and mount the thinnest section on a slide with a few drops of Benedict's reagent.
8. Examine and draw the cells under the microscope.
9. Heat the slide gently over a small flame until the tissue turns brown. Add water if the tissue looks like drying up.
10. Allow the slide to cool and then re-examine the cells.
11. Record your observations.
    (c) What changes have occurred in the cells?
    (d) Is sugar present in all the cells or only in certain ones?

Fehling's test for reducing sugars

Add $2cm^3$ solution of the reducing sugar to a test tube. Add $1cm^3$ of Fehling's solution A and $1cm^3$ of Fehling's solution B. Shake and boil. The mixture turns from blue to green to yellow till finally a brick red precipitate forms.

This test is not as convenient or as sensitive as the Benedict's test, but you should be familiar with it as you may come across it in textbooks.

Non-reducing sugar test

Sucrose (cane sugar) is a disaccharide, which does not reduce copper sulphate (non-reducing sugar). However, it can be detected by first hydrolysing the sucrose into its constituent monosaccharides and then testing with Benedict's reagent.

Boil 2 cm^3 of sucrose solution with $1cm^3$ of dilute hydrochloric acid. Neutralise with sodium hydrogen carbonate or sodium hydroxide (check with pH paper) then test with Benedict's reagent.

Cellulose stains purple with Schultz' solution

1. Put a drop of the stain onto a small piece of teased-out cotton wool and notice the reaction.
2. Mount a section of a plant tissue in Schultz' solution and examine and draw the cells. Note the colour reaction shown by the cell walls.

Lignin (wood) stains red with acidified phloroglucinol.

1. Put some phloroglucinol into a watch glass and add a few drops of concentrated hydrochloric acid.
2. Dip a matchstick into this mixture and note the colour reaction.
3. With a razor blade, cut thin, transverse and/or longitudinal sections of a woody stem.
4. Stain your sections in acidified phloroglucinol in a watch glass for five minutes and then mount in water, or (if you wish to keep them for long) in dilute glycerine.
5. Examine under low power and observe and draw the distribution of lignin in your section.

Practical 18 (a) – TESTING FOR THE PRESENCE OF LIPIDS

There are three tests to check whether a sample contains any fat. They are:

- **Smear test**
- **Sudan III dye test**
- **Emulsion test.**

Smear or grease spot test

Rub a small amount of sample on filter paper, if it becomes translucent when held up to light, it contains fat.

Sudan III dye test

Immerse the sample to be tested in the dye for five minutes. Wash the excess dye in water.
A pink stain will indicate the areas containing fat.
Alternatively, grind a small sample, transfer it to a test tube, and add about 1cm³ of water. Boil. Lipids will escape to the surface, then add a few drops of the Sudan III dye and shake. A red stained oil layer separates on the surface of the water, which remains clear.

1. Add a small amount of water to some olive oil in a test tube and shake it up with a few drops of Sudan III. On standing, the oil separates from the water and will be seen to have taken up the red stain.

Emulsion test

To about 2cm³ of sample add an equal volume of absolute ethanol and shake it for about 30 seconds. Add an equal volume of cold water. Mix well. Allow to stand. A milky white emulsion indicates presence of fat.

1. Shake some olive oil in a test tube with 5 cm³ absolute ethanol for one minute; add an equal volume of water. A cloudy white emulsion indicates lipids. The whiteness of the emulsion is proportional to the concentration of lipids in the substance being tested.
2. Grind caster oil seeds or peanuts in a mortar. Transfer to a test tube containing water, and boil. If lipids are present, oil droplets will escape from the tissue and rise to the surface of the water.
4. Add Sudan III and shake.
5. Allow the oil to settle and notice that, as before, it stains red. Try this on a fat containing seed such as sunflower or linseed.
6. Investigate the distribution of fat in different seeds and tissue by staining the tissue in Sudan III and then washing with several changes of water or 70 per cent ethanol. Any fat present will retain the red colour of the stain.
7. Section a castor oil seed longitudinally and investigate the distribution of fat in the same way.
8. Record your observations by drawing.

Practical 18 (b) – TESTING FOR THE PRESENCE OF PROTEINS

The peptide link in proteins —CONH— forms coloured complexes with copper salts in alkaline solution. This is called **biuret test** because biuret also contains the —CONH— group and forms the coloured complex.
Other compounds containing similar groups such as —$CSNH_2$, —$CNHNH_2$ and —CH_2NH_2 which are not proteins also give positive results with this test but generally a positive test is considered as indicative of likely presence of protein.
It is worth remembering that all enzymes are proteins but not all proteins are enzymes.

Biuret test for protein

This test is suitable for soluble proteins and is safer than Millon's test (below).
Add an equal volume of 5% potassium hydroxide to the protein solution; add a drop of 1% copper sulphate down the side of the test tube. Do not heat. A lilac ring at the surface of the solution indicates protein; on shaking, the lilac ring disappears and the solution turns lilac, pale violet or purple.

Caution: ***Millon's reagent is dangerous. Do not boil it for long, or inhale its fumes or get it on your skin.***

Millon's test for proteins

To about 2 cm³ of a solution or suspension of the protein, add about six drops of Millon's reagent, and boil. A brick-red colour on the surface of the substance being tested indicates protein.

1. Try this test on some egg albumen.
2. Next remove the testa from a pea and slice off a thin section of the testa and the seed.
3. Mount it in Millon's reagent on a slide, and heat gently to boiling. Add water if necessary.
4. Cool and examine under the microscope for the distribution of protein.
5. Carry out the protein tests on as many food substances as are available.
6. Record your observation in a table, with all colour changes observed.

By now you must have tested a range of food substances, plant tissues and organs for the occurrence and distribution of reducing and non-reducing sugars, starch, cellulose, lignin, fat and protein. In the case of a complex structure like an orange or a germinating seed, test different components (e.g. skin matrix, juice, pips, testa, embryo, cotyledon etc.) separately.

For consideration

(a) What happens to the albumen when you boil it? Explain your observations.
(b) How would you make these tests quantitative?
(c) What is the value of obtaining information on the occurrence and distribution of different substances in plants or animals?
(d) What are the physical properties of starch and cellulose, and how are the properties related to the functions of these two compounds in plant cells?
(e) How does knowledge of the chemical structure of starch and cellulose help explain their physical properties?
(f) Select one of the plant organs in which you have investigated the distribution of substances. Explain, as far as you can, how and why the various substances came to be located in their situations?
(g) Carbon is quadrivalent. Why does this make it ideal as a constituent of biological molecules? Illustrate your answer by referring to the structure of carbohydrates and proteins.

Practical 19 – ANALYSIS OF AMINO ACIDS BY PAPER CHROMATOGRAPHY

Chromatography is a technique used to separate a mixture into its various components. The technique depends upon the differential movement of each component in the mixture, through a stationary medium (chromatography paper,) under the influence of a moving solvent.

In this investigation you will determine some of the amino acids present in the protein albumen. The protein is first hydrolysed by treating it with the digestive enzyme trypsin; the amino acids are then separated and identified by paper chromatography as follows:

A strip of chromatography paper, with a concentrated spot of the mixed amino acids near the bottom edge, is suspended in the jar containing suitable solvent, so that its end dips into the solvent. The solvent moves slowly up the strip of paper, carrying the amino acids with it. As different amino acids travel at different speeds, they separate from one another. The paper is treated with a ninhydrin reagent, which stains the amino acids. The amino acids appear as pinkish/purple spots and can be identified.

Preparation of Tryptic Digest*–Breaking down the protein (this has been done for you)*

To 2g of albumen or 5.0 cm^3 of eggwhite add about 5 cm^3 trypsin solution (2g trypsin in 100 cm^3 of 1% sodium hydrogencarbonate). Add a crystal of thymol to kill any bacteria. Leave the mixture to incubate at 37°C for 48–72 hours.

Caution:

Ninhydrin is a poisonous irritant: Use it in a fume cupboard. Wash it off immediately if it gets onto your skin.

Solvents are highly volatile and flammable. Use a fume cupboard if available, if not make sure the room is well ventilated and that there are no naked flames.

Preparing the chromatogram

1. Pour the solvent into the jar/measuring cylinder to a depth of about 3 cm. Cover the open end of the jar so the atmosphere inside the jar becomes saturated with vapour.
2. Take a strip of chromatography paper, (holding it as lightly as possible from the edges, otherwise amino acids on your skin may get onto the paper), draw a pencil line across the strip about 4 cm from one end of the strip.
3. Write your initials on the other end and bend the strip so that it can be attached to the lid **Fig. 6.2** with adhesive tape.
4. Very carefully, using a fine capillary tube or a drawn out Pasture pipette place a small drop of the amino acid mixture in the centre of the pencil line. (Practice on a piece of filter paper first, because it is important to make the spot as small as possible. The smaller the spot, better the separation!)
5. Let the spot dry, use a hair dryer if available, and then place another spot on top of the first, and

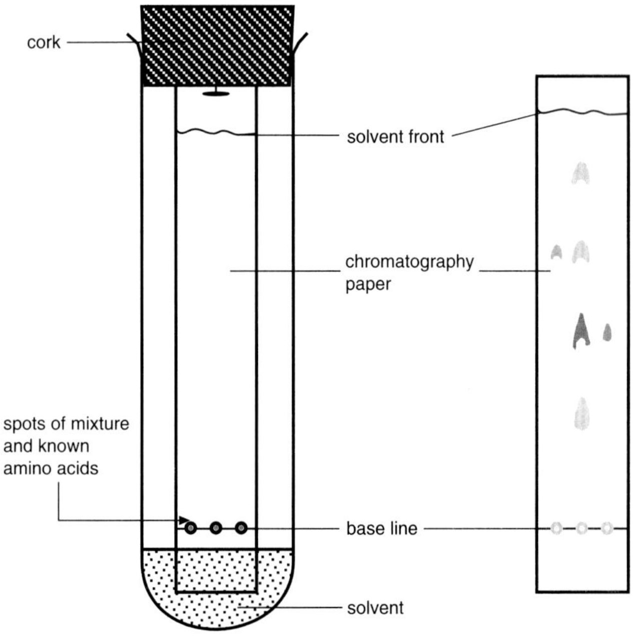

Fig. 6.2 Analysis of Amino Acid by Paper Chromatography

dry again. Repeat this about six times, to concentrate the mixture, keeping the spot as small as possible.

6. 'Spot' the paper with two different solutions of known amino acids, one on either side of the albumin spot, using a clean capillary tube each time. Concentrate it as before.
(Students can use different amino acids, and then pool class results.)
7. Lower the strip carefully into the glass jar, pencilled end first, taking care not to let the paper come into contact with the sides of the jar. Allow the bottom end of the strip to dip into the solvent, **ensuring that the spot is not submerged**.
8. Attach the bent top edge to the lid with adhesive tape. The solvent will ascend up the filter paper, carrying the amino acids from the tryptic digest with it. This will take several hours.
9. Keep an eye on the solvent moving up the paper strip. Make sure the solvent front does not run off the top edge of the paper. When it has reached about 2cm from the top edge of the paper, remove the strip from the jar.
10. Mark the highest point reached by the solvent (**solvent front**) at once, as this disappears once the solvent has evaporated.
11. Hang the strip to dry.

***Developing the chromatogram* (use disposable gloves).**

1. In a fume cupboard spray the chromatogram with ninhydrin spray (if available) or pour small amount of the ninhydrin reagent into a glass crystallising dish and slowly draw the chromatogram through the liquid. Ensure that the whole strip is thoroughly soaked.
2. Dry the strips either with a hair dryer or with the heat from an electric lamp bulb. Do not use a Bunsen flame, ***Ninhydrin is flammable!***
3. Purple spots should appear at points along the chromatogram. Continue heating until the spots are as dense as possible. Draw around each spot.

Interpretation of the chromatogram

Each purple spot represents one or more amino acids. Certain spots will be clear and easily identified; others are less distinct. To identify the amino acids, we make use of a measurement called the **R_f value**, which stands for **relative front**. This is the ratio of the distance moved by the spot to the distance moved by the solvent.

$$R_f = \frac{\text{Distance moved by the solute (spot)}}{\text{Distance moved by the solvent front}}$$

Draw a horizontal line through the centre of each spot and calculate its R_f value.

Compare your R_f values with those in **Fig. 6.3** and identify as many amino acids as possible.

Amino Acid	Concentration (%)	R_f value
Glutamic acid	16.5	0.30
Aspartic acid	9.3	0.24
Leucine	9.2	0.71
Serine	8.2	0.27
Phenylalanine	7.7	6.68
Valine	7.1	0.60
Isoleucine	7.0	0.72
Alanine	6.7	0.38
Lysine	6.3	0.14
Arginine	5.7	0.20
Methionine	5.2	0.55
Threonine	4.0	0.35
Tyrosine	3.7	0.45
Proline	3.6	0.43
Glycine	3.1	0.26

Fig. 6.3 The Amino Acids Present in Albumen Listed in order of Decreasing Concentrations.

Presentation of results

Attach your chromatogram to your notebook.
Write beside each spot its R_f value and its name.

For consideration

(a) How many different amino acids are present in your albumin sample?
(b) There are known to be 15 different amino acids present in albumin. Why did they not all appear in your separation?
(c) How could you extend the chromatographic technique in order to identify all of them?
(d) Would you expect albumin from different species of animals to contain all of these amino acids?
(e) How would increasing the temperature or the time of incubation of the tryptic digest affect your results?
(f) Why was trypsin used to breakdown the protein?

Separation by other more advanced techniques

Complete digestion of the polypeptide followed by chromatography only provides information about amino acid composition, and says nothing about the sequence. This was first achieved by Fredric Sanger in 1953 when he determined the sequence of insulin. His work was a landmark in biochemistry because it showed for the first time that a protein has a precisely defined amino acid sequence, which is now known to be genetically determined.

The primary structure of a protein can be determined by selectively splitting the polypeptide chain into smaller peptide fragments, with specific protease enzymes; the sequence can then be determined by further chemical techniques.

A protein will give a different set of peptide fragments depending upon which protease enzyme is used. This is useful for obtaining information about the primary structure as complete degradation will only provide information about amino acid composition and tells you nothing of the sequence.

For example, trypsin, cuts a polypeptide chain only at the carboxy side of lysine or argenine residue which obviously limits the extent to which the chain is degraded. This provides information about the primary structure of the protein. The fragments thus produced can be separated from each other and then sequenced. This is usually done by a combination of chromatography and electrophoresis, which provides a 'fingerprint' like the one shown **Fig. 6.4.** A more advanced method would be to use high performance liquid chromatography (HPLC).

Polyacrylamide Gel Electrophoresis (PAGE) Fig. 6.5

Electrophoresis is a modified form of chromatography used to separate charged molecules. An electric current is applied across a chromatography medium such that one end has a positive charge and the other negative. The molecules within the mixture move through the medium depending on their relative charge. Using **polyacrylamide gel** as a supporting medium, which also serves as a molecular sieve, thus separation on PAGE depends on charge as well as molecular mass, further modifying the separation technique.

The method requires only tiny quantities of proteins for analysis; (as little as 10μg is usually sufficient).

Proteins are first treated with a detergent sodium dodecyle sulphat (SDS), which uncoils and solubilises the protein molecules and attaches itself to the polypeptide chain, exposing negatively charged groups of SDS. The resulting negative charge on the denatured protein is proportional to the number of peptide bonds. On applying an electric current of about 200V, SDS treated molecules all move towards the anode, but in doing so, pass through the acrylamide gel's sieving effect bringing about separation on the bases of their size: small molecules pass relatively quickly towards the anode whereas larger ones take longer. A pattern of bands appears, as the gel is stained with coomassie blue. The distance moved by the protein is normally proportional to the molecular mass; consequently the molecular mass of 'unknown' proteins may be calculated, by comparison with molecules of known molecular mass, running alongside the unknown **Fig. 6.4**.

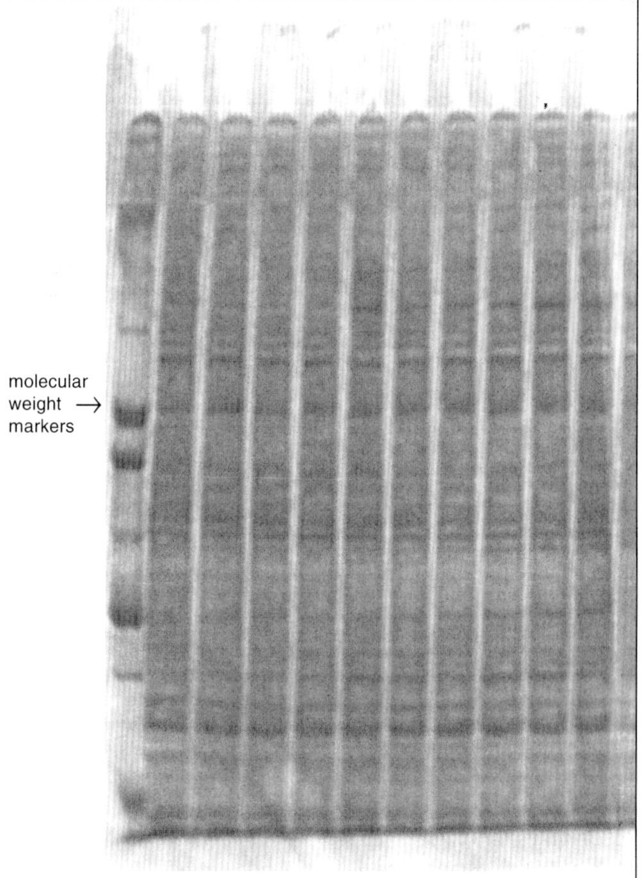

Fig. 6.4 Electrophoresis Gel showing Protein Mixture Separated according to Molecular Weight

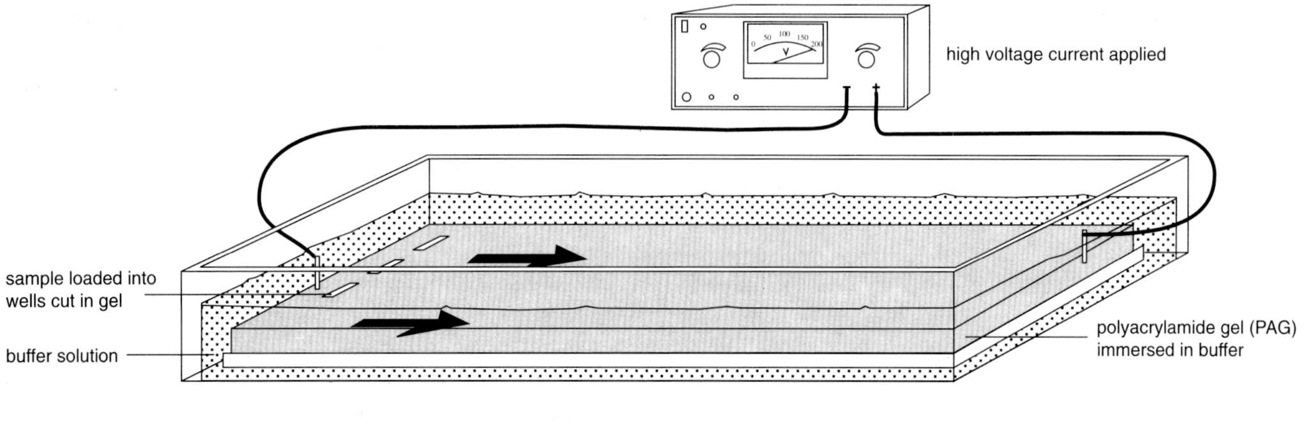

Fig. 6.5 Polyacrylamide Gel Electrophoresis (PAGE)

The technique is frequently used to separate fragments of DNA and RNA (genetic fingerprinting).

Separation according to the Isoelectric point of the protein

The technique is further modified to separate proteins according to their size or to relative amounts of acidic and basic groups that they contain.

pH affects the ionisation of $—NH_2$ and —COOH groups. The pH at which the protein molecule as a whole has a net charge of zero is called the **isoelectric point** of the protein. At this particular pH the two groups, $—NH_2$ and —COOH, are exactly equally ionised, so the molecule as a whole has a net charge of zero.

If a gel is made containing a pH gradient, the mixture of protein can then be applied to the gel and a potential difference set across the gel. Each protein moves across the gel until it reaches its isoelectric point.

Two Dimensional Electrophoresis

To get an even better separation of proteins the two methods can be combined. The protein mixture is first subjected to the method which separates according to isoelectric points in a vertical direction. The resulting gel is then placed on another gel, this time impregnated with SDS, and the potential difference is applied in the other direction. So the proteins first separate vertically according to their isoelectric points, and then according to their size. This is called **two-dimension** electrophoresis.

Redox Reactions

Oxidation is defined as the loss of electrons from a substance, and r**eduction** as the gain of electrons by a substance.

Many chemical reactions involve the oxidation of one substance and reduction of another. Oxidation and reduction always take place simultaneously, and a reaction in which this occurs is called a **redox reaction.** Electrons are lost by one substance and taken up by another. For example, during the light dependent reaction of photosynthesis, chlorophyll molecules lose electrons. **They are oxidised.** The electrons are taken up by an electron carrier, which is therefore reduced. The carrier passes the electrons onto another carrier, becoming oxidised. The electrons are passed from one carrier to the next eventually being taken up by oxidised NADH, which is therefore **reduced.**

$$\underset{\text{Oxidised NAD}}{NAD^+} + H^+ + 2e^- \rightarrow \underset{\text{Reduced NAD}}{NADH}$$

Reduced NAD can be oxidised to oxidised NAD by releasing hydrogen ions and electrons:

$$\underset{\text{Reduced NAD}}{NADH} \rightarrow \underset{\text{Oxidised NAD}}{NAD^+} + H^+ + 2e^-$$

If a substance has a strong tendency to take electrons from another substance, it is called an **oxidising agent.** If a substance has a strong tendency to donate electrons to other substances it is called a **reducing agent.**

Practical 20 – DESIGN AN INVESTIGATION TO SHOW THAT TETRAZOLIUM CHLORIDE IS A REDOX INDICATOR

Prepare a list of requirements and give to staff prior to the practical class.

Tetrazolium chloride (TTC) is a redox indicator, which is colourless when oxidised and pink when reduced. The indicator acts as an artificial hydrogen acceptor and is readily reduced in the presence of dehydrogenase enzymes.

Investigate the effect of at least four different temperatures between 10°C and 70°C on the dehydrogenase activity of yeast cells.

Place $10cm^3$ samples of yeast in a test tube and $1cm^3$ of TTC solution and measure the time taken to develop a definite pink colour.

For consideration

(a) Write a full report of your method and write any precaution taken.
(b) Record your results and present them as a graph.
(c) State your conclusion.
(d) Discuss the biological significance of your results.

Practical 21 – VITAMIN C CONTENT OF A LEMON

Vitamin C (ascorbic acid) is found in citrus fruits, such as oranges and lemons. It prevents the deficiency disease **scurvy**. Vitamin C is a powerful reducing agent, and decolourises the blue dye **dichlorophenolindophenol (DCPIP)**. The following investigation is based on this reaction.

Your colour test is standardised against a solution of ascorbic acid of known concentration.

Procedure

1. Add $2m^3$ DCPIP solution to a test tube.
2. Using a clean 1 cm^3 pipette or syringe add 0.1% ascorbic acid drop by drop to the DCPIP solution, until the solution is decolourised. Gently shake the test tube whilst adding the DCPIP, (vigorous shaking will result in oxidation of the ascorbic acid by oxygen in the air).

3. Note the volume of ascorbic acid required to decolourize 2cm^3 DCPIP solution.
4. Repeat this procedure twice more. Calculate the mean volume of 0.1 per cent vitamin C required to decolourise 2 cm^3 of DCPIP.
5. Calculate the mass of vitamin C in this volume of vitamin C solution. The vitamin C in this solution contains 0.001g vitamin C in 1.0 cm^3 water.
6. Now take a whole fresh lemon and work out its volume: Use a large (depending on the size of your fruit) measuring cylinder, half fill it with water. Note the exact volume. Immerse your lemon in it. Again record the volume, the difference in the two readings is the volume of your fruit. If a large measuring cylinder is not available, submerge it in water in a 100cm^3 beaker and mark the level at the base of the meniscus on the side of the beaker. Remove the lemon and add measured volume of water from a cylinder until the water level reaches the mark. The volume of water added is the volume of the lemon.
7. Cut the lemon in half; extract some juice in a test tube.
8. Using 1cm^3 of lemon juice extracted, record how much lemon juice is required to decolourise 2cm^3 of DCPIP solution as in steps 1–3.
9. Work out the mass of vitamin C in 1 cm^3 of lemon juice. Multiply by volume of the lemon in cm^3 to find vitamin C content of the whole lemon.

Reference: UCLES, Question 1, 2nd Nov. 1992.

Reference: UCLES, Question 1, 23rd May, 1995.

Reference: UCLES, Question 2, 21st May, 1996.

For consideration

(a) Discuss any sources of error in your investigation. How would you overcome them?

(b) Ascorbic acid is a derivative of hexose sugar. Why do you think it is so abundant in fruits and vegetables?

(d) Daily recommended intake of vitamin C is 30mg, intake of less than 10mg/day leads to scurvy. To what extent can a single lemon meet these requirements?

7 Enzymes

Enzymes

Different Enzymes

Effects of Change in Conditions on Enzyme Activity

Digestion of Starch by Salivary Amylase

Effect of Temperature on Catalase Activity

Effect of pH on Enzyme Activity

Digestion of Egg White

Design an Investigation to Observe the Effect of pH on Proteases

Effect of Bead Size on the Activity of Immobilised Yeast

Effect of Temperature on the Action of an Enzyme

Effect of Substrate Concentration on Enzyme Action

Hydrolysis of Sucrose by Sucrase

Enzymes

Background Summary

Enzymes are biologically active globular proteins produced by living cells. They take part in and control many important chemical reactions. They are vitally important because their absence in a cell would cause all reactions to proceed too slowly to sustain life. Enzymes are therefore **biological catalysts**; their three dimensional structure makes their action specific. Most enzymes catalyse only one reaction. They work by forming a temporary **complex** with the substrate molecule at the active site. (The **lock and key hypothesis**.) Once the reaction has occurred the complex breaks down into the product and the unchanged enzyme. The enzyme can then be reused for further reactions.

Various factors such as temperature, pH, presence of inhibitors and co-factors as well as allosteric effects alter the rate of enzyme catalysed reactions because the active site complex formation is prevented.

To initiate any chemical reaction e.g. the breakdown of sugar, **activation energy** must be supplied. Enzymes effectively lower the activation energy required to initiate the reaction. The energy required for the reaction comes from the reaction itself, yielding carbon dioxide, water, and energy (cell respiration). Usually a number of enzymes are required in a sequence to convert one substance into one or more products and a chain of reactions, referred to as metabolic pathway, takes place.

Different Enzymes

You are expected to be familiar with the action of various enzymes and the important ones are summarised below.

Carbohydrase

Types of reaction catalysed: hydrolysis of polysaccharides or disaccharide into shorter chains, or single monosaccharides e.g. amylase, sucrase, lactase and maltase.

Amylase:

This catalyses the hydrolysis of starch to maltose.
Detection: Its action can be detected by the disappearance of starch using iodine reagent or the production of reducing sugars using Benedict's reagent.
Occurrence: It is found in germinating seeds, or insect guts. In digestive tract – salivary and pancreatic.

Sucrase:

Catalyses hydrolysis of sucrose to glucose and fructose.
Detection: Its action can be detected by testing for the production of reducing sugar using Benedict's reagent. It is not appropriate to test for the disappearance of the non-reducing sugar, as reducing sugars will also give a positive test with the non-reducing sugar test.
Occurrence: Sucrase can be found in insect guts, plant storage tissues such as onion bulbs and carrot top roots. Also occurs in human digestive tract, for the digestion of sucrose.

Lipases

Types of reaction catalysed: hydrolysis of fats into fatty acids and glycerol.
Examples: In humans, it is involved in the digestion of fats in the elementary canal, in the break down of fats in adipose tissues and when it is used for respiration.

Protease

Types of reaction catalysed: hydrolysis of proteins and polypeptides into shorter chains or amino acids.
Examples: Pepsin and trypsin in human digestion of proteins. Also protease thrombin converts fibrinogen to fibrin.

Dehydrogenases or oxidoreductases

Types of reaction catalysed: These are a group of enzymes catalysing the oxidation (by removing hydrogen) of substrate and transferring the hydrogen atoms to co-enzymes.
Their activity can be detected by using artificial hydrogen acceptors, which changes colour on reduction. Commonly used acceptors are **methylene blue**, which becomes colourless when reduced and **tetrazolium chloride**, which is colourless becomes pink, and **dichlorophenolindophenol** (**DCPIP**), which is blue and turns colourless.
Examples: Dehydrogenase enzymes are involved in many metabolic processes including the Krebs cycle of aerobic respiration and are therefore provided with biological material as the enzyme source, such as actively respiring yeast culture, germinating seeds, or fresh milk.

Catalase:

Catalyses the breakdown of hydrogen peroxide to water and oxygen. It is the fastest enzyme known. Its activity can be detected by effervescence (indicating oxygen production) and a rise in temperature as the reaction is strongly exothermic.
Occurrence: It is found in all living tissues, hydrogen peroxide is a toxic by-product of metabolism. Absence of catalase activity indicates that the tissue is naturally inert or has been killed.

Transferase

Types of reaction catalised: removes parts of molecules and adds to another.

Examples: Live cells contain **aminotransferases,** which transfer amino groups from one molecule to another for conversion of one amino acid to another.

Ligases

Types of reaction catalised: link two molecules together.
Example: DNA ligase link together DNA molecules and is used in genetic engineering.

Nucleotidase

Types of reaction catalised: degradation of nucleotides into phosphoric acid, pentose sugars and organice bases.
Occurrence: Found in small intestine.

Effects of Change in Conditions on Enzyme Activity

You are required to investigate the effect of temperature, pH, substrate, enzyme concentrations and inhibitors on enzyme action and are expected to know the properties of enzymes. Some important points are outlined below.

Temperature

Generally the rate of reaction doubles with every 10°C rise in temperature. This is due to increased kinetic energy and the resultant increased rate of collision of the reactants. This is also true of enzyme reactions until the optimum is reached, after which the vibrations become too severe and the hydrogen bonds and the disulphide bridges break and hence the 3D shape of the molecule is lost, disrupting the active site and the enzyme is said to be denatured. Hence, all enzymes have an optimum temperature at which they work at their peak. Temperatures above or below this show a decline in enzyme activity.

pH

The shape of an enzyme molecule is crucial to its functioning. This shape depends upon chemical bonds holding the molecules together in its tertiary structure. Some of these are ion pairs, formed between basic and acidic side chains in amino acid residues. Residues at the active site may also be affected by pH. The pH change leads to an alteration in enzyme shape, particularly at its active site. If an enzyme encounters extremes of pH, then it will be denatured. Under conditions of constant temperature, every enzyme functions most efficiently within a narrow pH.
The optimum pH is that at which the maximum rate of reaction occurs. When the pH is altered above or below this value, the rate of enzyme activity diminishes. The optimum pH of an enzyme is not always the same as the pH of its immediate intracellular environment. This suggests that the enzyme's surroundings may be exerting some form of control over its activity.

Substrate Concentration

Enzyme activity increases proportionally with increased substrate concentration until the maximum

Effect of Temperature on the Rate of Reaction of Two Enzymes

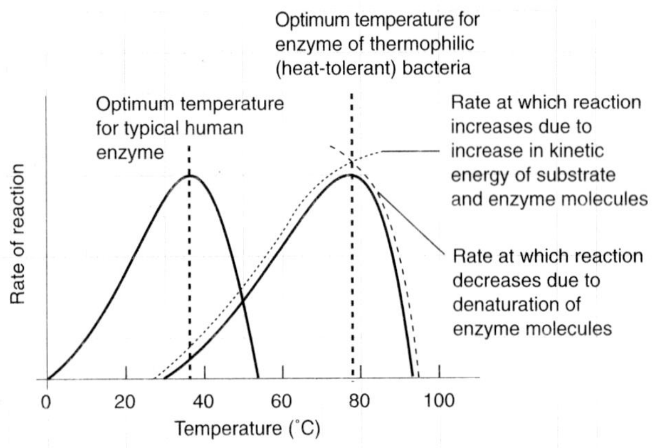

Effect of pH on the Rate of Reaction of Two Digestive Enzymes

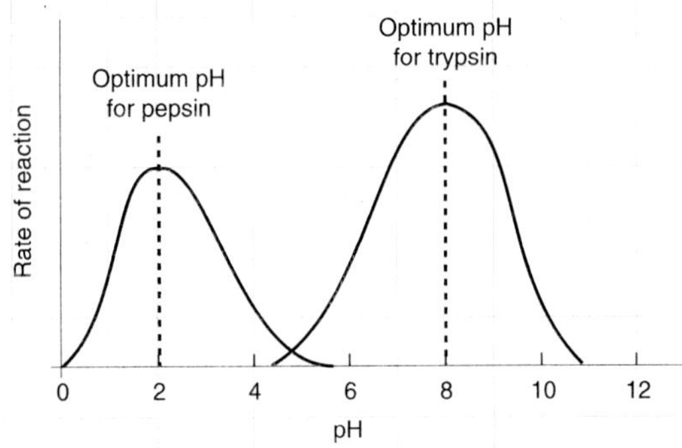

Effect of Substrate Concentration on the Rate of Enzyme-Controlled Reaction

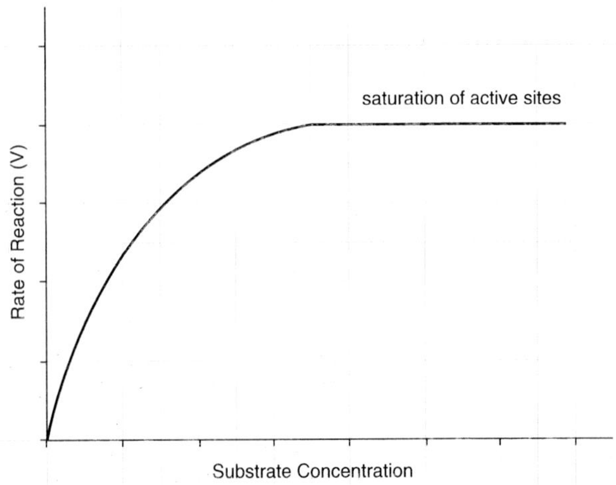

Effects of Change in Conditions on Enzyme Activity

turnover rate is reached. This is due to the increased chances of enzyme substrate collision. Once the maximum rate is reached no further increase is possible as the rate is limited by the availability of active sites.

Enzyme concentration

Activity also increases in direct proportion to enzyme concentration and increased collision rate increases the rate of reaction and the rate is eventually limited by the substrate availability.

Practical 22 – DIGESTION OF STARCH BY SALIVARY AMYLASE

Starch, a major source of energy is a polysaccharide. It has to be broken down into free sugar molecules before absorption can take place. This is achieved with the help of digestive enzymes amylases (salivary and pancreatic). The aim of this investigation is to show that saliva contains an enzyme, which breaks down starch to glucose, and to study the optimum conditions required for the enzyme to work. Starch is mixed with saliva under various conditions and after a given period of time the mixture is tested for starch with iodine solution and for reducing sugar with Benedict's reagent.

Procedure

1. Rinse your mouth with water. Collect 25 cm^3 of uncontaminated saliva in a measuring cylinder (chewing paraffin wax will help increase production of saliva).
2. Label three test tubes as **B** (boiled), **D** (denatured), and **S** (untreated saliva).
3. Transfer one quarter of the saliva to test tube B and place this in a boiling water bath for 15 minutes.
4. Transfer a further quarter to test tube D, add four drops of hydrochloric acid (1.0 mol dm^{-3}), mix well and leave for at least 15 minutes.
5. Keep the rest of the saliva untreated at room temperature in test tube S.
6. Now set up six pairs of test tubes as shown in the table. Label each test tube with its code number, using a marker pen as 1A, 1B, 2A, 2B etc. and arrange set A and set B in numerical order in the test tube rack.
7. To each test tube add the appropriate solutions as shown in the table.
8. Leave to stand for 10 minutes.
9. Carry out the starch test on set A by adding 2 drops of iodine solution to each tube.
10. Place a drop from test tube 4A, 5A and 6A in turn on a glass slide and observe the grains of starch under high power. Record your observations
11. Carry out the Benedict's test on set B by adding 2cm^3 Benedict's reagent to each test tube and heat them all together in a boiling water bath for at least 5 minutes.
12. Observe and record your results in a table, indicating which test tube gives a positive and which one a negative result for starch and sugar. It is possible that some may give a result in between, if so, then record.

Reference: UCLES Question 1, 9th Nov. 1993.
Reference: UCLES Question 2, 20th May, 1997.

For consideration

(a) What is the purpose of testing test tubes 1 to 3?
(b) Can you explain why you carried out the Benedict's test?
(c) Which test tubes, if any, support your explanation?
(d) Which test tubes provide information on the properties of the enzyme?
(e) What conclusions can you draw from your results about the chemical nature of the enzyme and what further experiments can be done to confirm these conclusions?
(f) Suggest a possible effect of boiling on the structure of starch to explain your observations.
(g) Suggest advantages and disadvantages of using a boiling water bath instead of boiling directly using a flame.

Test tube	**1A**	**2A**	**3A**	**4A**	**5A**	**6A**
Set A (Starch test)	4 cm^3 glucose	4 cm^3 starch	4 cm^3 saliva S	4 cm^3 starch + 2 cm^3 saliva S	4 cm^3 starch + 2 cm^3 saliva B	4 cm^3 starch + 2 cm^3 saliva D
Test tube	**1B**	**2B**	**3B**	**4B**	**5B**	**6B**
Set B (Benedict's test)	4cm^3 glucose	4 cm^3 starch	4 cm^3 saliva S	4 cm^3 starch + 2 cm^3 saliva S	4 cm^3 starch + 2 cm^3 saliva B	4 cm^3 starch + 2 cm^3 saliva D

Practical 23 – EFFECT OF TEMPERATURE ON CATALASE ACTIVITY

Catalase is an enzyme, which occurs in many plant and animal cells, catalysing the breakdown of hydrogen peroxide, to liberate water and oxygen gas as shown by effervescence:

$$2H_2O_2 \xrightarrow[\text{Catalase}]{} 2H_2O + O_2\uparrow$$

Hydrogen peroxide is a toxic by product of metabolism, which could kill the cell if not removed immediately. This is done extremely efficiently by catalase, which is one of the fastest enzymes known. At 0°C one molecule of catalase can decompose several million molecules of hydrogen peroxide per minute.

Procedure

1. Crush a fresh pea (or a soaked dry pea) on a white tile. Add a few drops of hydrogen peroxide solution. Observe carefully.
2. Take a small piece of meat in a watch-glass, add some hydrogen peroxide and observe. Repeat in clean watch-glasses with pieces of liver and kidney. Record your observations.
3. Remove the seed coats from two peas and test for catalase activity in both the seed coats and the cotyledons.
4. Place two test tubes labelled 1 and 2 containing about 5cm³ distilled water in a water bath at 40°C.
5. Boil two whole peas in another test tube, discard the water, and transfer the peas into test tube 1 in the water bath.
6. Place two whole unboiled peas in test tube 2 in the water bath.
7. Leave for about 10 minutes to allow enough time for the peas to reach the temperature of the water bath.
8. Test each pea for catalase activity.
9. Repeat the experiment at 50°, 60°, 70°, 80° and 100°C.
10. Record your observations and tabulate your data.

Reference: UCLES Question 1, 19th May, 1992.
Reference: UCLES Question 1, 9th Nov. 1994.
Reference: UCLES Question 1, 21st May, 1996.

For consideration

(a) What conclusion can you draw from these experiments and what further experiments could you do to test your hypothesis?

(b) Describe an experiment, which you can conduct to find out the precise temperature at which catalase is destroyed.

(c) Study **Fig. 7.1** carefully and comment on the shapes of the curves given for the enzymatic reaction at different temperatures.

(d) How could you make quantitative measurements of the rate of reaction?

Fig. 7.1 Time Course of Enzyme Reaction at Different Temperatures

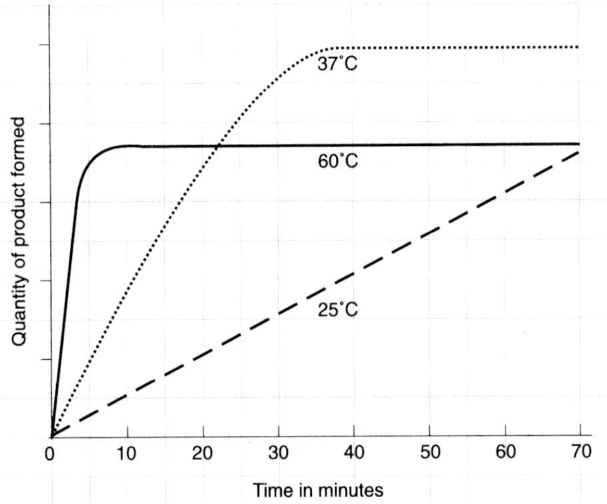

Practical 24 – EFFECT OF pH ON ENZYME ACTIVITY

This is a class investigation. The teacher should allocate pH buffers to each pair; for example 1 pair of students can work with pH 3, another at pH 5 and another at pH 7 etc. The class should test a range of pH 3–11 and then pool the results.
It is particularly important to read the whole procedure before you begin. Work in pairs. Organise yourself and work methodically.

Procedure

1. Rinse your mouth with about 5 cm³ of distilled water; discard the rinse in the sink.
2. Swill 10 cm³ of distilled water round your mouth for at least 1 min and then collect this liquid in a beaker and label it as salivary amylase.
3. Make up the volume of the salivary amylase to 40 cm³ with distilled water.
4. Test separately the salivary amylase, starch and buffer solutions for the presence of reducing sugar using Benedict's reagent.
5. Label a test tube **pH 3** and add 4 cm³ of starch solution and 4cm³ buffer solution pH 3 and mix well.
6. Label a test tube **BA** (boiled amylase), and another test tube **UA** (unboiled amylase).
7. Transfer 10 cm³ of salivary amylase solution to test tube BA and boil it.
8. Transfer 10 cm³ of salivary amylase solution to test tube UA and place both the tubes BA and UA in 40°C water bath and allow to equilibrate for a few minutes.
9. Place 11 test tubes labelled 1–11 in a test tube rack.
10. Add 1cm³ of Benedict's reagent to each of the 11 test tubes.

The following three steps must be carried out very quickly and carefully.

11. Add the buffered starch solution from test tube labelled pH 3 to the unboiled salivary amylase solution in test tube UA.
12. Mix the two solutions thoroughly and replace the test tube in the water bath. This is the reaction mixture and must be kept in the water bath after removal of 1 cm³ subsequent samples.
13. Start the stopclock and **immediately** remove 1cm³ of reaction mixture and place it in the test tube labelled 1.
14. Mix well, and replace the test tube in the rack.
15. After one minute, remove a second 1 cm³ sample, of the reaction mixture and place it in test tube 2 and replace the test tube in the rack.

16. Repeat the removal of 1 cm^3 samples of reaction mixture at one minute intervals until you have added reaction mixture to all 11 test tubes.
17. Carry out Benedict's tests on test tubes 1–11 and note the time of incubation at which a positive result (a brick-red precipitate) is first achieved.
18. Repeat the experiment using the boiled amylase solution from test tube BA.
19. Pool and tabulate class data.
20. Plot a graph of time taken for hydrolysis to occur against pH and comment on your results.

For consideration

(a) Explain the significance of steps 1 and 4.

(b) Why is pH control important in vivo?

(c) What sources of inaccuracy are there in this investigation?

(d) How could you improve this investigation?

(e) How could you take it a step further?

(f) Suggest why the enzymes work best at these pH?

Practical 25 – DIGESTION OF EGG WHITE

In the digestive tract proteins are hydrolysed by proteases, pepsin and trypsin. Pepsin is present in the gastric juice secreted in the stomach where conditions are markedly acidic. Trypsin, on the other hand, is present in the pancreatic juice secreted in the small intestine where conditions are alkaline. Presumably, these two enzymes work best at acidic (pH 2) and alkaline (pH 9) respectively. In this investigation we shall test this hypothesis, using egg white as the substrate for the enzymes.

Procedure

1. Label six boiling tubes **P2, P9** (pepsin), **T2, T9** (trypsin), and **C2, C9** (control).
2. Using separate pipettes or syringes for each solution set up test tubes as follows:

Test tube	**Enzyme**	**Solution**
C2 (control pH 2)	10cm^3 distilled water	1.0 cm^3 HCl
C9 (control pH 9)	10cm^3 distilled water	1.0 cm^3 Na_2CO_3
P2 (pepsin pH 2)	10 cm^3 pepsin	1.0 cm^3 HCl
P9 (pepsin pH 9)	10 cm^3 pepsin	1.0 cm^3 Na_2CO_3
T2 (trypsin pH 2)	10 cm^3 trypsin	1.0 cm^3 HCl
T9 (trypsin pH9)	10 cm^3 trypsin	1.0 cm^3 Na_2CO_3

3. Mix the contents of each tube and check the pH with pH paper, adjust it if necessary, using dilute acid or alkali, drop by drop.
4. To each tube add a strip of solid egg white (boiled egg). Leave the tubes in the incubator at 37°C overnight.
5. Observe the appearance of the egg white and the surrounding solution.
6. Record and interpret your results.

For consideration

(a) At which pH did the enzymes work best?

(b) Is this result what you expected?

(c) Why do you think boiled egg white was used rather than 'raw' egg white?

(d) Do your results support the hypothesis that pepsin and trypsin work best in acid and alkaline conditions respectively?

(e) How could you extend the experiment to determine the optimum pH for the action of each of these enzymes?

Practical 26 – DESIGN AN INVESTIGATION TO OBSERVE THE EFFECT OF pH ON PROTEASES

Egg whites contain several proteins – the most abundant being ovalbumin. When ovalbumin is mixed with water and boiled, a milky suspension is formed as the protein is rapidly denatured by heat. (This is just the physical state in which it would be in the stomach.)

Proteases such as pepsin and trypsin are enzymes that hydrolyse protein into smaller peptide fragments (pepsin is present in gastric juice and trypsin is present in pancreatic juice secreted into the duodenum). They work best on denatured proteins and can digest these solids to give a clear solution, because the peptides formed by the enzyme action are water soluble.

Design an experiment to investigate the rates at which the two enzymes turn an egg white suspension into a 'clear' solution using a range of pH buffer solutions.

Procedure

Work out and plan the procedure before you begin and show it to your teacher. Submit a list of requirements to staff prior to the practical class.

(1) You could try using 5 cm^3 of a 1% egg white suspension plus 5 cm^3 of a range of buffers from pH 2 to pH 8, and add 1cm^3 1% pepsin or trypsin solution to each.

(2) You may have to alter the quantity of enzyme, or the quantity of albumin solution. Alternatively, you could dilute your samples, but remember in order to get meaningful results you should only change one thing at a time, and remember to add some kind

of control to your investigation.
(3) Be methodical in your approach and make sure to apply the same conditions and procedure with all the different buffer solutions being tested.
(4) A water bath kept at about 40°C will replicate body temperature.
(5) If time permits, try other changes to your procedure that may give you better results.
(6) Tabulate your results.

Reference: UCLES Question 2, 2nd Nov. 1992.

For consideration

(a) At which pH value did the two proteases work best?
(b) Are the results consistent with what you expected? If not, explain.
(c) Was your plan effective for what you set out to do?
(d) If not, how did it falter and how could you improve your method to obtain better results?

Practical 27 – EFFECT OF BEAD SIZE ON THE ACTIVITY OF IMMOBILISED YEAST

Enzymes and micro-organisms such as yeast are commercially used in industry but their use is limited by the fact that they are readily denatured and are very expensive. This has been overcome by entrapping or immobilising the enzyme in a solid support, such as **alginate beads** (a polysaccharide extracted from seaweed). By doing so, the beads can be easily replaced, recovered, counted, or handled, and can be cleaned with distilled water for reuse which greatly reduces costs. Another advantage of immobilising the enzyme is that this process makes them more stable possibly by protecting the molecule from external conditions such as changes in temperature, solvents, pH and restricting the change in the shape. For example, glucose isomerase immobilised in polyacrylamide beads is stable almost for a year at 65°C, whereas it will denature in a matter of hours at 45°C unsupported.

In this investigation we shall entrap yeast in alginate beads of different sizes, and use the rate of production of carbon dioxide gas as a measure of the rate of respiration. Similarly, we could immobilise catalase in beads and measure the effect of bead size on the production of oxygen when the enzyme catalyses the breakdown of hydrogen peroxide.

Caution: ***Take care when handling the fragile, delivery tubes.***

Procedure

Work in pairs.

1. Add 1.0g sodium alginate to 25 cm^3 distilled water, and stir until a viscous mixture of even consistency is formed.
2. In another beaker stir 1g of yeast into 20 cm^3 distilled water.
3. After about five minutes, mix the two solutions together, using a glass rod.
4. Place 100 cm^3 of 1.4 % calcium chloride solution in another beaker.
5. Using a glass tube with a rubber teat attached or a dropper with a large aperture, draw about 10 cm^3 of the mixture and practice forming beads by dropping the mixture from a height of about 10cm into the beaker of calcium chloride. A bead of about 5mm is required. This may take some practice!
6. When you manage to start producing beads of similar size, make enough beads to cover the bottom of the flask to about three layers deep.
7. Repeat this procedure twice more using different sized glass tubes and with different beakers of calcium chloride solution. Try and produce three sets of beads of different sizes in separate beakers.
8. Allow the beads to stand in the calcium chloride solution for twenty minutes.
9. Transfer the beads from one beaker into a Petri dish. Discard all deformed, broken, or beads that float.
10. Using a hand lens and a ruler measure and record the average diameter of the beads.
11. Transfer enough well formed beads of equal diameter to the fermentation flask to cover the base of the flask to about two layers deep.
12. Repeat the same procedure with the other two sets of beads.
13. By now you should have three fermentation flasks with beads of different sizes in each, covering the base of the conical flask to about two layers deep.
14. Add enough 3% sucrose solution to cover the beads (equal volumes in all three flasks).
15. Carefully set up three fermentation flasks as shown in **Fig. 7.2** (*caution: the delivery tubes are very fragile*), and investigate the relative rates of reaction.
16. If time permits, estimate and record the number of beads in each flask.
17. Record your observations.

Reference: UCLES Question 1, 6th Nov. 1996.

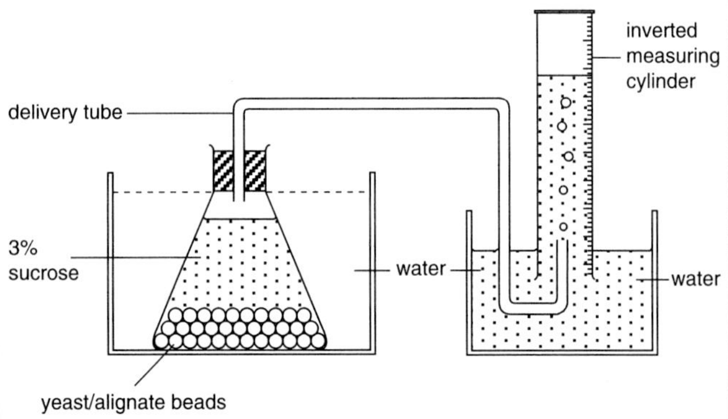

Fig. 7.2 Effect of Bead Size on Immobilised Yeast

For consideration

(a) Estimate the total surface areas of the beads in each solution, and the distance from the surface of a spherical bead to the centre.
(b) Compare the rate of reaction in the three flasks.
(c) Explain your results in terms of the ease with which sucrose enters a bead, the distance the molecules have to diffuse and the average distance of the yeast cell from the surface of the bead. Consider molecular size.
(d) Would the rate of reaction be affected in any way, if a very large molecule were to react with the entrapped enzyme?
(e) Why do enzymes in free solutions work much faster than immobilised enzymes?
(f) Why do you think beads that float were discarded?
(g) How could you improve this procedure to give better results, and to take this investigation further?

Reference: UCLES Question 1, 20th May, 1997.

Practical 28 – EFFECT OF TEMPERATURE ON THE ACTION OF AN ENZYME

Enzymes are proteins and are easily denatured by temperature. In this investigation you will observe the effect of temperature on enzyme action. This is easily achieved by exposing the enzyme to various temperatures and observing its effect on enzyme action. Samples of diastase are incubated at various temperatures; the time taken for the enzyme to hydrolyse a sample of starch is noted by the action of iodine on the starch solution at regular intervals.

Procedure

1. If constant water bath are available set them up at 40°, 60°, 80°C. If not, use boiling water to set up the appropriate water baths into large beakers. Use ice to obtain the lower temperatures.
2. Label six test tubes 0°, 20°, 40°, 60°, 80° and 100°C.
3. Add 5cm^3 of diastase solution to each test tube.
4. Leave the first test tube in iced water.
5. Place all other tubes in the appropriate water bath for exactly five minutes.
6. After five minutes of incubation remove the test tubes from the water baths and place them in iced water.
7. Add 5 cm^3 of starch solution to each test tubes, and mix thoroughly.
8. Immediately start the stopwatch and with a separate dropper for each test tube remove a drop at one-minute intervals from each test tube. Place the drop on a white tile, add a drop of iodine to the drop of reaction mixture, and record your observations.
9. Continue to take samples at one-minute intervals until addition of iodine stops indicating the presence of starch, (not longer than ten minutes).
10. Present your results in a way in which they are easy to understand.

For consideration

(a) How could you improve this technique and take it further?
(b) Explain your observations keeping in mind all you know about enzyme structure.
(c) What type of bonds would you expect the enzyme to have?
(d) How could you make this method quantitative?

Practical 29 – EFFECT OF SUBSTRATE CONCENTRATION ON ENZYME ACTION

In 1913 Leonor **Michaelis** and Maud **Menten** put forward a theory to explain how enzymes work. They had noticed that, at low substrate concentration, the rate is proportional to concentration, but as concentration increases, the rate levels off until a maximum value is achieved. This rate can only be increased on further additions of enzyme **Fig. 7.3.**

From their work Michaelis–Menten defined two important properties of enzymes:

i. **K_m the Michaelis constant is the substrate concentration at which half the maximum enzyme velocity (V_{max}) is reached.**
ii. **A low value of K_m means that the enzyme has a high affinity for (binding tightly to) its substrate.**

To demonstrate this theory we will look at hydrolysis of hydrogen peroxide by catalase.

$$2H_2O_2 \xrightarrow{\text{Catalase}} 2H_2O + O_2\uparrow$$

Hydrogen peroxide is a toxic by product of metabolism,

Fig. 7.3 Effect of Substrate Concentration on the Rate of Enzyme-Controlled Reaction

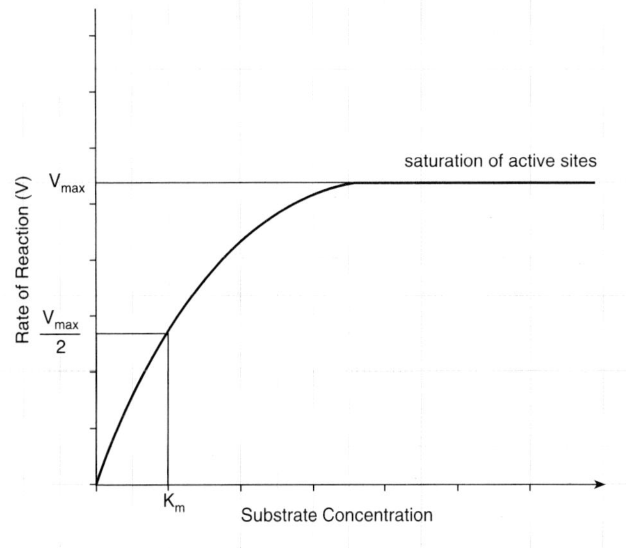

which could kill the cell if not removed immediately. This is done extremely efficiently by catalase, which is one of the fastest enzymes known. At 0°C one molecule of catalase can decompose several million molecules of hydrogen peroxide per minute. Catalase is particularly abundant in the liver.

Procedure

Preparation of enzyme extract

(To save time this has been prepared for you).

The liver was homogenised (liquidised) in 10 cm^3 of buffer. It was filtered through several layers of muslin and made up to 200 cm^3 with buffer.

1. Add 15cm^3 hydrogen peroxide and 10cm^3 buffer to the conical flask.
2. Set up the flask as shown in **Fig. 7.4.**
3. Push in the gas syringe plunger.
4. Fill a syringe with 2cm^3 enzyme extract, attach a needle to the syringe and add to the Büchner flask (side arm flask) through the rubber seal.
5. On shaking the flask, oxygen is produced, which pushes out the plunger.
6. Measure the volume of oxygen produced in 15 seconds. (If the volume of oxygen produced is not between 40 and 60cm^3 adjust the volume of enzyme accordingly.)
7. Repeat steps 1–6.
8. Repeat the procedure with a range of hydrogen peroxide concentration, obtained by adding 12, 10, 8, 6, 4, 2, 0 cm^3 of hydrogen peroxide to buffer, always keeping the total volume in the flask at 25cm^3 by altering the volume of buffer added accordingly.
9. A control should be carried out, by substituting the enzyme with water. If gas is produced in 15 seconds, subtract this volume from your readings.
10. Plot the rate (volume of oxygen produced divided by time) against concentration (20 volume hydrogen peroxide is 1.74 M).
11. Plot the graph you would expect if you doubled the enzyme concentration.

For consideration

(a) Explain the shape of your graph. Do the results support the Michaelis-Menten model? If so record V_{max} and K_m.

(b) Why was it necessary to work with buffered solutions?

(c) Which factors were kept constant in this experiment, and why was it necessary to keep them constant?

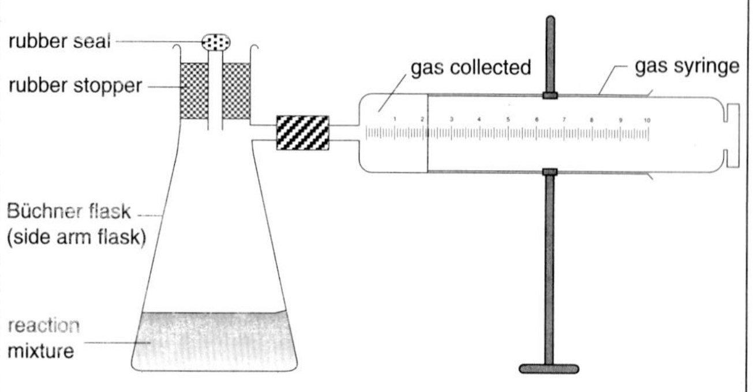

Fig. 7.4 Effect of Substrate Concentration on Enzyme Controlled Reaction

Practical 30 – HYDROLYSIS OF SUCROSE BY SUCRASE

A convenient way to demonstrate the effect of substrate and enzyme concentration on the rate of reaction is exhibited by hydrolysis of sucrose by sucrase (invertase) to glucose and fructose:

$$\underset{\text{Sucrose}}{C_{12}H_{22}O_{11}} + H_2O \rightarrow \underset{\text{Glucose}}{C_6H_{12}O_6} + \underset{\text{Fructose}}{C_6H_{12}O_6}$$

(To avoid any confusion, in this investigation we will refer to sucrase as invertase.)

To determine the effect of enzyme concentration, you will need to vary the enzyme concentrations, but maintain equal volume of substrate concentration.

To investigate the effect of substrate concentration, a standard concentration of enzyme needs to be added to different concentration of substrate. **Remember there should be only one variable at any one time.**

The progress of the reaction can be followed either by testing for the disappearance of the substrate or the appearance of the products. Sucrose is the substrate and it is a non-reducing sugar and gives a negative test with Benedict's solution, but glucose and fructose, the product both test positive and produces a yellow/brown or red precipitate.

It is important to measure the initial rate of the reaction, that is, the reaction over a short period of time, say 30 seconds. This is because the rate of reaction decreases with time, and if you continue the experiment for a longer time, the effect of the decline of the reaction rate becomes confused with the effect of the enzyme or the substrate concentration.

Procedure

1. Test both sucrose and invertase solutions for reducing sugar individually.
2. Label eight test tubes 1–8.
3. Add 1 cm^3 of Benedict's solution to tubes 1–8.
4. Add 5 cm^3 of 2% sucrose solution to another clean labelled test tube.
5. Add 5 cm^3 of 1% invertase solution to another labelled test tube.
6. Place both test tubes in a 38°C water bath; allow about five minutes to equilibrate to this temperature.

It is important to proceed quickly and systematically in the following steps.

7. Start the stopclock and immediately add the invertase solution to the sucrose solution, mix well and return the test tube to the 38°C water bath.
8. After 30 seconds remove $1cm^3$ of this reaction mixture and add to test tube 1.
9. Using a clean syringe or a pipette for each, repeat this at 30 seconds intervals, adding the reaction mixture to test tube 2–8.
10. Place test tubes 1–8 in 50°C water bath for 5 minutes.
11. Record the amount of precipitate formed in each tube.

Effect of enzyme concentration can be investigated as follows:

(i) Repeat steps 1–10, twice, once using 0.75% and once using 0.5% invertase solution with 2% sucrose solution.

Effect of substrate concentration can be investigated as follows:

(ii) Repeat steps 1–10 twice using 0.25%, 0.5% and 1% sucrose solutions respectively, with 1% invertase each time.

Reference: UCLES Question 1, 3rd Nov. 1997.

For consideration

(a) Examine your results. What relationship is there between the initial rate of reaction and either enzyme or substrate concentration?

(b) Explore ways of making your results into figures, which can be plotted on a graph. For example, if you calculate the rate of reaction as 1/reaction time for the first reducing sugar to be detected, you may then be able to plot reaction time (vertical axis) against enzyme or substrate concentration (horizontal axis).

(c) Do you think that Benedict's solution affects the reaction in any way?

(d) Explain your results in term of the interactions between enzyme and substrate molecules.

(e) Why do you think sucrose tests negative with Benedict's solution whereas the two sugars of which it is composed both give a positive test?

(f) What effect, if any, would increasing the temperature from 30°C to 60°C have on the investigation?

8 Cell Division

Cell Division

Background Summary

Cell division is responsible for **reproduction** and **growth**. Nuclear division occurs either by **mitosis** or **meiosis.** Mitosis is associated with growth and asexual reproduction. It can be observed in plant endosperm meristematic tissue. A cell normally contains two of each type of chromosomes – **diploid state.**
Meiosis is associated with sexual reproduction. It may be seen in developing spores, pollen grains, embryo sacs, eggs or sperms. Meiosis results in the daughter cells containing only one of each type of chromosome – **haploid state.**

Both types of cell division involve the orderly movement of chromosomes on the fibres of the **spindle apparatus.** This is a continuous process but for convenience it is divided into five stages: **Fig. 8.1**
In **interphase** the cell gets ready for division, and the genetic material (DNA) replicates, the nucleoli become prominent.
In **prophase** the chromosomes appear as distinct bodies, chromatids become visible.
In **metaphase** the chromosomes arrange themselves on the equator of the spindle.
In **anaphase** the chromosomes separate and move towards opposite poles of the spindle.
In **telophase** as the chromosomes reach the two poles, the cell finally divides – **cytokinesis.** The nucleus divides first, followed by the cytoplasm.
The interval between cell divisions is known as **interphase.** At interphase the cell is not resting but the chromosomes instigate the control of growth, development and functioning of cells by controlling protein synthesis.

Practical 31 – OBSERVING CELL DIVISION

The chromosomes can be selectively stained with a dye such as aceto-orcein, to observe stages in mitosis and meiosis in cells where division is taking place. **Mitosis** can be observed in the **meristematic tissue** located in the zone of cell division, in the tip of the growing lateral root of an onion or broad bean. **Meiosis** can be observed in immature anthers that are still enclosed inside the flower bud. Within such anthers diploid pollen mother cells may be found dividing meiotically to form haploid pollen grains. Young anthers, pale creamy in colour generally have meiotic stages in them. To observe meiosis in plants *Tradescantia virginiana* or onion flower buds can be used.

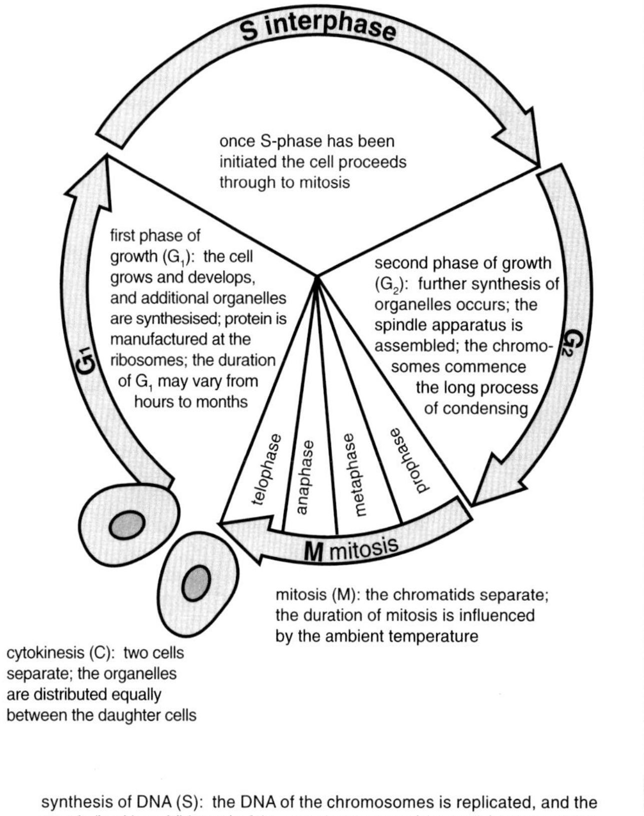

Fig. 8.1 Generalised Cell Cycle of Eukaryotic Cell

Procedure

Mitosis in onion root tips

1. Set up a boiling water bath in a $100cm^3$ beaker.
2. Cut off about 5 mm from the apical root tip of an onion.
3. Place the root tip in a watch glass; add 40 drops of aceto-orcein stain and 4 drops of concentrated hydrochloric acid to help macerate the cells.
4. Place the watch glass on top of the boiling water bath, and turn off the Bunsen burner.
5. Keep the watch glass on top of the water bath for about 3-4 minutes; making sure the stain does not evaporate dry. Add more stain if necessary.
6. Place the root tip on a clean glass slide; add a drop of cold stain.
7. Without interfering too much with the arrangement of the cells, break the root tip either with a mounted needle or crush it with the back of a glass rod so as to spread it out as thinly as possible.

8. Place a coverslip on top of the macerated tissue and, wrap the slide in several layers of filter papers.
9. Place the slide on a flat surface and squash firmly with your thumb, without allowing the coverslip to slide.
10. Carefully remove the filter paper and warm the slide by quickly passing it through the blue flame of the Bunsen burner. This will intensify the stain. The slide should be warm, but not too hot to touch the back of your hand.
11. Examine under high power of the microscope.
12. If you are lucky you will see almost colourless cytoplasm with red/purple nuclei **Fig. 8.2**. Look for chromosomes at various stages of mitosis.
13. If the cells appear uniformly pink you have overheated the slide. You may have to repeat the procedure several times before getting the desired results.
14. Using **Fig. 8.3** to help you, identify and make annotated drawings of as many stages of mitosis as you can see. Bear in mind that the chromosomes will not be as neatly arranged in your preparation, as are shown in the diagrams and that experts prepare textbook photographs after a lot of hard work. However, there is no reason why you should not see most of the stages in mitosis in your preparations.
15. Supplement the information obtained from your own slide by observing mitosis in prepared slides.
16. If you have been unable to find dividing cells in your preparation, make drawings from a prepared slide of mitosis.
17. Compare with mitosis in prepared animal cells e.g. *Ascaris*.
18. Watch a film or video recording of cell division if available. Notice in particular that cell division is a continuous process, dividing it up into various stages is purely for our convenience.

Meiosis in Flower Buds of Tradescantia

1. The youngest flower buds are at the apex; the flower buds at the base are the most advanced. Make slides of both and of intermediate buds between the two extremes.
2. Cut away open flowers and flower buds that have open clusters, select a flower bud only 2-3 mm long from the apex. Place it on a clean microscope slide and using a mounted needle tease out the anthers, discard all other parts of the flower.
3. Follow steps 6–18 in the above procedure. Prepare anther squash slides and instead of the cold stain use acidified acetio-orcein.
4. Compare your preparation with prepared sections of anther squash slides and with slides of mammalian testis.
5. Under oil-immersion look for bivalent homologous chromosomes, chiasmata and centromeres.
6. Make a table of similarities and differences in mitosis and meiosis.

For consideration

(a) Sometimes, no dividing cells are visible in a root tip or in an anther squash no matter how carefully you prepare the slide. Suggest possible reasons for this. (I sincerely hope that you have not been unlucky today!)

(b) In what situation apart from those studied here would you expect to find mitosis taking place in animal and plant cells?

(c) What can you say about the chromosome number of the plant from which the root was obtained?

(d) Which particular events in mitosis ensure that the diploid state is preserved?

(e) If possible, work out approximately the proportion of cells dividing at each stage.

(f) Which stage of mitosis appears to take the longest?

(g) Why was it suggested that you choose anthers from the apex of the inflorescence?

(h) Which particular event in meiosis ensures the reduction of chromosomes from diploid to haploid?

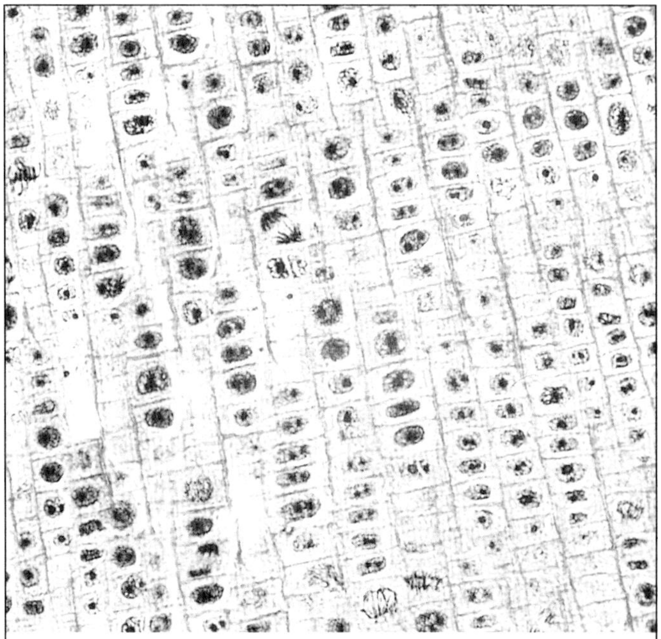

Fig. 8.2 Mitosis in Onion (*Allium*) Root Tips

In **mitosis**, the **homologous chromosomes** do not pair up with each other. They appear as **chromatids,** held together at the **centromeres**, the nuclear membrane breaks down and a **spindle** becomes visible. The fibres of the spindle pull the chromatids apart to form the basis of new nuclei at opposite ends of the cell. End result being that **the daughter cells have the same chromosome and genotype make up as the original cell.**

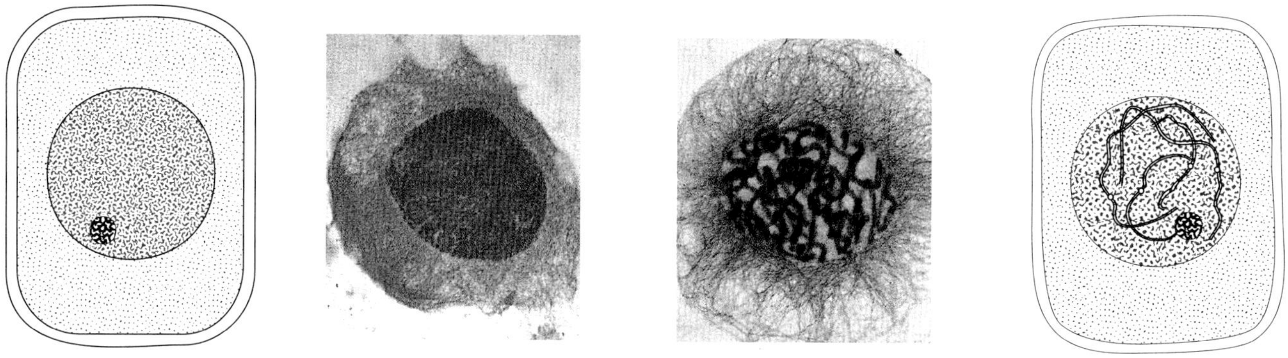

1. Interface (before mitosis)
Chromosomes indistinct, nuclear membrane intact.

2. Prophase
Condensed chromosomes appear as long, thin threads, each thread has already replicated into two chromatids, but the chromatids are tightly held together and still appear joined at the centromere. Nuclear membrane begins to disintegrate.

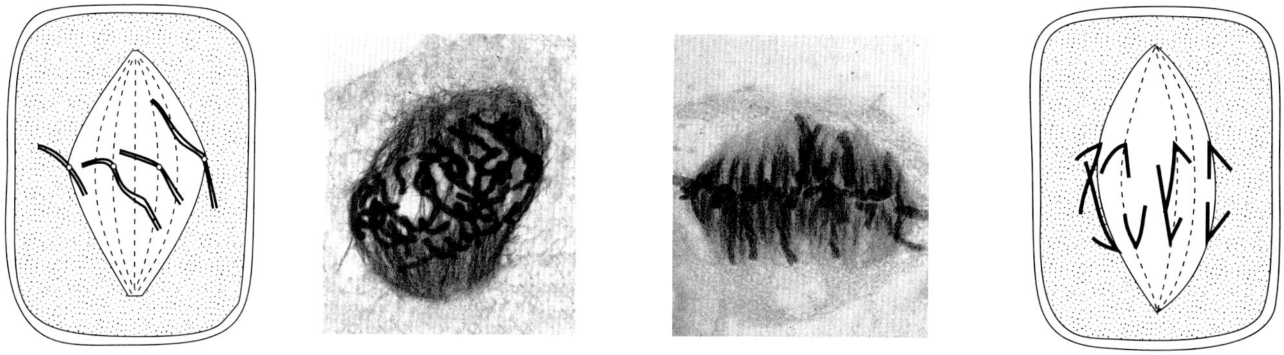

3. Transition to Metaphase
Nuclear membrane breaks down; each chromosome attaches to the spindle fibres at the equator of the spindle by its centromere.

4. Metaphase
All chromosomes line up at the equator of the spindle and are now very condensed.

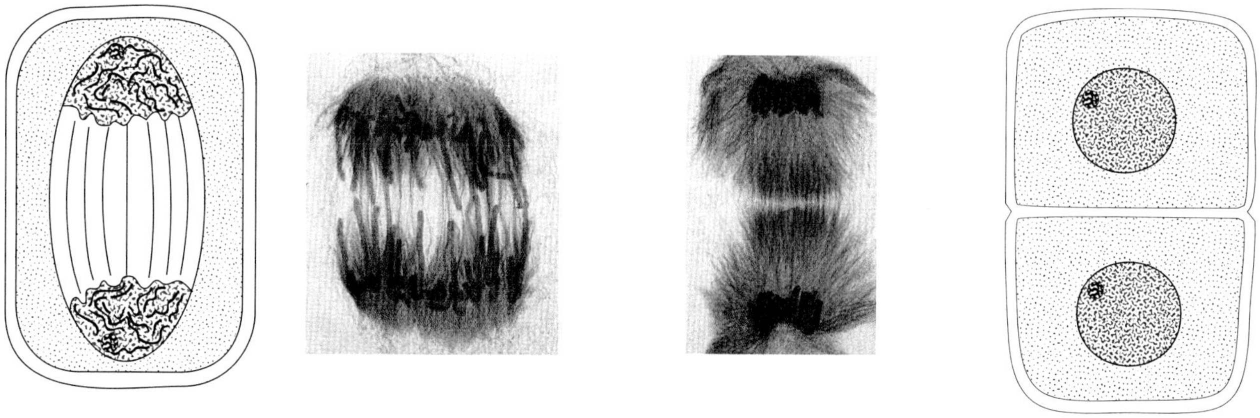

5. Anaphase
Attachment between the two sister chromatids of each chromosomes breaks; the two are now chromosome in their own rights. They move to opposite poles. Nucleolus and nuclear membrane reappear.

6. Telophase progressing to interphase
Chromosomes decondensed. Nuclear membrane reforms. Chromosomes appear as chromatin granules.

Fig. 8.3 Mitosis in Onion (*Allium*) Root Tips
(most species of Allium have 16 chromosomes but, for simplicity, only four chromosomes are shown in the diagram)

In **meiosis**, the nucleus divides twice to eventually form four nuclei. Each of these divisions is organised into phases very similar to those in mitosis. The four non- identical nuclei formed contain an assortment of the maternal and paternal **chromatids**, and also **recombination** of various parts of individual chromatids due to crossing over during meiosis. Meiosis is associated with sexual reproduction, and the four cells produced are totally different in genotype.

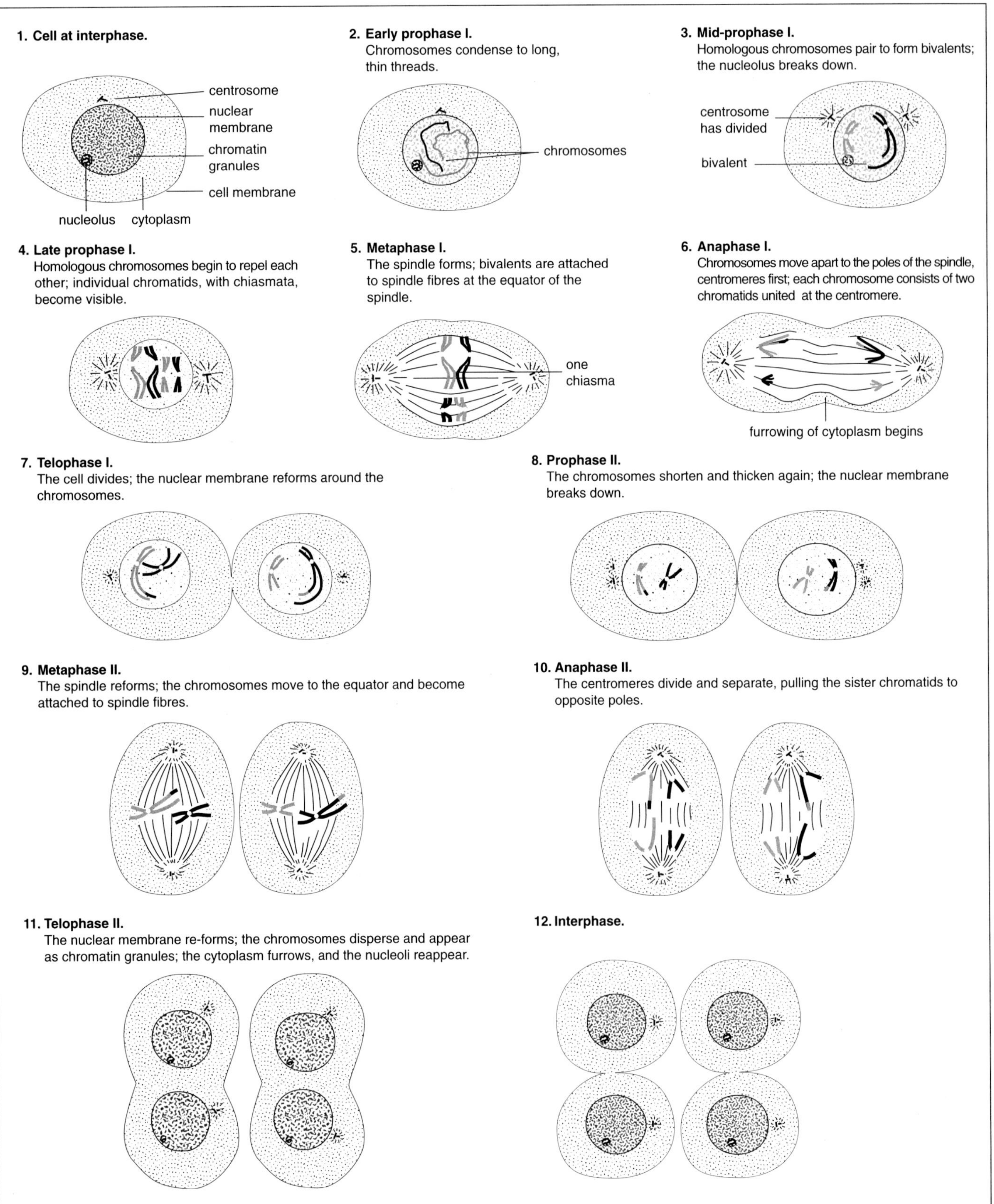

Fig. 8.4 Meiosis in an Animal Cell

9 Energetics

Autotrophic Nutrition

Factors Affecting Photosynthesis

Destarching a Plant

To Test a Leaf for Starch

To Investigate the Need for Light

To Investigate the Need for Carbon Dioxide

To Investigate the Need for Chlorophyll

To Investigate Evolution of Oxygen

Effect of Light Intensity on the Rate of Photosynthesis

Design an Investigation to Test the Effect of Carbon Dioxide Concentration on the Rate of Photosynthesis

Nutrient Requirements for Healthy Plant Growth

Photosynthetic Pigments

Extraction of Photosynthetic Pigment

Demonstration of Fluorescence

Measurement of the Absorption Spectrum

Hill's Reaction

Synthesis of Starch

Formation of Starch in the Green Leaf

Autotrophic Nutrition

Autotrophic nutrition, the synthesis of organic compounds from relatively simple inorganic raw materials such as water, carbon dioxide and energy takes place by **photosynthesis** in plant leaves. Inside the leaf are cells containing **chloroplasts**, where light energy is trapped by the **chlorophyll** to produce carbohydrates; **oxygen** is the waste product.

Photosynthesis is of great **ecological, economic** and **environmental importance** to living things because the survival of all life depends on photosynthesis. All non-photosynthesising organisms obtain their nutrients directly or indirectly, from green plants. In nature only a tiny portion, about 1% of the total energy of sunlight is fixed, the rest is lost by various processes. Incidentally, not all-autotrophic organisms use light energy; certain autotrophic bacteria synthesise organic compounds from inorganic raw materials, a form of **chemosynthesis**. Chemosynthetic bacteria are important in the nitrogen cycle.

Photosynthesis and chemosynthesis play a vital role in the **carbon cycle**. Nearly all carbon dioxide released each day (from respiration and combustion) is removed from the atmosphere and is built up as complex carbon compounds by photosynthesis and chemosynthesis. It is later released back into the atmosphere via respiration. Plants release all the oxygen as waste product in our atmosphere at present about 21%.

The chloroplasts are mainly in the **green leaf** of the terrestrial plants; an organ specialised for photosynthesis, whose anatomy is well adapted for its functions. In the upper layers loosely packed photosynthetic cells (**palisade and spongy mesophyll**) carry out photosynthesis whilst the lower epidermis is pierced by numerous **stomata** for gas exchange. Other tissues are responsible for structural support and transport.

The most important single factor controlling photosynthesis is light and plants exhibit a wide variety of adaptation in securing maximum illumination. The **absorption spectrum** for the photosynthetic pigments and the **action spectrum** (indicates amount of photosynthesis) for the process of photosynthesis both show that these are responsible for the absorption of light which initiates photosynthesis. The absorption spectrum of chlorophyll indicates that red and blue light are absorbed the most **Fig. 9.1.**

Chromatography reveals that chlorophyll is a mixture of pigments, which are **chlorophyll a** and **chlorophyll b** plus accessory pigments **xanthophyll** and **carotene**. A further pigment **phaeophytin** is a breakdown product of chlorophyll. As you can see the absorption spectrum, chlorophyll a and chlorophyll b absorb primarily violet-blue and red light respectively, the function of the accessory pigments is to increase the range of wavelengths in photosynthesis from which plants can gather energy.

Photosynthesis is a multi-stage process consisting of a **light stage,** requiring light and an enzymic **dark stage,** which is able to proceed in the dark. In the light reaction, ATP is produced, water is split (**Hill's reaction**), oxygen is released as a bi-product, and hydrogen atoms are released for the following reduction of carbon dioxide in the dark reaction. In the subsequent dark stage carbon dioxide is reduced to carbohydrate via the **Calvin cycle**. This is known as the C_3 pathway, since the first product is a three carbon compound.

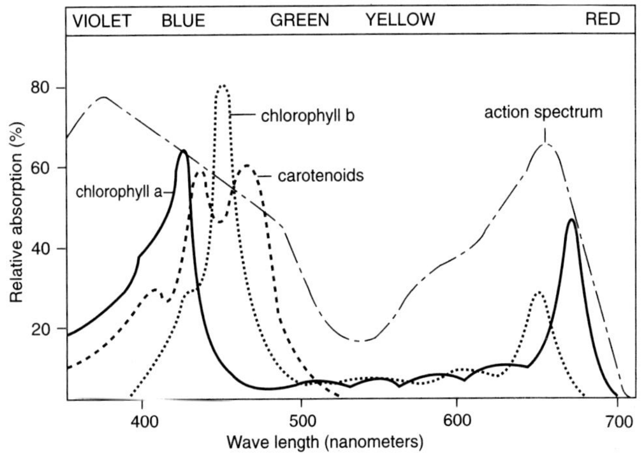

Fig. 9.1 Absorption Spectrum

Practical 32 – FACTORS AFFECTING PHOTOSYNTHESIS

The rate of photosynthesis is influenced by various factors such as carbon dioxide concentration, temperature and light intensity. An understanding of these factors is important in agriculture as it affects crop yield and can lead to improvement in crop production.
Presence of starch, the end product of photosynthesis, can be taken as an indication that photosynthesis has occurred, provided that the precaution is taken of starting the experiment with a destarched leaf or plant.

Destarching a plant

Leaving a plant in complete darkness for 24–48 hours will destarch it. Prior to starting the experiment check that destarching is complete before attempting the experiment. If not, leave for a further 24 hours. Geranium (*Pelargonium*) is suitable for this purpose.

To test a leaf for starch Fig. 9.2

Caution: avoid naked flames, ethanol is highly inflammable.

Procedure

The leaf has to be decolourised because the green colour of the chlorophyll in the leaf masks the colour change in the starch test.

1. Immerse the leaf in boiling water for a few minutes to soften it.
2. Transfer it in a test tube of 90% ethanol in a boiling water bath.
3. Carefully take the brittle leaf out of the ethanol and dip it in hot water to soften it. Spread it out on a white tile. Add a few drops of iodine solution (I_2/KI). Blue/black colour is indicative of presence of starch.

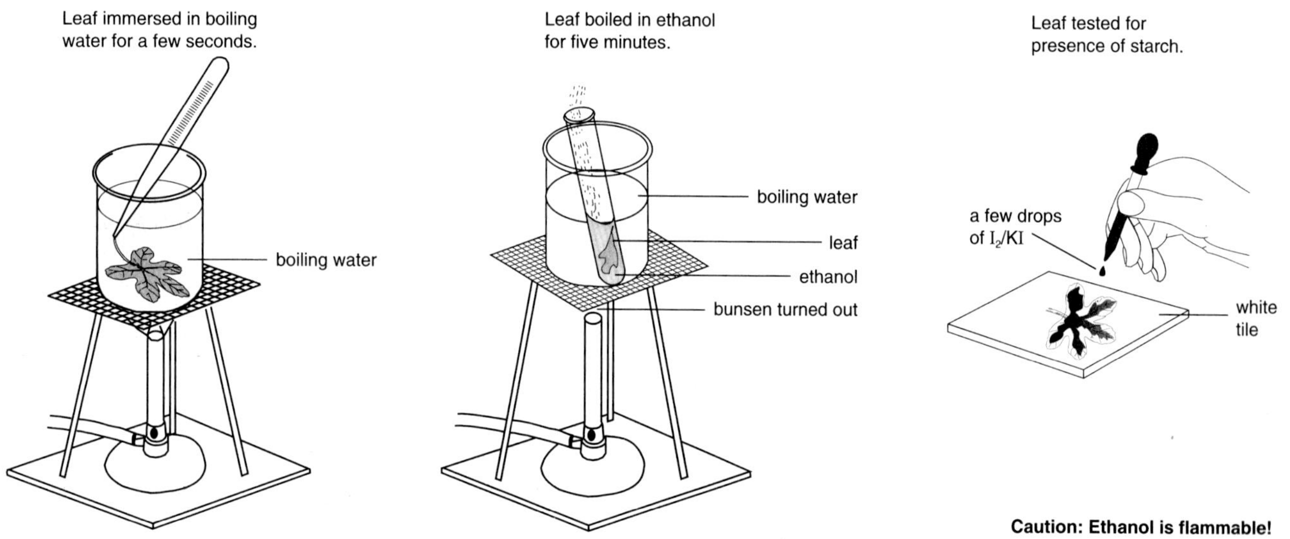

Fig. 9.2 Testing a Leaf for Starch

To investigate the need for light

Procedure

The destarching process itself demonstrates the need for light, but this can be further demonstrated by placing a strip of black paper or metal foil over a destarched leaf and exposing it to light for several hours **Fig. 9.3.** After which the leaf is tested for starch.

For consideration

(a) How would you criticise the experimental design and how would you modify the experiment taking into account your criticisms?

To investigate the need for carbon dioxide Fig. 9.4

Procedure

1. Destarch two potted plants by keeping them in a cupboard for at least 48 hours.
2. Test a leaf from each plant to make sure destarching has occurred (if not, leave in the dark for a further 24 hours).
3. Place some soda lime (this absorbs CO_2 from the air) in a suitable container on the pot and enclose the plant in a clear transparent plastic bag, with an elastic band.
4. Place a dish of saturated sodium hydrogencarbonate (this gives off CO_2 around the plant) on the other plant and enclose it in a plastic bag.

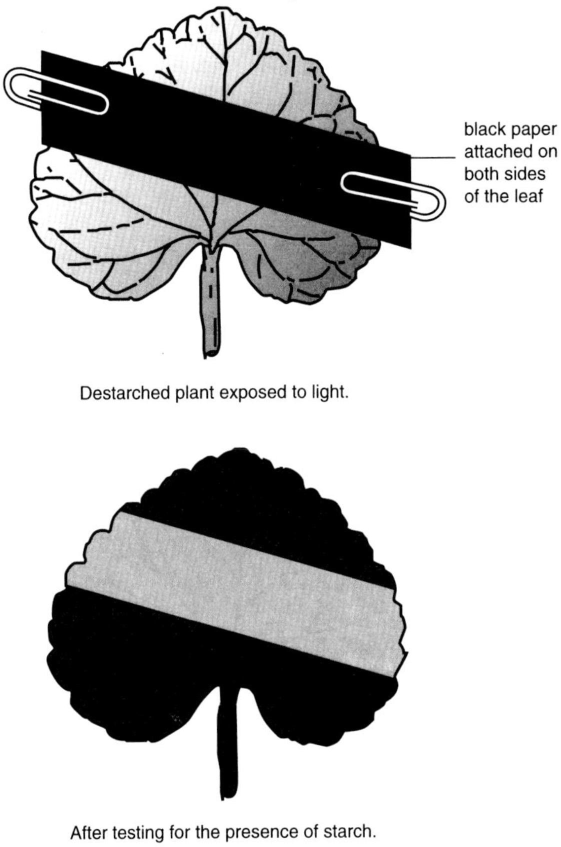

Fig. 9.3 To Demonstrate the Need for Light

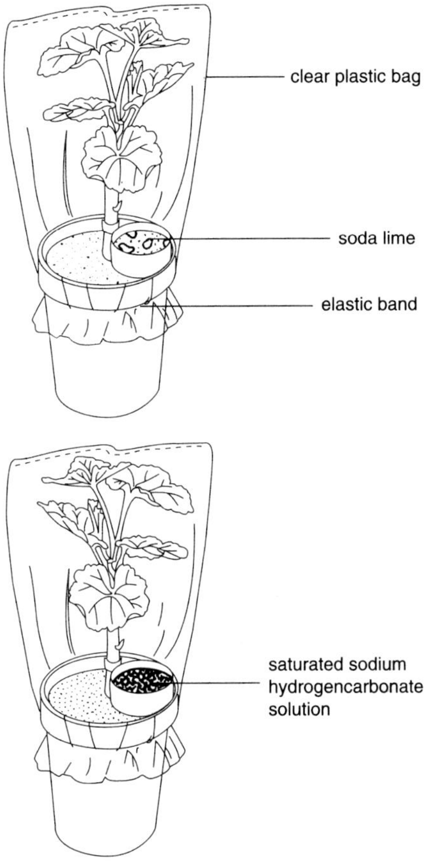

Fig. 9.4 Demonstrate need for Carbon Dioxide

5. Place both plants in bright sunlight for 6–12 hours.
6. Test a leaf from each plant for the presence of starch.

(b) Design a control for this investigation.

The importance of carbon dioxide has been demonstrated by use of labelled $^{14}CO_2$ (radioactive carbon dioxide).

To investigate the need for chlorophyll **Fig. 9.5**
Destarch a potted plant with variegated leaves such as *Bougainvillea Variegata* that has green leaves with yellow/ white patches which are areas having no chlorophyll. Trace the leaf, marking out the non-green areas. Carry out the starch test on the leaf.

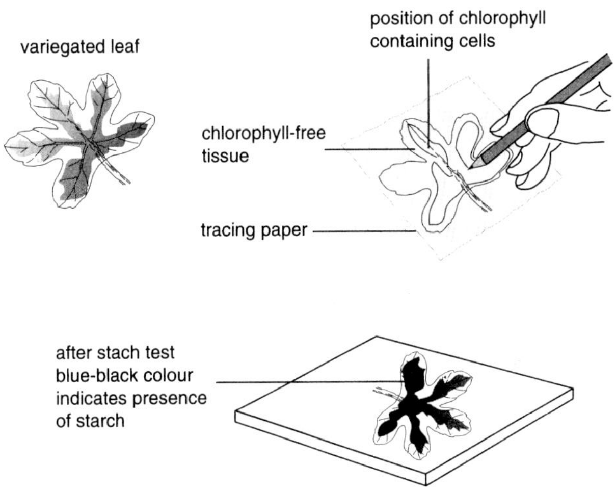

Fig. 9.5 Demonstrate the Need for Chlorophyll

To investigate evolution of oxygen
Procedure

1. Place some well-illuminated aquatic plant, such as *Elodea* or *Hydrilla* under a funnel in pond water as shown in **Fig. 9.6.**
2. Fill a test tube with pond water and invert it over the funnel.
3. Add a spatula full of sodium hydrogencarbonate to the solution to enrich carbon dioxide content of the water.
4. Illuminate the plant with a bright light for several hours.
5. Note the collection of gas at the top of the test tube.

Practical 33 – EFFECT OF LIGHT INTENSITY ON THE RATE OF PHOTOSYNTHESIS

The effect of light intensity on the rate of photosynthesis can be measured by the evolution of oxygen from an aquatic plants such as Canadian pondweed, *Elodea*, or *Hydrilla* at different levels of illumination. A very simple but tedious method of doing this is to count the evolution of the number of bubbles per unit time. A more precise and sophisticated method is to use a **photosynthometer Fig. 9.6**.

In this investigation, the volume of gas given by *Hydrilla* in a given time, at various light intensities, is measured using a photosynthometer.

This investigation can also be carried out with an oxygen electrode, monitoring changes in dissolved oxygen in the medium over several hours. An oxygen sensor and probe in conjunction with the Data Capture Equipment and Data Loggers DL Plus 32 Datadisc PRO and a microcomputer (Philip Harris, UK) can be used to record oxygen liberated by the pondweed under varying conditions of light intensities.

Procedure

(Use pondweed that has been well illuminated over several hours.)

1. Cut a piece of fresh looking pondweed about 10cm in length.
2. Place the pondweed; cut end at the top, in a test tube of pond water.
3. Fill the photosynthometer with pond water containing a pinch of sodium hydrogencarbonate, making sure it is completely filled with water, without any air.
4. Place the flared end of the photosynthometer in the test tube, under water so that any gas that evolves from the plant enters the apparatus **Fig. 9.6.**
5. Place the test tube in a beaker of water to maintain a fairly constant temperature.
6. Illuminate from the side using a 60V lamp from a distance of 5cm from the plant.
7. Wait for a few minutes to allow the plant to come to equilibrium with this light intensity.
8. Allow to proceed for 5–10 minutes.
9. Collect the gas from the capillary tube into the syringe, by pulling on the plunger, and measure its volume.
10. Record the volume of gas evolved per minute together with distance from the plant.
11. Replace the water in the beaker and repeat the whole process with increasing distances from the plant e.g. 10, 20, 30, 40, 50, 60, 70 and 80cm.
12. If time permits, repeat the procedure decreasing the distance, gradually moving the light source nearer to the plant.
13. Tabulate your data.
14. Plot a graph to show how the rate of photosynthesis varies with light intensity, using the following information:
    i. Light intensity is inversely proportional to the square of the distance between the source and the object being illuminated. In other words, doubling the distance between the plant and the lamp does not halves the light intensity received by the plant, but quarters it.

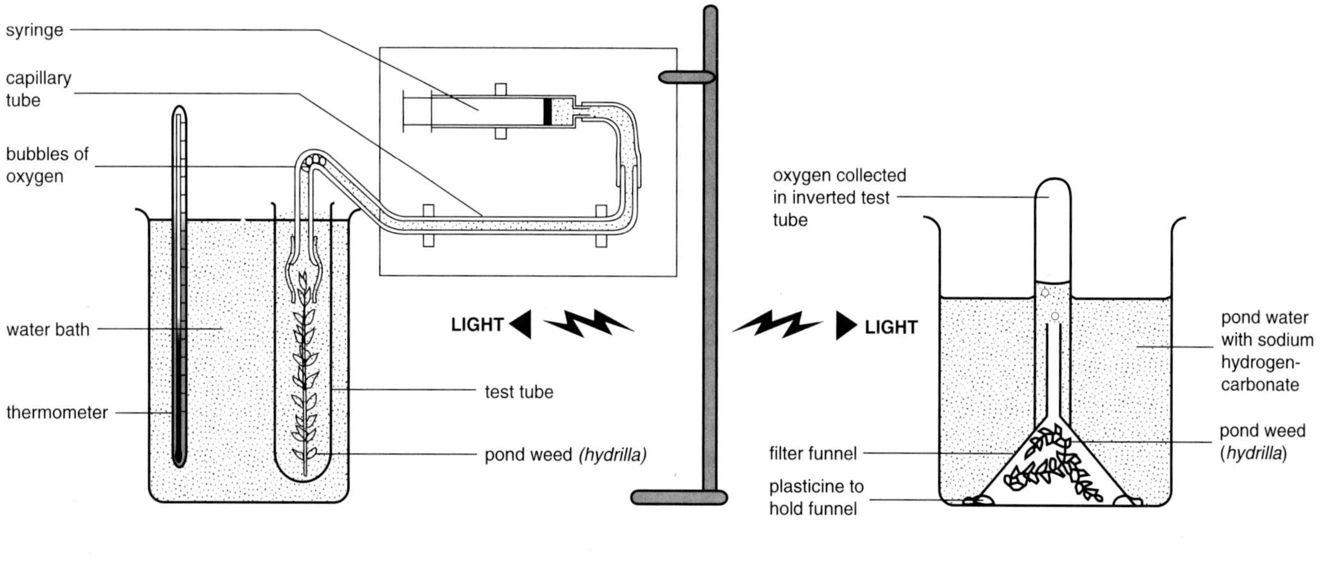

Fig. 9.6 Evolution of Oxygen during Photosynthesis

$LI \times \frac{1}{d^2}$

where:

LI is the light intensity and

d is the distance between the object and the light source.

ii. The rate of photosynthesis is the volume of oxygen produced divided by the time taken to produce it.

Plot your results on a graph, putting light intensity on the horizontal axis (as $1/d^2$ or, more conveniently, $1000/d^2$), and the amount of oxygen evolved (as length of bubble in mm) on the vertical axis.

For consideration

(a) Comment on the shape of your graph.

(b) Did you face any difficulties in carrying out this investigation? If so, how did you overcome them?

(c) Why did you add sodium hydrogencarbonate to the pond water?

(d) What variables other than light intensity might have changed and influenced your results?

(e) What measures could you take to make sure they remain constant if you were to repeat the investigation?

(f) Why was the distance between the light source and the plant first increased and then decreased?

(g) Is the volume of gas produced an accurate measure of the rate of photosynthesis?

(h) How could you modify the procedure to investigate the influence of carbon dioxide concentration on the rate of photosynthesis?

(i) Could you use pondweed to investigate whether or not photosynthesis obeys the law of limiting factors? If so how?

Practical 34 – DESIGN AN INVESTIGATION: TO TEST THE EFFECT OF CARBON DIOXIDE CONCENTRATION ON THE RATE OF PHOTOSYNTHESIS

Write down your procedure stepwise and show it to your teacher before you begin.

Prepare a list of requirements and give to staff prior to the practical class.

Set up as shown in **Fig. 9.7**. The pondweed absorbs CO_2 from the medium, which should be a dilute solution of sodium hydrogencarbonate made up with pond water.

You will require a range of solutions, starting perhaps with a 0.1 mol dm^{-3} stock solution of sodium hydrogen carbonate, ($NaHCO_3$); Na=23, H=1, C=12, O=16) and dilute it to give solutions of 0.05, 025, and 0.0125 mol dm^{-3} sodium hydrogencarbonate. Use a $20cm^3$ glass-gas syringe if available. Grease the plunger.

The pondweed should be fresh and in the pond water.

Make sure to include a control in your investigation.

Further investigation.

Try and analyse the gas collected.

40 % Potassium hydroxide solution, and pyrogallo, pyrogallic acid (Benzene1, 2, 3-triol) are provided.

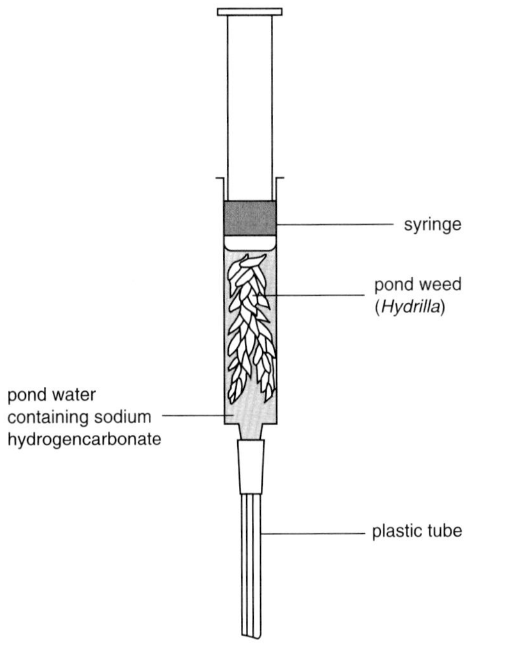

Fig. 9.7 Evolution of Oxygen during Photosynthesis

Practical 35 – NUTRIENT REQUIREMENTS FOR HEALTHY PLANT GROWTH

(Investigation proceeds over several weeks)

By growing plants (such as chickpeas, peas, sunflower or barley seedlings) with their roots immersed in aerated solution we can discover which ions are essential for normal healthy plant growth **Fig. 9.8**. The technique is a form of hydroponics and can be adapted to use seedlings grown in boiling tubes.

Procedure

Use plants of the same species. If there is a short supply of suitable plants to work with you can work in groups or the investigation can be set up by the teacher for the whole class and the observations made by the students.

Setting up the hydroponics experiment

i. complete culture medium (CCM) contains a mixture of all the soluble salts required by the plant;
ii. CCM minus nitrogen;
iii. CCM minus sulphur;
iv. CCM minus phosphorus;
v. CCM minus potassium;
vi. CCM minus calcium;
vii. CCM minus magnesium;
viii. CCM minus iron;
ix. distilled water

1. Label 10 boiling tubes 1–10.
2. Fill the boiling tubes to about 1 cm from the top with the appropriate culture solution (or distilled water).
3. Count out five healthy plants of equivalent size into each boiling tube. Make sure the roots are dipping in the solution. Add more solution if required.
4. Plug them upright with a cotton wool plug and leave them all together, near a window where they can receive good even illumination.
5. Allow the experiment to proceed for several weeks. If some of the medium evaporates after some weeks, add distilled water to bring back the volume to the original level.
6. Examine the plants about twice each week and note any deficiency symptoms.
7. For each boiling tube, record the following numerical information:
   (a) the number of live plants;
   (b) the number of green leaves;
   (c) the number of dead leaves (those turning yellow or white);
   (d) the length of the longest root. Record once a week (or alternate weeks, depending on the growth rate).
8. Present your observation in a table.

For consideration

(a) Explain what is a complete culture medium.
(b) With reference to the table and your observations try and explain the deficiency symptoms in relation to the culture medium in which the plant was growing.
(c) How do the essential substances such as nitrates, phosphates and sulphates enter the plant?
(d) You may notice that nitrogen deficiency symptoms only appear in the oldest leaves, why?

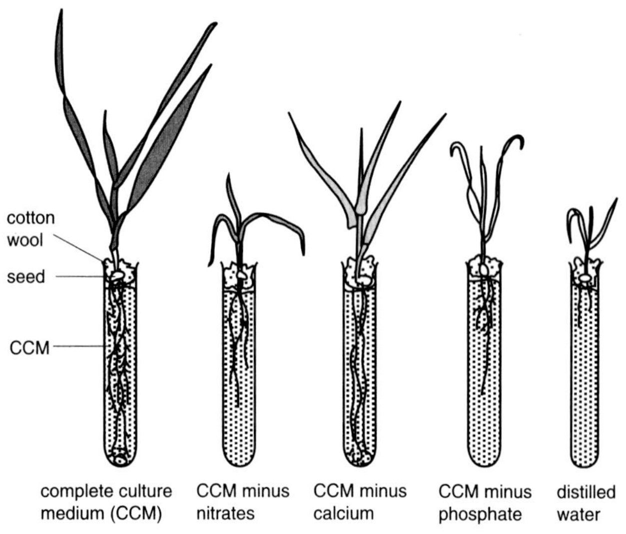

Fig. 9.8 To Demonstrate Nutrient Requirements for Healthy Plant Growth

Substance (amount/mg ℓ^{-1})	Example of functions
ammonium nitrate (1650)	nitrogen source
calcium chloride (440)	enzyme cofactor
magnesium sulphate (370)	enzyme cofactor
potassium nitrate (1900)	nitrogen source
copper sulphate (0.025)	component of cytochromes
manganese sulphate (22.3)	enzyme cofactor
potassium iodide (0.83)	enzyme cofactor
iron sulphate (28.8)	enzyme cofactor
sucrose (30 000)	carbon and energy source
potassium dihydrogen-phosphate (170)	buffer

Table showing the Nutrient Requirement for Healthy Plant Growth

(e) Calcium deficiency in plants leads to structural malformations, explain why?
(f) Explain the role of magnesium ions in green plants.
(g) Describe an experiment you could perform to determine which mineral elements are required for the growth of healthy plants, and in what form?

Practical 36 – PHOTOSYNTHETIC PIGMENTS

Chlorophyll pigments occur in green plant cells, in the **grana** of the **chloroplasts**. Chlorophyll is in fact, a mixture of **chlorophylls** and **carotenoids** (**see page 85**) and it is largely insoluble in water, but may be extracted with organic solvents. Such an extracted solution absorbs light energy, but cannot photosynthesise. The light energy absorbed by chlorophyll in solution is in fact re-emitted as red fluorescence.

The photosynthetic pigments can be separated and identified by chromatography **Fig. 9.9.**

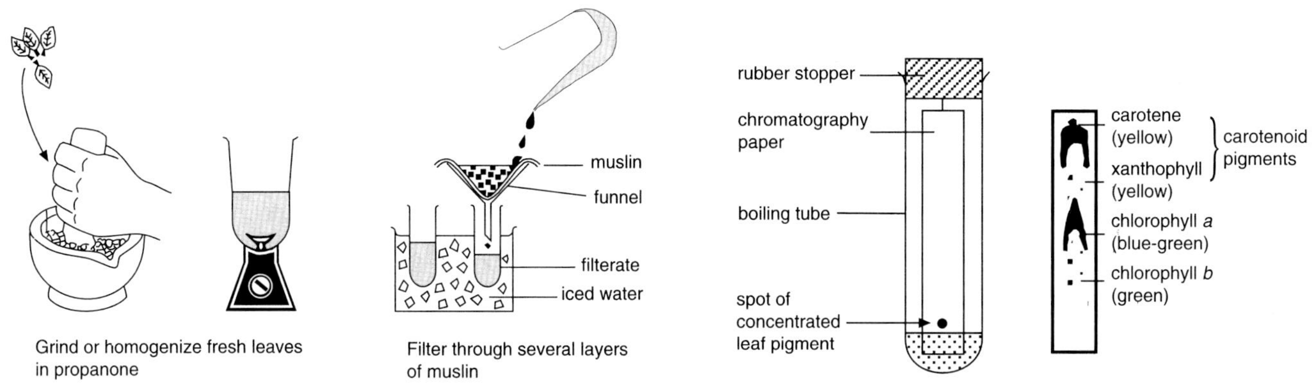

Fig. 9.9 Separation of Pigment by Paper Chromatography

Chromatography literally means 'writing with colour'. It is one of the most important techniques in biochemistry for separation and purification of mixtures of pigments and proteins (**see page 60**). The mixture to be separated is applied to an absorbent material (chromatography paper) which is then placed in contact with a solvent. As the solvent ascends the absorptive paper, it carries the various components of the mixture with it at rates that differ according to their solubility. The process leads to separation of its various components.

An alternative technique

A quicker and more complete separation of photosynthetic pigments can be achieved by thin layer chromatography (**TLC**). Instead of absorptive paper, a glass or plastic slide or an aluminium sheet coated with silica gel can be used. Use these if available.

Extraction of photosynthetic pigment
(To save time this has been done for you).

1. Dip about 10–15g fresh spinach, grass, green cabbage or nettle leaves into boiling water.
2. Chop the leaves finely, removing the midribs and petioles and grind them with clean sand in $20cm^3$ propanone in a pestle and mortar, or liquidised in a food processor.
3. Filter the extract through several layers of muslin. If available, centrifuge briefly.
4. Store in the dark in a stoppered test tube on ice.
5. Once extracted, the chlorophylls are quite unstable and need to be carefully handled. Keep on ice in the dark.
6. Extract flower pigments as above, but instead of propanone use acidified methanol. Various flowers such as geranium, chrysanthemum, roses etc. can be used.

Demonstration of fluorescence
Procedure

1. In a darkened laboratory set up a strong light source (such as a slide projector).
2. Place the glass tube containing the chlorophyll extract in the light beam against a dark background. A ruby-red glow of florescence will appear at right angles to the beam.

Measurement of the absorption spectrum

This can be carried out with a colorimeter with a set of coloured filters.

1. Switch on the colorimeter and allow to warm up for 10 minutes before taking readings.
2. Transfer the chlorophyll solution to a glass cuvette, and read it against a cuvette of propanone using different filters as follows:
   i. Place the first colour filter into the colorimeter.
   ii. Place the cuvette with propanone in the colorimeter and adjust to zero absorbance.
   iii. Place the cuvette with the chlorophyll solvent in the colorimeter and record the absorbance.
3. Repeat the procedure with each filter in turn, noting the colour and code number of each filter. Using the chart provided with the colorimeter, note down the wavelength of peak transmission (nm) of each filter.

Procedure

Caution: ***organic solvents are highly flammable and their vapours may be harmful. Work in a fume cupboard if available, otherwise make sure there are no naked flames and the room is well ventilated.***

1. Cut a strip of chromatography paper or filter paper, of sufficient length to reach almost the bottom of a large test tube and of such width that the edges do not touch the sides of the tube. Handle the paper from its edges, as perspiration from your hand will appear on the chromatogram.
2. Pour solvent A (a mixture of propanone and petroleum ether) into the boiling tube to a depth of about 15 mm.
3. Seal the tube with a stopper for about 10 minutes so the atmosphere inside becomes saturated with vapour.

4. Draw a pencil line across the strip about 1 cm from one end of the strip of the paper. Write your initials on the other end and bend the strip so that it can be attached to the stopper.
5. Very carefully, using a fine capillary tube or a drawn out Pasture pipette place a small drop of the chlorophyll extract in the centre of the penciled line. Practice on a piece of filter paper first, because it is important to make the spot as small as possible. The smaller the spot, better the separation!
6. Let the spot dry, use a hair dryer if available, and then place another spot on top of the first, and dry again. Repeat this about six times, to concentrate the mixture, keeping the spot as small as possible.
7. Lower the strip carefully into the test tube, pencilled end first, taking care not to let it come into contact with the sides of the test tube. Allow the bottom end of the strip to dip about 5 mm into the solvent, making sure the spot is not submerged.
8. Attach the bent top edge to the stopper either with adhesive tape or with a drawing pin.
9. Repeat steps 1–8 with flower pigments, use solvent B (glacial ethanoic acid, HCl and water).
10. The solvent will travel up the filter paper, carrying the pigment extract with it. This will take about 10–15 minutes.
11. Keep an eye on the solvent ascending the paper strip. Make sure the solvent front does not run off the top edge of the paper. When it has reached about 2cm from the top edge of the paper, remove the strip from the jar.
12. Mark the highest point reached by the solvent (**solvent front**) at once, as this disappears once the solvent has evaporated.
13. Hang the strip to dry.
14. Encircle each spot and measure the distance from the pencil line to the leading edge of each clearly detectable pigment, and work out the **R*f*** value (**see page 61**) for each one.
15. Identify the pigments according to their colours and **R*f*** values with reference to the table.

$$R_f = \frac{a}{b}$$

Where

a = distance moved by substance from its original position

b = distance moved by solvent from same position.

Name	R_f
Photosynthetic pigments (in solvent A)	
Carotene	0.95
Phaeophytin	0.83
Xanthophyll	0.71
Chlorophyll a	0.65
Chlorophyll b	0.45
Flower and fruit pigments (in solvent B)	
Pelargonidin	0.70
Malvidin	0.60
Cyanidin	0.50
Petunidin	0.45
Delphinidin	0.30

Table showing R_f Values of Pigments

For consideration

(a) Compare your results with the information given in the table above.
(b) How can you ascertain if there are more pigments present in a leaf than the ones you have already identified?
(c) What is the functional significance of the fact that there are several pigments, not just one?
(d) How could you attempt to improve the clarity of your chromatogram?
(e) What factors might cause the Rf value to differ from the published values?
(f) Which pigments would you expect to find in autumn leaves and why?

Practical 37 – THE HILL'S REACTION

You may recall that photosynthesis involves **light** and **dark reactions**. In the light reaction **photolysis** takes place, causing the splitting of water to liberate oxygen and hydrogen (as NADPH) for the subsequent reduction of carbon dioxide. It also provides ATP for the subsequent synthesis of carbohydrate in the dark reaction. Thus the role of the light reaction is to synthesise ATP and NADPH resulting in release of oxygen, using light energy. This takes place in the **grana membranes** of the chloroplasts.

In 1965 Robert Hill first produced biochemical evidence about the reactions involved in the complicated process of photosynthesis. Hills' work showed beyond any doubt that:

i. isolated chloroplasts could be made to liberate oxygen in the presence of a suitable oxidising agent (electron acceptor);
ii. the light reaction of photosynthesis takes place entirely in the chloroplast;
iii. that oxygen evolution could occur without reduction of carbon dioxide, providing evidence for separate light and dark reactions and the splitting of water.

In the following investigation instead of the naturally occurring electron acceptor NADPH, a blue dye DCPIP (dichlorophenolindophenol) is used which becomes colourless when reduced.

(a) The reduction of the DCPIP dye is represented by the equation:

$$2DCPIP + 2H_2O \rightarrow 2DCPIPH_2 + O_2$$

Isolation of chloroplasts Fig. 9.10

(To save time this has been prepared for you.)

Note: all glassware must be extremely clean and rinsed with distilled deionised water. It is important to carry out the procedure quickly and at 0°C.

1. Cut 50g of chilled spinach or green cabbage leaves into small pieces, avoiding midribs and petioles.
2. Grind in a blender with 120cm³ of iced cold buffer solution for 10-15 seconds at low speed, and then for 5 seconds at high speed.
3. Filter through several layers of muslin.
4. Centrifuge at low speed for two minutes. Discard pellet, recentrifuge at high speed.
5. Discard the supernatant and use a paint brush to resuspend the pellets in 15cm³ of iced cold buffer.
6. Store in stoppered test tubes at 0°C in the dark.

The Hill's Reaction

Switch on a colorimeter (if available) to warm up in readiness for the second part of the practical. If a colorimeter is not available, visually record your observation after 15–20 minutes.

Carry out the following treatment to the tubes, preparing each mixture **one at a time** and adding the chloroplast suspension last of all.

Tube	Chloroplast suspension	DCPIP	Distilled water	Treatment
1	0.5	5.0	0.0	Leave in bright light
2	0.5	5.0	0.0	Leave in bright light
3	0.5	5.0	0.0	Place in the dark at once
4	0.5	5.0	0.0	Place in the dark at once
5	0.5	0	5.0	Control

Reaction mixtures for investigation of Hill's reaction/cm³

1. If a colorimeter is available use a red or yellow filter. Transfer the mixture from test tube 5 (control) to a cuvette and adjust the colorimeter to zero.
2. Set up tube 1 and immediately transfer the mixture from the tube to a cuvette. Follow the progress of the reaction by recording at 30s intervals, the decrease in absorption as the blue colour of the DCPIP dye is oxidised to a colourless state. This takes about 10 minutes.
3. Once the reduction has taken place, record the absorbance of tubes 3 and 4.
4. Similarly check for reduction in tube 2.
5. Plot a graph of change in absorbency (y-axis) against time (x-axis) and record your observations in each tube.

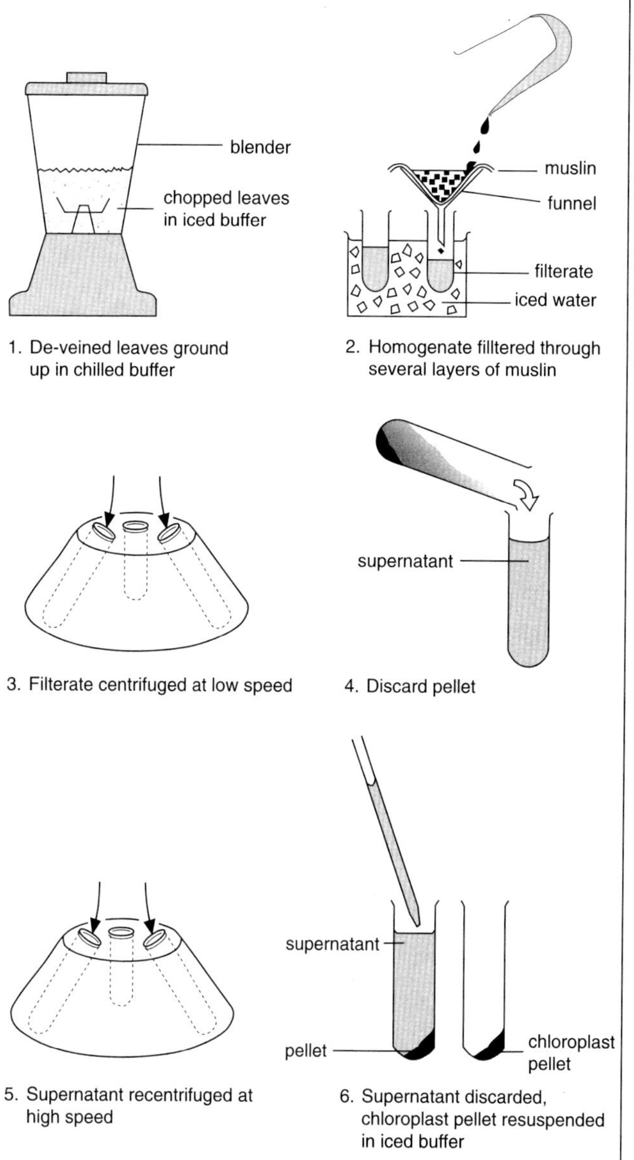

Fig. 9.10 Isolation of Chloroplasts (Hill's Reaction)

Note: If the reaction does not take place within about 15 minutes you may need to alter the volume of DCPIP so that the colorimeter will read on scale.

For consideration

(a) What are the electron donors and electron acceptors in the Hills reaction?

(b) What conditions are necessary for DCPIP to be decolourised in this experiment?

(c) It was particularly important to use extremely clean glassware for this investigation. Why?

(d) What was the purpose of tubes 2 and 4?

(e) Certain steps in the investigation were carried out at 0°C, whereas for the actual experiment, the reaction tubes were allowed to be placed in the light and dark at room temperature. Why?

(f) Why was an isotonic pH buffer used for the suspension of the chloroplasts rather than distilled water?

Practical 38 – THE SYNTHESIS OF STARCH

Starch synthesis in plants is indicative of photosynthesis even though the immediate products of photosynthesis are sugars. Potato tubers contain an enzyme which catalyses the synthesis of starch from simple sugar glucose. Sugars formed in photosynthesis are transported to every organ and cell, and may be deposited as starch almost anywhere in the plant.

In this investigation you will study starch synthesis in plant cells from three possible substrates: **glucose, glucose-1-phosphate and maltose**. Glucose-1-phosphate is formed from a reaction between glucose and ATP and maltose is a disaccharide formed from two molecules of glucose.

Extraction of starch phosphorylase
(To save time this has been prepared for you)

A crude preparation of starch phosphorylase, the enzyme that catalyses the conversion of glucose to starch, can be made from a potato. (In the in tact potato the enzyme catalyses the breakdown of starch.)

1. Peel a good sized potato and chop it into tiny pieces.
2. Grind them to pulp using a blender (or a pestle and mortar).
3. Squeeze the juice through several layers of muslin.
4. Centrifuge the juice extracted for a few minutes at 5000 rpm, to remove suspended starch grains and all other solids.
5. Decant the supernatant into a clean tube labelled *starch phosphorylase* place it in a iced water bath.
6. Test the supernatant for the presence of starch, if it tests positive re-centrifuge to make sure all the starch is removed.

Synthesis of Starch
Procedure

1. Label four test tubes A–D and prepare reaction mixtures as indicated in the table, but **add the starch phosphorolase last, just when you are ready to make your observations.**
2. In test tube A add 5cm^3 of glucose solution. In test tube B add 5cm^3 of glucose-1-phosphate. In test tube C add 5cm^3 of maltose and in test tube D add 5cm^3 of distilled water.

Solutions(cm^3)	Tube A	Tube B	Tube C	Tube D
Glucose (3% w/v)	5	0	0	0
Glucose-1-phosphate (3% w/v)	0	5	0	0
Maltose (3% w/v)	0	0	5	0
Distilled water	0	0	0	5
'Starch phosphorylase'	5	5	5	5

3. Add 5cm^3 of starch phosphorylase to test tube A and mix thoroughly.
4. Using a clean glass rod withdraw a drop from the reaction mixture and test for starch on a white tile.
5. Repeat step 3 at three minute intervals for the next fifteen minutes.
6. Record the presence or absence of starch and the time taken for the starch to be formed in a table.
7. Repeat steps 3–6 with test tubes B, C and D.
8. If a colorimeter is available, plan and carry out steps 3 and 4 quantitatively. Remember you will need to increase the volume of the reaction mixture as you will need about 3cm^3 in the cuvette at each time interval.

For consideration

(a) Study the structure of the three substrates and try and work out what structural features might be recognised by the starch synthesising enzyme.

(b) In the potato tuber the same enzyme is responsible for the break down of starch, why then in this investigation the conditions favoured starch synthesis?

(c) The process of starch synthesis requires ATP, where do you think it comes from?

(d) Were there adequate 'controls' in your procedure?

(e) What steps could you include in your procedure to show that an enzyme is involved in the reaction?

(f) Why was the enzyme kept at 0°C?

Practical 39 – FORMATION OF STARCH IN THE GREEN LEAF

Caution: ***sodium chlorate is an irritant, avoid contact with it.***

The plant has been destarched for you as follows:

A healthy potted plant of geranium *Pelargonium* (or any other suitable plant) was placed in the dark for at least 48–72 hours to destarch it completely.

A leaf was tested for starch, to make sure it is completely destarched.

Procedure

1. Using a small cork borer (or a plastic straw) cut out 40 discs from the **youngest** healthy green leaves from the destarched plant and soak them in sodium cholorate solution to sterilise them.
2. Remove the plunger from a 20 cm^3 syringe, transfer about 10 leaf disc at a time into the syringe.

3. With a finger placed on the nozzle pour about 10 cm^3 of sodium hydrogencarbonate solution into the syringe. Replace the plunger, and expel all the air from the syringe.
4. Keeping the finger firmly on the nozzle pull the plunger back as far as possible. Hold for about 10 seconds, remove the finger from the nozzle. The procedure expels air from the discs.
5. Repeat step 4 twice more. The discs should sink at this stage.
6. Repeat steps 2–4 with all the other discs to remove air from them.
7. Label six beakers A–F.
8. In beakers A and B pour 20 cm^3 3% **degassed** glucose solution carefully pouring on the side of the beaker to avoid getting any air into the solution.
9. In a similar manner pour 20 cm^3 **degassed** distilled water into beakers C and D and 20 cm^3 **degassed** sodium hydrogencarbonate solution into beakers E and F.
10. Transfer 6 leaf discs, right side up into each of the six beakers.
11. Cover each beaker with a watch glass and very carefully place beaker A, B and C into a dark cupboard and beaker D, E and F under a bright light so that they all receive equal illumination. Leave them overnight in a place where they will not be disturbed.
12. Note the position of the discs.
13. Test each leaf disc, one by one for the presence of starch, by placing it on a white tile and adding a drop of iodine solution.
14. Tabulate your results.

For consideration

(a) Why do you think the leaves were sterilised?
(b) Explain any variations in the behaviour of the discs in differing solutions and conditions that you have observed.
(c) If starch synthesis has occurred, under what condition did it occur?
(d) What are the advantages to the plant for storing excess sugar as starch?
(e) Were there adequate controls in your procedure?

10 Gaseous Exchange

Gaseous Exchange

Respiration is the requirement of all living organisms to release energy as ATP from food substances to facilitate all cellular activities. Cellular respiration requires oxygen (**aerobic respiration**) where sugar is oxidised to carbon dioxide, water and energy.

$$C_6H_{12}O_6 + 6O_2 \rightarrow 6CO_2 + 6H_2O + 38 \text{ ATP} \quad \Delta G = -2280 \text{ kJ mol}^{-1}$$

However, some micro-organisms such as yeasts and bacteria are able to carry out **anaerobic respiration** (in absence of oxygen) partially oxidising sugar to carbon dioxide and ethanol or lactic acid and a small amount of energy.

$$C_6H_{12}O_6 \rightarrow 2C_2H_5OH + 2CO_2 + 2\text{ATP} \quad \Delta G = -210 \text{ kJ mol}^{-1}$$

For respiration to take place, gaseous exchange with the environment is essential. In plants this takes place inside the leaf where the respiratory structures are the stomata, and in animals are the lungs.

Practical 40 – GASEOUS EXCHANGE IN LEAVES

Photosynthesis results in evolution of oxygen and uptake of carbon dioxide. In respiration, oxygen is used and carbon dioxide is produced. When light intensity is gradually increased from zero at dawn the rate of photosynthesis increases accordingly. There comes a point, when photosynthesis and respiration exactly balance each other, with no net exchange of oxygen and carbon dioxide. This is called the **compensation point**, or more accurately the **light compensation point**, that is light intensity at which net gaseous exchange is zero.

Since the rate of photosynthesis is affected by the carbon dioxide concentration there is also a **carbon dioxide compensation point.** At this carbon dioxide concentration the net gaseous exchange is zero for a given light intensity. The rate of photosynthesis increases with increasing concentration of carbon dioxide. For most temperate plants the carbon dioxide compensation point is 50-100ppm (parts per million), beyond which photosynthesis exceeds respiration.

In the following investigation hydrogencarbonate indicator is used. This indicator changes from cherry red to purple in alkaline conditions and to orange to yellow in acidic conditions.

Note: The hydrogencarbonate indicator (bicarbonate indicator) solution should be freshly aerated with air from outside the laboratory until it turns cherry red. The indicator is supplied as a concentrated solution and has to be diluted x10. The colour of the indicator solution at this stage is deep red but appears orange-red in the test tubes. This takes about 20–30 minutes.

Procedure

1. Rinse four test tubes with the indicator solution and label them 1–4.
2. Rinse a 2cm³ syringe with a little of the indicator solution and add 2 cm³ of the indicator solution to each of the four tubes. Do not touch the open ends of the tubes, as the acid in the sweat will affect the indicator. Also avoid breathing over the tubes.
3. Cover the outside of tubes 1 and 3 with aluminium foil.
4. Using a 1cm cork borer cut discs from freshly picked leaves.
5. Using a pair of forceps, insert a small ball of cotton wool into all the test tubes **Fig. 10.1.**

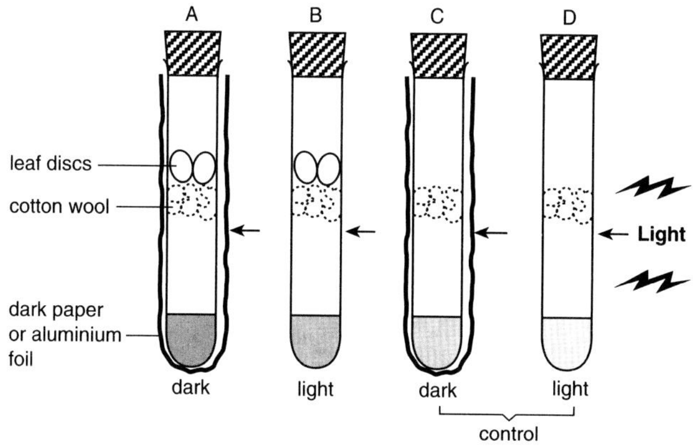

Fig. 10.1 Gaseous Exchange in Leaves

6. Place two leaf discs in tubes 1 and 2.
7. Arrange the tubes in such a way that a bench lamp illuminates them all equally.
8. Place the tubes in a beaker of water to minimise the increase of temperature during the investigation.
9. Note the colour of the indicator in the tubes.
10. Shake the tubes gently and leave for at least 2 hours or more, preferably overnight.
11. Hold the tubes against a white tile and observe and record the colour of the indicator.

12. Interpret the results using the following guide to colour changes.

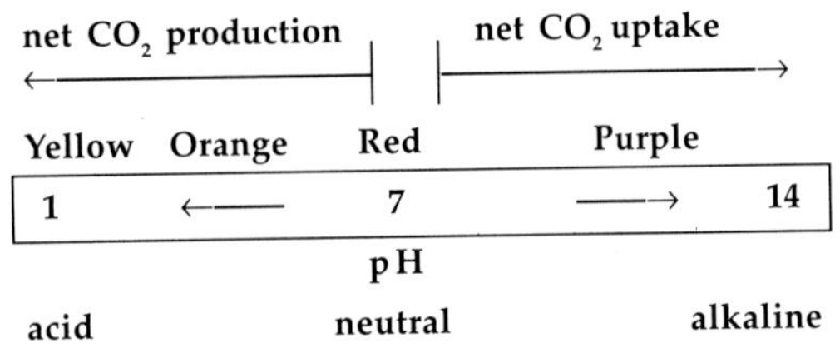

If conditions become more acidic, this can be assumed to be the result of carbon dioxide being produced and dissolving in the indicator solution. Lowering of the carbon dioxide concentration would be indicative of less acidity.

Modification of this Investigation

To measure the light compensation point, a microcomputer linked to Data Capture Equipment and Data Loggers (e.g. Philip Harris oxygen sensor meter, oxygen electrode and DL Plus 32, Datadisc PRO) will give more accurate results. The software and the set up is available from Philip Harris (UK).

Further investigations can be carried out:

i. Using leaf discs from old and young leaves on the same plant, leaves in shade (deep lower down the plant) and in bright light (at the top of the plant) yellow and green areas of variegated leaves, leaves from different species;
ii. Varying the light intensity;
iii. Using water plants such as *Hydrilla,* or *Elodea* instead of leaf discs. If water plants are used they should be thoroughly washed to remove all micro-organisms. The plants should be immersed in indicator solution to cover them. The solution does not effect the plants.
iv. To compare the rate of photosynthesis the colour of the indicator could be measured using a colorimeter at regular intervals during, or at the end of the investigation.

Reference: UCLES, Question 1, 20th May, 1997.

For consideration

(a) What is the purpose of tubes 3 and 4?
(c) What is the name given to the equilibrium point where there is no further net uptake or production of carbon dioxide by the leaf discs in tube **B**?
(d) How could you improve this investigation?
(e) Would you expect the compensation point of a sun plant to differ from a shade plant? If so, how?
(f) Why is it necessary to wash off all the micro-organisms from water plants and why must the plants be submerged in the indicator?

Practical 41 – MULTIPLICATION OF YEAST CELLS IN AEROBIC AND ANAEROBIC CONDITIONS

(This investigation proceeds over a week)

Cell division, like all vital activity, requires energy, and the rate at which cells divide depends on the amount of energy available. Much more energy is produced by aerobic respiration than by anaerobic respiration.

$$C_6H_{12}O_6 + 6O_2 \rightarrow 6CO_2 + 6H_2O + 38\ ATP \quad \Delta G = -2280\ kJ\ mol^{-1}$$

$$C_6H_{12}O_6 \rightarrow 2C_2H_5OH + 2CO_2 + 2ATP \quad \Delta G = -210\ kJ\ mol^{-1}$$

We would therefore expect cell division to proceed faster in aerobic than in anaerobic conditions. The following experiment is designed to test this hypothesis.

A **haemocytometer (see page 30)** can be used to take actual cell count, but this method is tedious.

A photometric method employing the use of **colorimeter** is relatively easier. As the number of cells are increased less light passes through the sample. The amount of light blocked by the yeast suspension is called **absorbance**.

Procedure

Pre-incubation (to save time this has been done for you)

1. Label three conical flasks of the following sizes: 50 cm^3, 150 cm^3, and 500 cm^3.
2. Pour 50 cm^3 of cider or clear apple juice into each flask. (Keep some apple juice or cider to use as blank, to adjust the colorimeter to zero, if optical density is to be recorded.)
3. Mix the suspension of yeast thoroughly to ensure even distribution of cells, and add a drop of yeast suspension to each flask.
4. Cover the flasks with four layers of muslin, and leave in a cupboard for one week.

Estimation of cell concentration

5. After a week's incubation, mix the contents of each flask and estimate the cell concentration in each flask, using a haemocytometer (**see page 30**). If a colorimeter is available measure the absorbance of each flask using apple juice or cider to adjust the colorimeter to zero (blank).
6. To obtain accurate results take several individual readings both with the haemocytometer and/or the colorimeter, and work out the mean reading.
7. Calculate the concentration of yeast cells in each flask as number of cells per cm^3.

For consideration

(a) Is the hypothesis that cell division proceeds more rapidly in aerobic than anaerobic conditions confirmed or disproved with your results? Explain.
(b) Summarise the conditions in the three flasks with reference to the availability of oxygen; take into consideration the size of each flask, the depth of the medium and the surface area exposed to oxygen.
(c) Are there any other possible explanations for the different cell concentrations in the three flasks apart from availability of oxygen?
(d) If you consider each flask as an *organism* can you from your results explain the need for development of complex respiratory systems in larger organisms.

Practical 42 – RESPIRATION IN YEAST AND THE EFFECT OF TEMPERATURE

Yeasts such as *Sacharomyces* can grow anaerobically, converting glucose to carbon dioxide and ethanol. The rate of production of carbon dioxide is indicative of the rate of respiratory metabolism. In this investigation, you will observe the effect of temperature on this process.

Pre-incubation of yeast
(to save time this has been done for you)

Dried yeast (*Sacharomyces cereviside*) is usually available as granules consisting of dormant cells bound with inert filler (normally starch). In suitable conditions, the cells begin to be metabolically active in a matter of 30 minutes or so.

Add 3g of dried yeast to 100cm^3 warm water in a conical flask. Add 3g glucose, and place a loose cotton wool plug. Leave in a 37°C water bath for about an hour.

Procedure

1. If constant water baths are available set them to 10°, 20°, 30°, 40° and 50°C. If not, then label 5 large beakers and set up water baths of 10°, 20°, 30°, 40°, and 50°C mixing hot water with cold water to obtain the desired temperature.
2. Place 5 test tubes labelled 10–50 in the appropriate water bath, and add 15 cm^3 of yeast suspension in each (make sure to mix the yeast suspension thoroughly before taking the sample).
3. After about five minutes when the yeast has equilibrated with the temperature of the water bath, using a teat pipette completely fill a fermentation tube with yeast suspension from one of the test tubes. Carefully invert the fermentation tube back into the same test tube, sliding the full fermentation tube gently. Make sure there is no air trapped inside the inverted fermentation tube. If air does get inside the fermentation tube, take it out and try again **Fig. 10.2.**
4. Place the test tube with the inverted fermentation tube back into the appropriate water bath. Make a note of the time.
5. Repeat this procedure with all the other temperatures.
6. At five minute intervals carefully take out the tubes from the water bath and measure the length of the air bubble in each tube.
7. Plot a graph of the length of air bubble, against time for each of the temperatures.

Reference: UCLES, Question 1, 26th May, 1993.

For consideration

(a) Explain your results, with regards to the effect of the temperature in each tube.

(b) Many yeasts are able to respire both aerobically and anaerobically, if for some reason the culture starts to respire aerobically what effect, if any, would you expect it to have on the volume of gas production?

(c) Suggest ways by which you could further improve your set up.

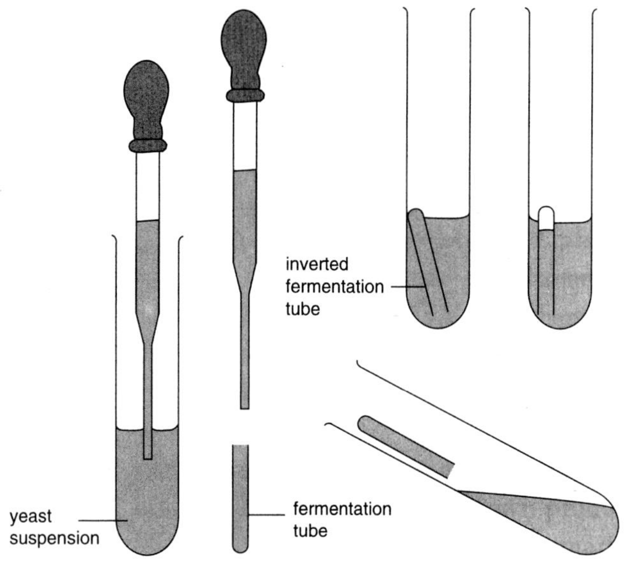

Fig. 10.2 Respiration in Yeast and the Effect of Temperature

Practical 43 – THE EFFECT OF TEMPERATURE ON THE RATE OF RESPIRATION

Small invertebrates such as woodlice, maggots and plants cannot control their own body temperatures, their temperature fluctuates with that of the environment. The respiration rate of such organisms changes accordingly. The rate of respiration can be measured by using a differential **respirometer Fig. 10.3.** The respirometer consists of two identical manometers attached to boiling tubes. One of the tubes contains living organisms such as germinating mung beans (moong daal), broad beans, woodlice, or maggots. The other contains an equal volume of dead organisms (boiled mung beans) or an inert material such as glass beads which is the control.

It works on the principle that if a group of organisms is oxidising glucose by aerobic respiration, the volume of oxygen uptake is equal to the volume of carbon dioxide produced. In a closed system containing respiring organisms, the concentration of oxygen will decrease and the concentration of carbon dioxide will increase. If soda lime, a compound which absorbs carbon dioxide, is placed inside the closed vessel, the respiring organisms will continue to take up oxygen, but all the carbon dioxide produced is absorbed by the soda lime. The rate at which the pressure falls is indicative of the oxygen taken up.

This is a difficult set up, either work in pairs, or carry out a class investigation. Each pair can work at a different temperature (10°–50°C), and then pool the results. The teacher should allocate a specific temperature to each pair.

Setting up the Respirometer

(To save time this has already been set up for you.)

1. Set up the respirometer as follows: Label two boiling tubes L (live) and D (dead). Place germinating seeds (or other suitable living organisms) in tube L and the equivalent number of boiled seeds, or the same volume of inert material in tube D.
2. Add 5g soda lime into the tubes, then a cotton wool plug and then the seeds on top **Fig. 10.3.**
3. Carefully (**the manometer tubes are extremely fragile**) pour coloured water into the reservoir of one of the manometers. If air bubbles appear in the capillary tube of the manometer, use a pipette filler to blow air down the long arm of the manometer tube to remove them.
4. Without creating air bubbles in the fluid, fit the long arm of the manometer tube into the rubber tubing attached to one of the rubber stoppers. Fit the rubber stopper securely into one of the boiling tubes (take care!).
5. Repeat the last two steps with the other manometer tube and rubber stopper. Clamp the two boiling tubes vertically in the water bath, making sure that both spring clips are open.

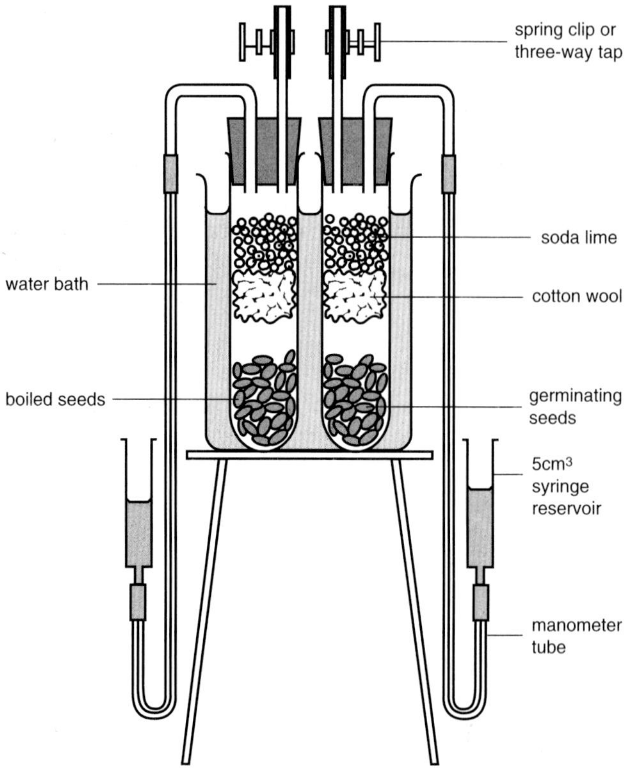

Fig. 10.3 Differential Respirometer

Measuring the Rate of Respiration

1. If constant temperature water baths are available, set them at various temperatures between 10°–50°C, to use later. Use crushed ice to obtain the lower temperatures.
2. If constant temperature water baths are not available use boiling water mixed with cold water to obtain the desired temperature. Adjust your set up so that the test tubes are immersed in a large beaker of water at a temperature allocated to you by your teacher. Record the temperature of the water.
3. Make sure both spring clips are open. Mark the level of the menisci of the coloured fluids in both manometer tubes. Close both the spring clips. Note the time.
4. Record the level of the fluid in both manometers, at regular intervals, after 5, 10 and 15 minutes. If the level of the manometer fluid attached to boiling tube L does not change, check carefully for leaks and start again.
5. If no problems are encountered and you have obtained the manometer readings at this temperature you can try to take readings at another temperature as well.
6. Proceed by opening both spring clips. Place the set up in the next temperature water bath. Allow at least ten minutes for the set up to equilibrate to the new temperature, and for the volume of air in the tubes to settle.
7. Repeat the procedure.
8. Repeat also at 10°C. Add ice to tap water until the water is at 8°C. Allow ten minutes for the set up to equilibrate at this temperature and for the volume of the air in the boiling tubes to stabilise. By this time the water in the beaker should have reached about 10°C. Repeat steps 3 and 4 at this temperature.
9. Calculate the rate of oxygen uptake (obtain data from other groups so that you have the data for each temperature tested).
10. Plot a graph to show the volume of oxygen consumption against time for each temperature.

Reference: UCLES, Question 1, 20th May, 1994.
Reference: UCLES, Question 1, 19th May, 1998.

For consideration

(a) What is the effect of an increase in temperature on the rate of respiration on the organism?

(b) The rate of the reaction doubles with a 10°C increase in temperature and is referred to as Q_{10}. Q_{10} is slightly over 2 for a large number of enzyme controlled reactions. Are your results in agreement with this?

(c) Explain in terms of molecular behaviour why the rate of an enzyme-controlled reaction doubles with a 10°C increase in temperature.

(d) If you have used soaked germinating seeds they may have been respiring anaerobically as well as aerobically. How would this affect your results?
(e) Why was it necessary to use boiled seeds or inert beads as control?
(f) What kind of experimental errors might have affected your results? How would you overcome them?
(g) If you encountered problems carrying out this investigation how did you try to overcome them?

The Respiratory Quotient

In a given time the volume of carbon dioxide produced during respiration of carbohydrates is equal to the volume of oxygen consumed.
This is quite clear from the generalised equation of respiration:

$$C_6H_{12}O_6 + 6O_2 \rightarrow 6CO_2 + 6H_2O + \text{energy}$$

The ratio of volume of carbon dioxide produced to the volume of oxygen absorbed by an organism is called the **respiratory quotient (RQ)**. Knowledge of the RQ values is indicative of the type of food being respired and the kind of metabolism taking place.

$$RQ = \frac{\text{Volume of } CO_2 \text{ evolved}}{\text{Volume of } O_2 \text{ absorbed}}$$

For the metabolism of carbohydrates respiratory quotient is 1.0

$$RQ = \frac{CO_2}{O_2} = \frac{6}{6} = 1$$

However if instead of glucose fats are being used, for example, steric (octodecanoic) acid is used in respiration:

$$C_{17}H_{35}COOH + \mathbf{26}O_2 \rightarrow \mathbf{18}CO_2 + 18H_2O$$

The respiratory quotient is 18/26 = 0.69.
During anaerobic respiration in muscular tissue CO_2 is not produced, whereas organisms such as yeast and plant tissues respiring anaerobically to ethanol do produce CO_2, in which case the respiratory quotient is very high.
In reality there is always more than one substrate being metabolised at any one time, and most organisms simultaneously carry out both aerobic and anaerobic respiration. The extent to which aerobic or anaerobic respiration is taking place can be worked out from their respiratory quotient.

RQ	Substrate
> 1.0	Carbohydrate plus some anaerobic respiration
1.0	Carbohydrate
0.9	Protein
0.7	Fats, e.g. tripalmitin
0.5	Fats associated with carbohydrate synthesis
0.3	Carbohydrate with associated organic acid synthesis

Practical 44 – DESIGN AN INVESTIGATION TO MEASURE THE RESPIRATORY QUOTIENT OF GERMINATING BROAD BEANS

Prepare and give a list of requirement to the staff prior to the practical class.
Using a modified respirometer such as the one used in the previous investigation 43, **Fig. 10.3** the respiratory quotient of an organism can be determined. Respiration in humans is usually observed using a spirometer **Fig. 10.4**.

Some guidelines

Use germinating broad beans:
i. soaked in water for 48 hours;
ii. soaked for 42 hours and exposed to air for 6 hours;
iii. soaked for 36 hours and exposed to air for 12 hours.

1. Set up a respirometer with the test tubes immersed in a water bath maintained at a constant temperature.
2. Add soda lime in one test tube only; replace the soda lime with an equal volume of inert material in the other test tube, so that the volume of gases is maintained equally in both the test tubes.
3. Use equal mass of respiring broad beans in each test tube.

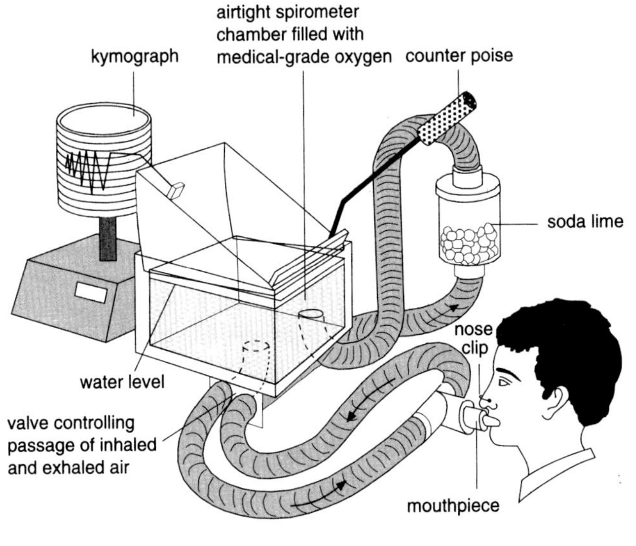

Fig. 10.4 Spirometer

In the tube containing soda lime all the carbon dioxide in the test tube will be absorbed, any movement observed in the manometer fluid will be due to the oxygen uptake. The other tube measures net gas exchange. The carbon dioxide output is the difference between these readings. A fall is negative and a rise is positive.

For consideration

(a) Explain your results with regards to the soaking procedure.

(b) What is the RQ when glucose is respired anaerobically to ethanol and carbon dioxide?

(c) Why is the RQ for humans between 0.7 – 1.0?

(d) Why is it important to use a constant temperature water bath?

(e) What is the RQ in the following equation?

$$2C_{51}H_{98}O_6 + 145O_2 \rightarrow 102CO_2 + 98H_2O$$

(tripalmitin)

11 Ecology

Ecology

Background Summary

Ecology is the scientific study of interaction between organisms and their environment. It is one of the most important components of modern biology because living things can only be understood fully in context of their natural environment.

The tiny habitable portion on earth is referred to as the **biosphere**. An **ecosystem** is a natural ecological unit, consisting of living things – **biotic components** (all the organisms that are part of the particular environment) within their physical environment – **abiotic components** (such as temperature, light, water and nutrients). Organisms are not only affected by their environment, but by their very presence they also change the environment. The most dramatic change brought about by the organisms on their environment occurred when micro-organisms started to photosynthesise.

The energy source for all living things is the **Sun**. Green plants use this energy to manufacture food from inorganic substances and are therefore **primary producers**. All other organisms including animals rely on them for food and are therefore **consumers**. Other organisms, which feed on dead plants and animals, are called **decomposers** and **recycle** the nutrients on which all living things depend. The transfer of energy from one consumer to the next forms a **food chain**. In nature food chains are interconnected to form **food webs** illustrating the interdependence of all living things.

The seashore, forests, woodlands and lakes are all examples of terrestrial ecosystems and are affected by **abiotic factors** such as **climate**, **topography**, and **edaphic** (soil) factors. The interaction of living things in the ecosystem is known as the **biotic factors**, which also play a key role in distribution of the organisms. The biotic factors include competition for resources between members of the same species (**intraspecific competition**) and different species (**interspecific competition**), **predation** and browsing on vegetation by animals, and **symbiosis**. Symbiotic relationships range from **commensalism**, **mutalism** to **parasitic** relationships.

Organisms can be seen to be occurring in **populations** of the same species and in **communities** of different species, present in the ecosystem. In an individual community birth rate, death rate, immigration and migration will determine the size of the population. Fluctuating about a set point, populations are generally held fairly constant by a homeostatic mechanism involving feed back. However, sudden changes may occur in a population if some factor of the environment changes suddenly. The study of communities and ecosystems is known as **synecology.**

One of the most powerful influences on the environment is by humans. Pollution, indiscriminate use of pesticides herbicides, radioactive contamination, urbanisation and exploitation of natural resources are ways in which we affect and destroy our environment.

Ecological Investigations

Ecological investigations are generally more difficult, complex and time consuming than laboratory work because of the numerous variables involved which are often out of our control. For example, you may wish to investigate the diversity of minibeasts-small organisms in a particular habitat and set out traps to capture them overnight. The sudden change in climatic conditions are totally beyond our control – it may rain, or a farmer may turn up before your collection time in the next field, using a tractor which drives the small creatures away.

Even when you manage to collect the required data it is often very difficult to analyse and presents great challenges. However, do not let this deter your planned course of ecological study. The key to success is **planning**. Plan your investigations with extreme care, taking into account every possible problem that might arise. Work out exactly what sort of information you will collect and exactly how you will collect it, taking into consideration methodology and techniques involved, but be prepared to modify your plans as and when required. This will help you to collect useful and meaningful data without wasting time.

There is a tremendous amount of published material available on various ecological investigations, and techniques that can be carried out in different habitats. Here, we will only deal with some very basic **synecological** (involving **abiotic** and **biotic**) elements associated with a defined terrestrial natural ecosystem. Investigations which are simple, meaningful, less time consuming and within the scope of most students to carry out will be discussed. For best results the study should be carried out as a project lasting several days, but if that is not possible day trips can also be of great importance in giving you the gist of the exercise.

Planning your ecological trip

(a) Decide exactly what sort of data you wish to collect and to what accuracy. It may be easier to divide the class into small groups so that each group is responsible for carrying out a particular part of the whole study, and later class data could be pooled and analysed. If such is the case, select a group leader for each group and utilise different abilities of your classmates. Some students may be particularly good at identifying animals, or plants, then they can be responsible for identifying and recording which organisms are found. Others may be very good at chemistry; they can carry out chemical analysis on the soil etc.; those who are very capable practically can carry out the practical work and so forth.

(b) To make the ultimate use of your ecological trip meticulous **pre-planning** is essential. Decide exactly what type of investigation you wish to carry out (this will depend on the site you choose to visit). Choose the location carefully. Decide what sort of habitat you wish to study. It could be a most enjoyable learning experience outside the classroom, where you can all participate in different ways.

If you live near the coast you may wish to study seashore ecology; if you are near a river you may wish to study fresh water habitats. You could make an expedition to a nearby wood; an uncultivated field or even a hedge can provide you with a wealth of information.

(c) Map the area and habitat(s) in plan view and if necessary in profile **Fig. 11.1.**

Note the topography – position of nearby rivers, fallen trees, paths, ponds, factories, residential areas, farms, etc. (in fact any thing that may affect your study).

(d) Decide on the sampling techniques so that relevant equipment can be collected.

(e) Make sure you have all the equipment you require, such as sample jars (empty jam jars), plastic bags, measuring tape, quadrat squares, Sellotape, sticky labels, string, wooden pegs, large hammer, portable pH meter or litmus paper, magnifying lens, markers pens etc. are useful.

(f) Know EXACTLY what each individual is supposed to do before you depart for your trip.

(g) Prepare data sheets of all data you intend to collect. This will save valuable time and avoid confusion as to exactly what information is to be collected at each station. It may be possible to revisit your location later but certain information such as temperature, light intensity etc. has to be recorded at the time of sample collection. It may be useful to look up in reference books and photocopy illustrations of common organisms you may find, prior to your trip to help identification on the spot. You can, however, collect samples of each organism for identification later (be very careful not to disturb the habitat more than is necessary and usually one sample for the whole group is quite sufficient, it may be possible to free living specimens after examination).

(h) Identify the species (it is easier to work with plants than with animals) and estimate the number present.

(i) Measure the abiotic (possibly collect and analyse) factors within the habitat(s).

(j) Finally analyse the data collected in depth.

(k) Write up as a project.

The overall aim of such an investigation is to determine the quantitative and qualitative relationship between the plant and animal population within the area being studied and the possible interaction between biotic and abiotic factors. With this information it should be possible to determine the nature and extent of the factors governing the number and distribution of organisms in terms of food web and, pyramid of numbers, standing crop, biomass and energy.

The limit to the depth of your investigation is endless and depends upon how much time you can allocate to this part of your course. In the following program we will simply touch the subject of ecology to give you a feel of what it involves.

Mapping an area

1. Select the exact area to be studied, for example, an uncultivated field, grassland, or a wood.
2. Mark out with poles and measure a base line A-X.
3. From the base line mark out and measure perpendicular distance selected for study A-Y **Fig. 11.1.**
4. Divide the base line A-X into equal number of sections and lay out perpendicular string transects. Repeat the procedure for A-Y.
5. Record all this information on squared paper in an appropriate scale.
6. Mark any prominent features such as trees, ponds, rivers or vegetation zones within your area of study on your plan.
7. Note directions using a compass.

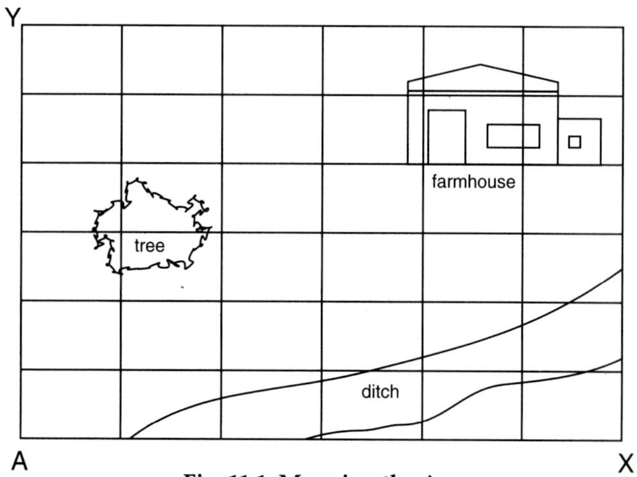

Fig. 11.1 Mapping the Area

Measuring the abiotic factors within the habitat(s)

Direct measurements of abiotic features of the environment should be made at regular intervals, or samples should be taken for subsequent analysis later. The main environmental factors that should be recorded are type of soil, topography and climatic effects.

i. Soil (edaphic) profile

Soil is a vital link between biotic and abiotic components of terrestrial ecosystems. It varies tremendously in pH, water content, air content, composition and texture.

A soil sample should be taken at each station using a **soil auger Fig. 11.2** which is an elongated cork screw instrument. Various colours and textures of clearly differentiated bands should be noted, and then samples removed from each of these bands (horizons) for on the spot analysis, and/or to be analysed later.

Soil texture should be carefully checked for particle size, moisture, and composition. Soil testing kits are also available which will determine mineral content, soil pH, soil air, soil water and humus content as well as soil temperature and dissolved substances.

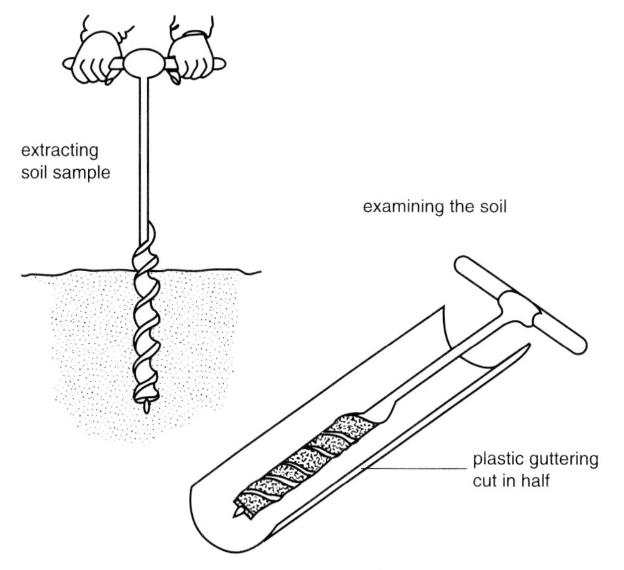

Fig. 11.2 Soil Auger

ii. Topography (terrain or relief)

Topography exerts its influence mainly due to **altitude**, **steepness of slope** and **aspect**. Altitude will affect the climate while steepness has a marked affects on both drainage and soil type. For example, on steep slopes drainage is good but at the base of the slope, soil is progressively higher in water retention, whereas in valleys it will be progressively waterlogged which has a distinct affect on vegetation and organisms. On the slopes, the soil tends to be a little thinner and drier due to water run off which carries soil with it, and due to gradual response to gravity. This leads to xeromorphic vegetation on steep slopes, and total absence of vegetation on slopes in excess of 35°.

Another effect of topography is aspect; in the Northern Hemisphere south-facing slopes receive more sunlight, and therefore have higher temperature and more light than north-facing slopes and bottom of valleys. The reverse is the case in the Southern Hemisphere. This has a distinct effect on the vegetation and land use for cultivation.

iii. Climatic factors

The main climatic factors are light, temperature, water and wind. It is known that light is essential for photosynthesis and therefore the sustenance of life but light intensity, wavelength and light duration (photoperiod) all have different effects. Light intensity is affected by the angle of incidence of the Sun's rays on the Earth's surface, varying with latitude, season, time of day and aspect of the slope.

(a) **Photoperiod** varies according to the latitude causing photoperiodic response that synchronises with seasons, such as time of flowering and germination in plants, hibernation, migration and reproduction in animals. Also, competition for light affects plant development such as plant height, density and size of a leaf etc. and thus determines differing ecosystems. Take this in consideration when you analyse your data.

(b) **Light intensity** should be recorded using a photographic light meter or a light sensor meter linked to a microcomputer at each station at regular intervals and whenever you think it may have altered. Alternatively, Ozalid papers can be used to record the cumulative sensitivity to light. Light intensity, temperature, humidity and pH can be continuously recorded over a period of time using a microcomputer linked to sensometers and to Data capture equipment, DL Plus 32, Datadisc PRO (Philip Harris, UK) **Fig. 11.3**.

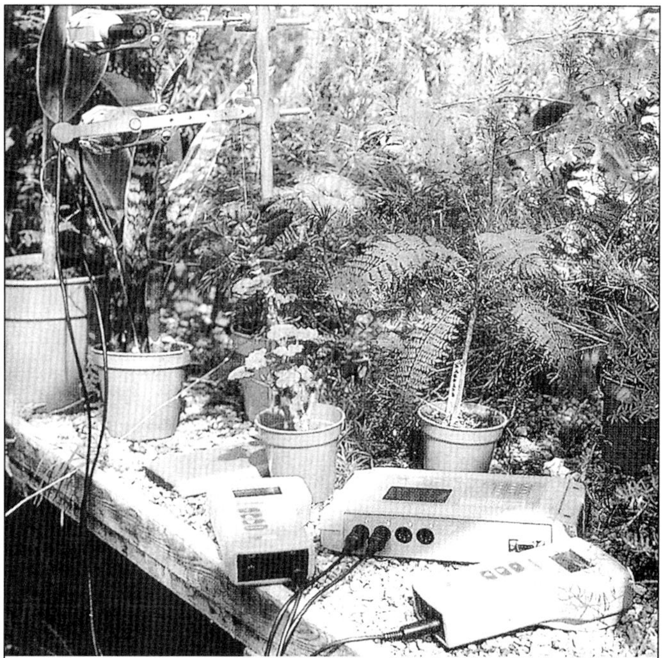

Fig. 11.3 Data Capture Equipment

(c) **Temperature** also affects the development of ecosystems as all living organisms survive within a narrow range of temperature. Most organisms can exert some degree of control over their temperature by various methods and adaptations but beyond a certain extreme they perish. As is light, temperature is also dependent on latitude, season, time of day and aspect of day. An ordinary mercury thermometer is too fragile to be used in the field, an electronic field thermometer is ideal and readings should be taken at each station at regular intervals and when any change is noted.

(d) **Water** is vital for life and a limiting factor for terrestrial ecosystem. It is continuously recycled by the water cycle, precipitating as rain from the atmosphere. The roots of the plant absorb water, so the water content of the soil has a profound affect on the type of vegetation that develops. High tolerance plants are called **xerophytes**, medium tolerance **mesophytes** and **hydrophytes** are low tolerance water plants.

(e) **Salinity** may also be important in terrestrial habitat; if evaporation exceeds precipitation, soil may become saline. It may be possible to record the rainfall over a period of time, but if this is not possible you may be able to obtain this information from your meteorological office.

(f) Interaction of **wind** with other environmental factors has a profound affect on vegetation. It can alter the water vapour in the atmosphere and affect the transpiration rate and has a physical affect on certain trees, for examples trees may have stunted or distorted growth on the exposed side. It also aids seed and spore dispersal in plants and helps migration of airborne animals. Wind speeds can be judged subjectively using **Beaufort scale** of wind force or measured accurately with a **flowmeter** or an **anemometer**.

Making biotic analysis

In all ecological studies it is essential to study the **community structure**, identify and estimate the number of organisms within a certain habitat. The method employed varies according to the size and mode of life of the organism, and to the area size under investigation. It is obviously not possible to count all the individual organisms present because of the time limitations. Direct counting can be carried out relatively easily of small, slow moving animals or the number of plants in a particular area using simple sampling techniques. However, special sampling techniques such as **line** or **belt transect,** and **systematically frame quadrat sampling, random quadrat sampling** etc. have to be employed to give an accurate indication of the numbers present in the whole area of interest.

Decide on the method of sampling. This depends on the kind of data you have decided to collect and the type of vegetation within your chosen area of study. Fast moving organisms require special techniques such as **removal method, capture** and **recapture methods** or **photography** can also be employed e.g. of a herd of animals or a flock of birds.

Methods of sampling

Quadrat frame. A metal or wooden frame, preferably light and collapsible to facilitate carriage. It forms a square of known area such as 0.5m^2 or 1.0m^2. The size of the quadrat depends upon the nature of the organisms to be studied **Fig. 11.4**.

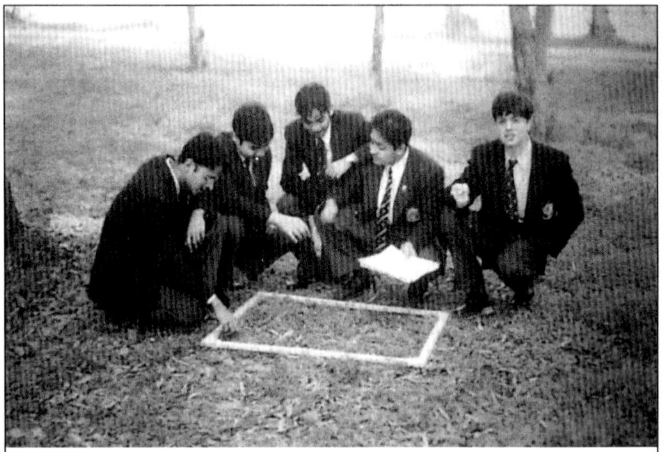

Fig. 11.4 Quadrat Frame

The structure of the quadrat can be modified according to the demands of the investigation; for example it can be subdivided with strings to assist in counting or when counting an abundance of species **Fig. 11.5**.

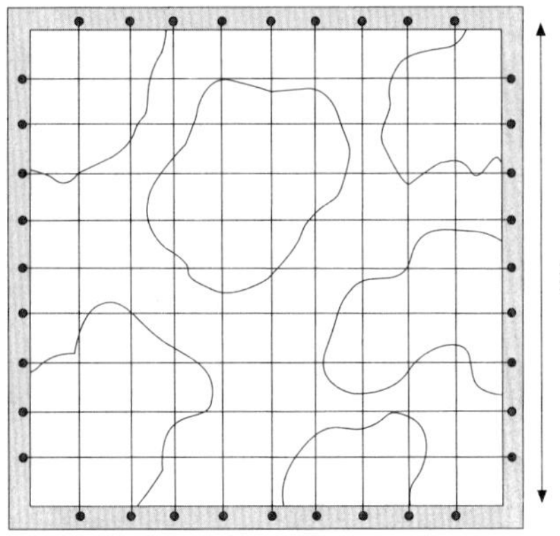

Fig. 11.5 Quadrat with Strings

It may be used systematically alongside a belt transect, or randomly (thrown over the shoulder) when sampling a fairly uniform habitat. This has to be repeated several times to obtain meaningful results. This method provides a means of calculating aspects of species distribution, and is a useful method of sampling where communities are relatively uniform over a given area.

Using a quadrat frame

1. Systematically sample the area, and identify and estimate the number of each species present.

2. Data should be recorded directly on to prepared data sheets, best kept on a clip-board in a large plastic bag (in case it rains), along with a pencil. Species are identified using a key and the numbers of organisms are either counted or estimated within a previously decided range (eg. 5< or 5> etc.) or the five point DAFOR scale can be used which is:
   ≥5 = **D**ominant
   ≥4 = **A**bundant
   ≥3 = **F**requent
   ≥2 = **O**ccasional
   ≥1 = **R**are
3. On the spot identification of most organisms is best, using keys if necessary (identification can be limited to order or class unless greater precision is necessary). If that is not possible, samples can be collected for identification later, but do take care not to take more samples than is necessary. Try to keep all animals alive and return them to their habitat after identification. Keep different animals in separate jars, and record as much information as is possible at the time of collection, such as exactly where the organism was taken from, (e.g. from under a stone, log, roots of a particular plant etc.) This information will help to construct possible food chains and food webs.

Following quantitative assessments can be made with a quadrat

Density–the number of organisms per unit area; the total number of individuals within the quadrat need not be counted. It can be estimated by counting the number of individuals in randomly thrown quadrats. It is an accurate method and enables different areas and different species to be compared and provides an accurate measure of abundance but it is time consuming and tedious.

Abundance–a subjective assessment of abundance, such as the five point DAFOR scale given above can be used.

Species frequency–this is the measure of the probability (chance) of finding a given species with any one throw of a quadrat in a given area (expressed as a percentage). For example, if the species occurs once in every ten throws the species frequency is 10%. This measure is recorded as the presence or absence of the species in the randomly thrown quadrats. (Evidence suggests that if five consecutive throws fail to show new species, chances are that all the species present have been recorded). This method is quick and easy and especially useful in large areas of vegetation, but has the disadvantage that the quadrat size, plant size, and spatial distribution all affect species frequency.

Species cover–this is the method of measuring the percentage ground covered by the species. This is a useful method of estimating plant species, especially grasses, where individuals are difficult to count and are not as important as cover. However, this is a slow and tedious task.

Pin frame–this is a frame with holes through which a needle such as a knitting needle can be passed **Fig. 11.6.**

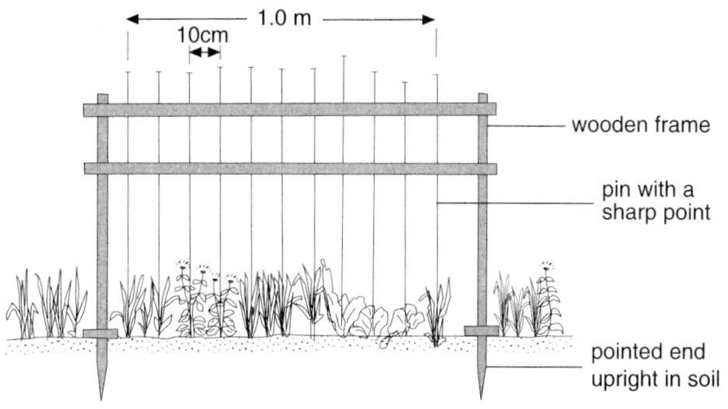

Fig. 11.6 Pin Frame Quadrat

To avoid errors due to subjective estimations of cover, a pin frame can be used for objective estimations. It is particularly useful with transect studies of overgrown habitats where several species may overlap. All species touched by the pin are recorded.
When studying an area which shows a trend of variation in a particular direction, for example due to change in topography or abiotic conditions, other methods of sampling such as transects have to be employed.

Transects–are a means of sampling both biotic and abiotic data at right angles to the unidirectional physical forces.

Line transects–a tape or string running on the ground between two poles along the area to be sampled indicates the transect. Sampling is carried out at regular intervals, and only those plants that are actually touching the string are recorded. Line transects should be repeated several times as a single transect does not give an adequate sample.

Belt transects–this is again a strip in a straight line of chosen width say 0.5–1.0 m, between which sampling is carried out. An easier method of obtaining both qualitative and quantitative data is to use a quadrat frame along the belt transects at regular intervals.

Collecting Organisms

Estimation of animal population is a little time consuming, and is difficult to achieve on a day trip. For best results it has to be carried out over several days. However, even if you are on a day trip, you can try and collect some small animals to learn how it is done and can observe what type of organisms are present in your field of interest as well as to help in identification. Which method you adopt for capturing the organism depends on the type of animal, its mode of life, its habitat and obviously the time available.

Pitfall traps **Fig. 11.7**

Small animals such as woodlice and other crawling animals can be caught in pitfall traps. A jam jar buried in the soil so that its neck is flush with the soil surface, with a piece of glass placed on top, and balanced on stones to keep the rain out, is ideal. This has to be left for several days, with daily visits, as carnivores eat each other.

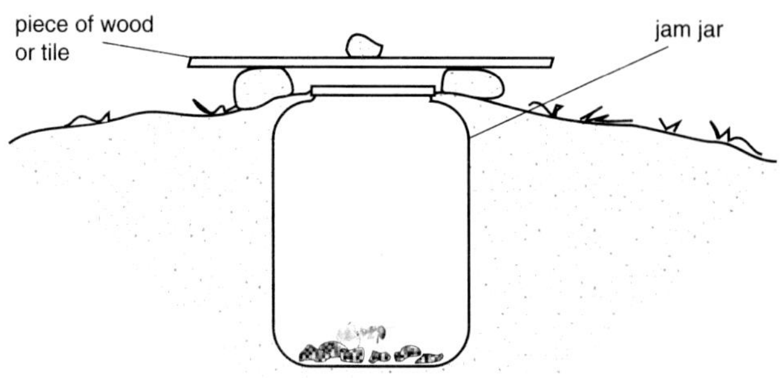

Fig. 11.7 A Pitfall Trap

Sticky traps

For flying insects, a tube covered with sticky tape or preferably honey or syrup can be used. Hang it in the insects flying path.

Sweeping air nets

Nets can be used to catch flying insects.

Beating tray method

A large sheet is held under a branch of a tree and the branch is then hit with a stick repeatedly. Small non-flying animal such as spiders, caterpillars etc. will fall into the sheet and can be collected for study.

Capture and recapture method

Small animals such as insects, mammals etc. can be caught, marked in some way that does not harm the animal, for example by using nail varnish or correction fluid, and then released to resume their normal life. The animals are again captured and population estimated using the Lincoln index:

$$\text{Estimated total population} = \frac{\text{Nos. of organisms in initial sample} \times \text{Nos. of organisms in second sample}}{\text{Nos. of marked organisms recaptured}}$$

Recording and presenting data

Data should be recorded directly on the data sheet, such as the one shown, best kept on a clip-board in a large plastic bag (in case it rains), with a pencil.

Once all the data has been collected, it is often more useful to pool class data, especially if the class was divided into groups collecting different information. The data should then be analysed fully, presented in tables, graphs, histograms, kite diagrams, trophic pyramids and charts. The study should be first discussed as a group and then written up as an project.

Suggested format of data recording sheet.

Date.................. **Exact location of site...**

Station no .... **Special features ....**

Biotic components

Animal species A and abundance .... Notes..

Animal species B and abundance.. Notes..

Animal species C and abundance etc. .... Notes..

Plant species A and abundance .... Notes..

Plant species B and abundance.. Notes..

Plant species C and abundance etc. .... Notes..

Abiotic components

Soil sample taken.........Y/N .... pH of soil ....

Type of soil ....

Traps laid out for later collection.........Y/N .... Notes..

Climate

Temperature .... Cloud cover ....

Time of day .... Light intensity ....

Wind direction .... Relative humidity ....

Topography

Direction .... Height above sea level ....

Land use ....

Drainage ....

This data sheet is only to give you an idea and will have to be modified according to your planned area of study and to the type of investigation you have decided to carry out.

12 Plant Structure and Functions

Transport in Plants

Background Summary

Materials are constantly transported to and from individual cells. Water is continually being drawn up from the soil and transported to all parts of the plant. Most of the water travels via the **apoplast** (cell walls), the vacuole and the water filled lumen of the **xylem vessels,** generally by-passing the cytoplasm. The **Casperian strip** diverts water and solutes through the **symplast** (cytoplasm and plasmodesmata).

The bulk of the water entering the plant from its root system is lost through **transpiration**. Transpiration also provides the driving force for water movement from the roots to the leaves through the **transpiration stream**. The water evaporates in the leaves into the **sub-stomatal** air chambers in the **mesophyll**, from where it diffuses to the atmosphere through the stomatal pores in the lower epidermis of the leaves. **Guard cells** surround these pores and are controlled by an **osmotic mechanism**, dependant on the **active transport** of potassium ions. These ensure that the stomata remain open during the day and close at night. Gaseous exchange between the leaf and the environment also takes place through these pores. The rate of transpiration depends on temperature, relative humidity, air movements, atmospheric pressure, light and water supply. Some structural features of plants appear to prevent excessive transpiration.

The stem is well adapted for carrying the transpiration stream from roots to the leaf. Water, mineral ions and salts are transported in the **lignified xylem** (**vessels** and **tracheids**) within the **vascular bundles**, continuous with the vascular tissues of the roots and the leaves. Bordered pits permit lateral movement.

Movement of **water** from soil to vascular tissues occurs by **osmosis** aided by **root pressure** and **active transport.** Waterflow through the plant is maintained by a water **potential gradient**. The water potential is highest in the soil surrounding the roots and is lowest in the atmosphere outside the leaves. Water column is prevented from breaking or falling back by **adhesion** and **cohesion** forces developed in the anatomical elements involved. The roots are adapted for the uptake of water.

Mineral and **salt** uptake however, is a **selective process** via **active transport** in which energy from respiration is used. Ions occur in the soil solution, mostly at very low concentrations, and it is from here that plants accumulate them. The natural reserves of minerals are limited. The essential nutrients are involved in biochemical cycles, of which the **water**, **carbon**, **nitrogen**, **sulphur** and **phosphorus cycles** are important examples.

The element **nitrogen**, which makes up 80% of our atmosphere as nitrogen gas (N_2), is only useful to plants in a combined form (for example, as nitrate NO_3^- or ammonium ions NH_4^+). Plants growing where nitrates are absent or at very low concentrations have evolved elaborate mechanisms to obtain nitrogen from specialised sources. These methods include exploitation of nitrogen-fixing bacteria living in root nodules and the digestion of animal protein by carnivorous plants.

Organic compounds, mainly sugar, manufactured in leaves are **translocated** to the rest of the plant via the **sieve tubes** in the **phloem** within the vascular tissues. The structure of the **sieve elements** is well adapted for this function. The exact mechanism of translocation is not yet fully understood but it may take place by means of **mass flow, active transport, electro-osmosis**, and **surface spreading** or **streaming** in protein filaments.

Practical 45 – GENERAL STRUCTURE OF THE FLOWERING PLANT

Procedure

External Structure

1. Examine an entire dicotyledonous plant such as Geranium *(Pelargonium)*, sunflower (*Helianthus*), tomato (*Lycopersicon esculentum*). Observe the relationship between the main stem and other structures **Fig. 12.1** such as the roots, leaves and the flowers.
2. Make a drawing of the generalised structure of the plant and label the **axillary buds, node, internode** and the arrangement of the leaves, buds and flowers on the stem.

Structure of the Stem

Note the colour of the stem and observe if the stem is smooth or hairy.

3. Peel off a piece of the epidermis from the stem, examine under the microscope, and record your observations by drawing.

Stems have three major functions:

i. to lift the flowers and leaves to an elevated position,
ii. to conduct water and mineral salts from the roots to the rest of the plant,

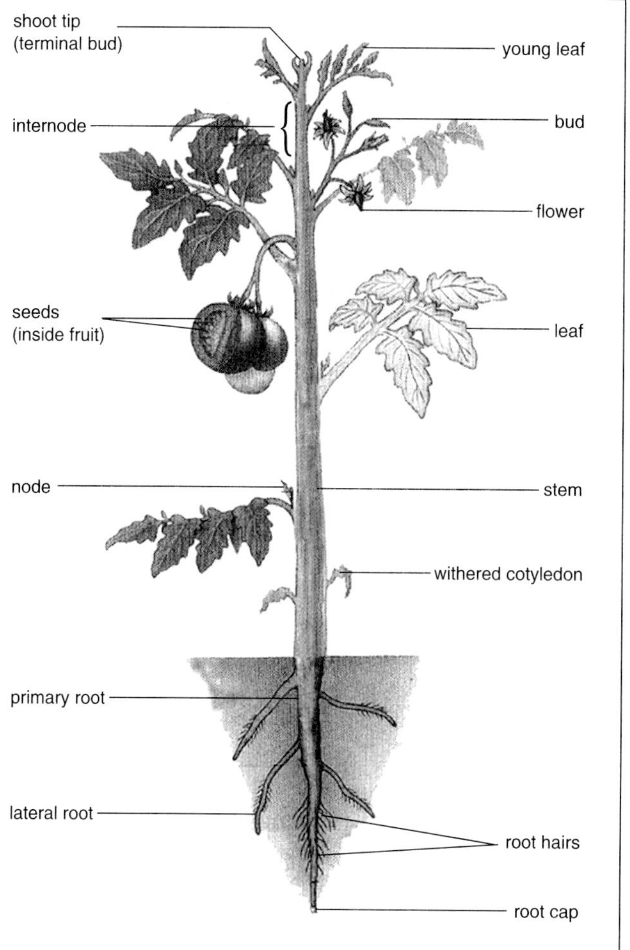

Fig. 12.1 General Structure of a Flowering Plant

iii. to translocate synthesised food from the leaves to all parts of the plant.

As with all structural features of an organism, the stem of the plant has been modified in different plants according to its habitat, for example succulents in xerophytes (swollen stem for water storage, leaves reduced to spines), large air spaces in stems of hydrophytes.

Internal Structure of a Dicotyledonous Stem

4. Select a firm piece of stem from the internode. Using a sharp blade cut thin transverse and longitudinal sections. If only soft, flexible stem is available insert a short length of the stem into a vertical slit made down the centre of a piece of elder pith or carrot tuber as shown in **Fig. 12.2.** Cut smoothly and rapidly thin sections keeping the stem and the blade moist. Transfer the sections to a dish of water.
5. Select the thinnest section and stain it with acidified phoroglucinol, (stains lignin red) for about five minutes.
6. If other stains are available stain sections with iodine solution (stains starch blue/black). Schultz's solution, (stains lignin yellow) toludine blue (stains lignin blue, cellulose purple). FABIL (xylem elements will stain brown, sclerenchyma pink, cellulose pale blue, cytoplasm and nuclei dark blue, starch black).
7. Mount in glycerine, observe and make labelled drawings under low and high power of the microscope with reference to **Figs. 12.3** and **12.4**.

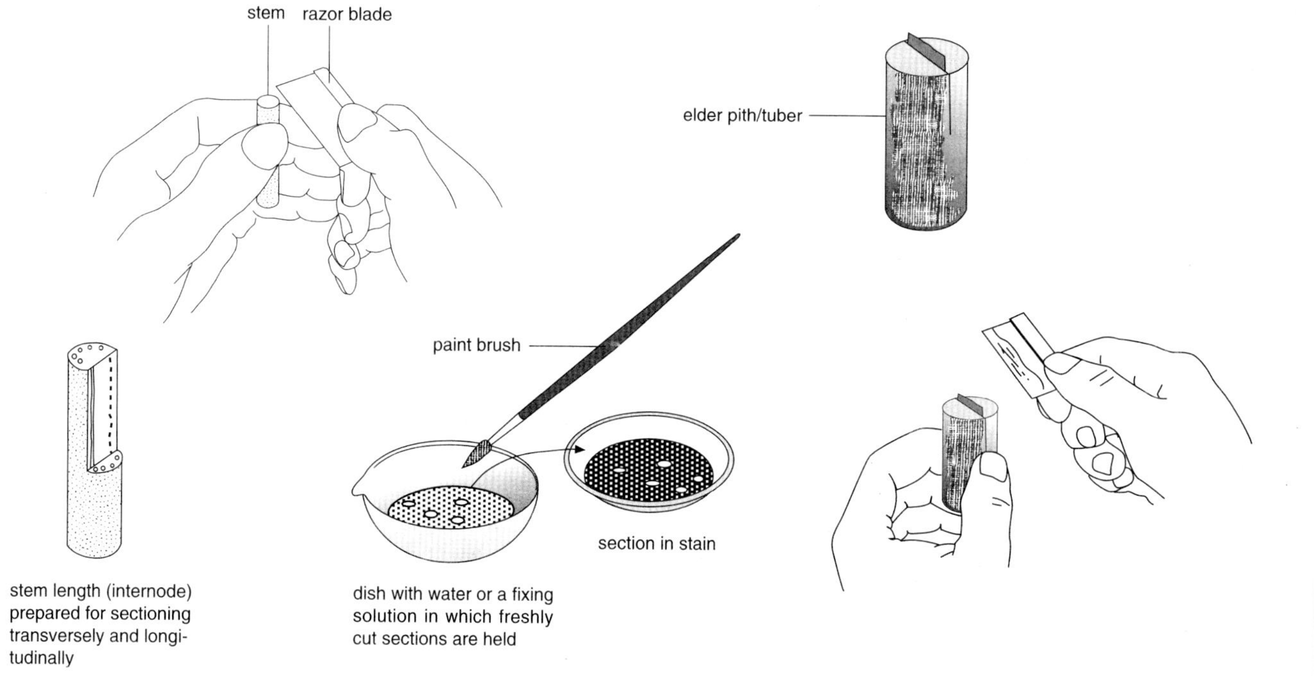

Fig. 12.2 Cutting Thin Sections

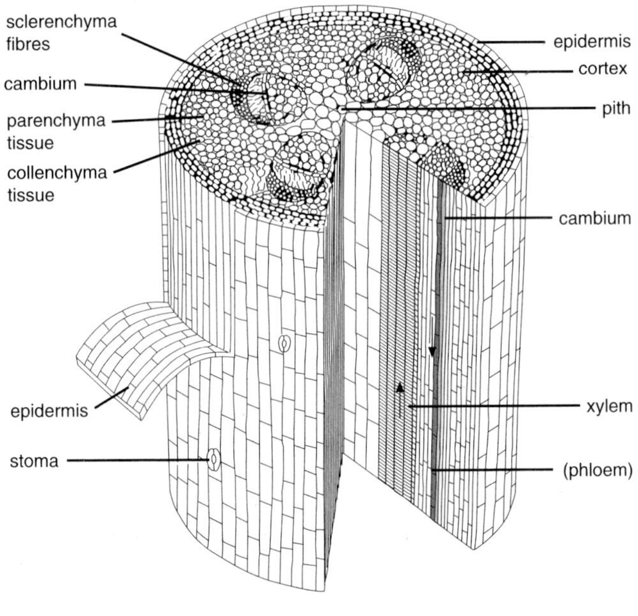

Fig. 12.3 Internal Structure of a Dicotyledonous Stem

Observing from the outside to the centre of the stem:-

Cuticle: present as the outermost layer. Some cells bear multicellular hairs. Stomata may be present, chloroplast always absent.

Epidermis: consisting of tangentially flattened cells, closely linked with each other on the radial walls.

Cortex: in the mature plant the cortex is differentiated into three layers:

i. Hypodermis–outermost region of cortex, with few layers of closely packed collenchyma cells.
ii. General cortex–consisting of several layers of parenchyma cells. Intercellular spaces present.
iii. Endodermis–innermost layer of the cortex, consisting of barrel shaped closely packed cells. The cells contain starch granules.

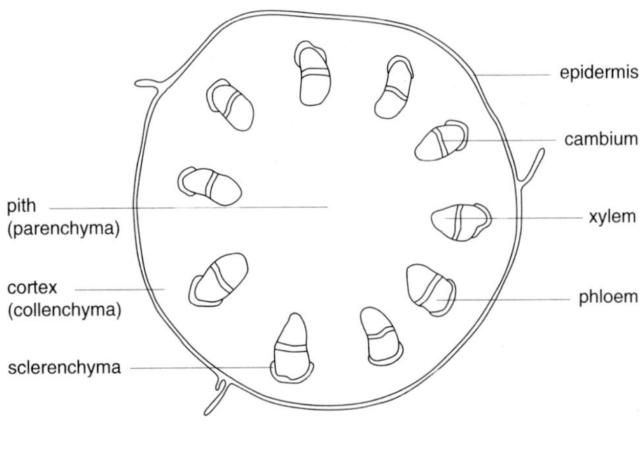

Fig. 12.4 TS of a Mature Dicotyledonous Stem

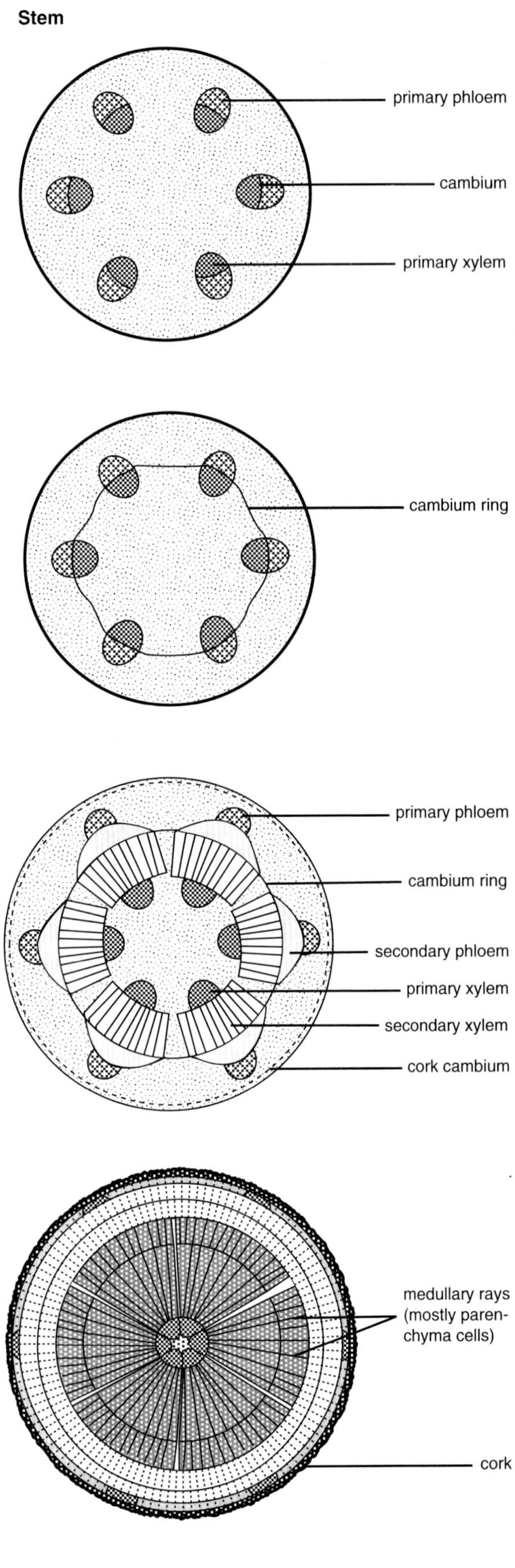

Fig. 12.5 Stages in the First Year of Secondary Growth in a Dictotyledus Stem

Vascular bundles: are arranged in a ring consisting typically of xylem, phloem and cambium.

Pith: this is the central part of the stem, consisting of parenchyma tissue.

8. Note the distribution of starch, cellulose and lignin in your section.
9. Macerate the tissue by adding a few drops of 5% chromic acid (*very corrosive*!) to the tissue section on a glass slide. The chromic acid dissolves the cement (middle lamella) that holds the cells together, but the cell walls remain intact. Examine under low and high power to see tracheids and vessels in detail. Record you observations with drawings. See **Figs. 12.15–12.21**.

Comparison with Monocotyledonous Stem

10. Cut, stain and mount section of monocotyledon stem such as maize, iris or lily.
11. Examine and make plan drawing of a complete section under low power. Notice and compare the arrangement of the vascular bundles to those of the dicotyledonous stem **Figs. 12.4–12.6**. Note that the monocotyledonous stem is very similar in the general composition of the tissue but the vascular bundles are scattered throughout the ground tissue. They are smaller and more numerous to the periphery of the stem **Fig. 12.7**. The arrangement of the xylem vessels is sometimes refered to as 'monkeys face' **Fig. 12.19** with two large metaxylem vessels (pitted) and smaller protoxylem vessels (annular and spiral). In the phloem tissue, only sieve tube and companion cells are present, phloem parenchyma is generally absent.
12. Examine and draw an individual vascular bundle under high power. Notice that it is similar to that of the dicotyledon **Fig. 12.18**; phloem towards the outside of the stem, xylem towards the inside. Note the absence of the cambium.
13. Examine young and mature stem slides and observe stages of primary and secondary growth development **Figs. 12.3–12.6**.

For consideration

(a) What is the function of the epidermis and hairs on the stem?

(b) How does the structure of dicotyledonous stem differ from that of a monocotyledonous stem, and of what significance are these differences to the plant?

(c) What is the significance of the absence of the cambium in the monocotyledonous stem?

(d) How is the structure of the xylem and phloem adapted to its functions?

(e) Why do dicotyledonous stems get taller and support heavier masses than monocotyledonous stems? Relate your answer to the structure of the stem.

(f) Explain the presence of cellulose, lignin and starch in each location and comment on its significance at the particular location.

(g) Explain the significance of the different types of lignification in the tracheids.

Reference: UCLES, Question 2, 19th May, 1992.

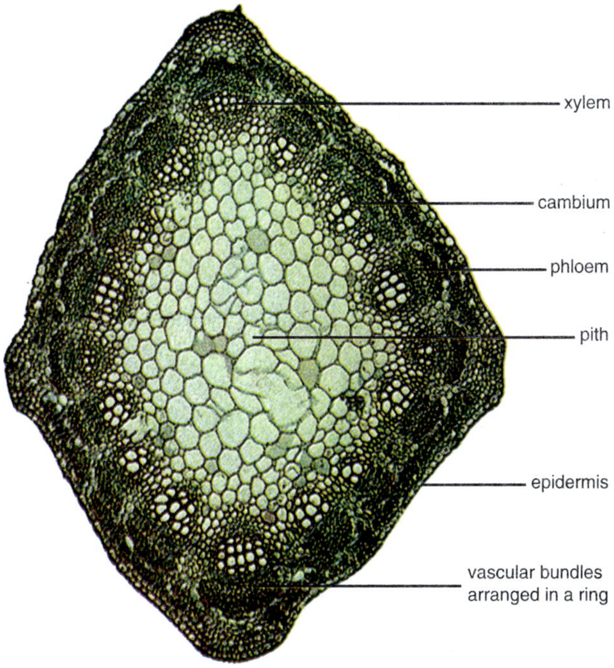

Fig. 12.6 Structure of Dicotyledon Stem TS

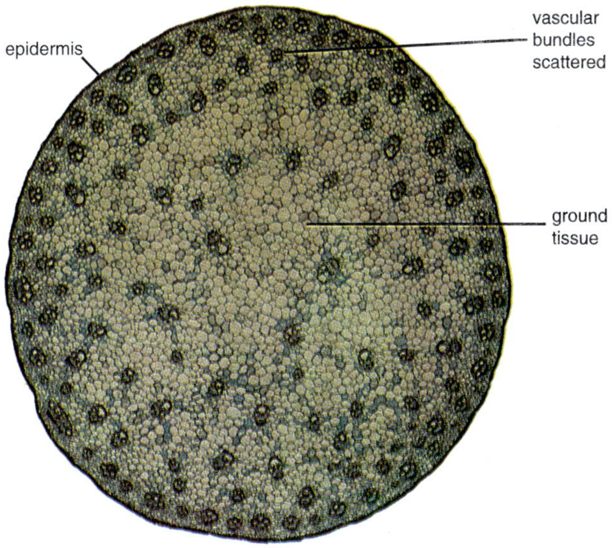

Fig. 12.7 Structure of Monocotyledon Stem TS

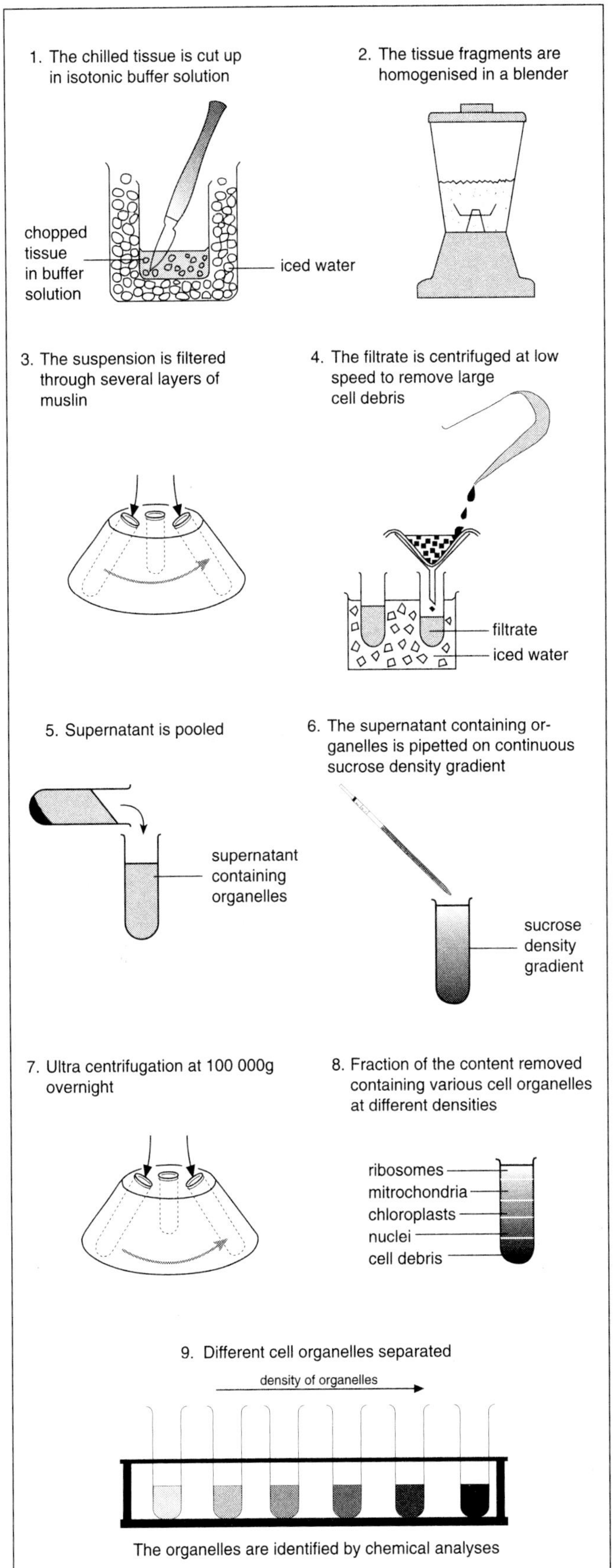

Fig. 2.5 Cell Fractionation to Isolate Cell Organelles
All steps are carried out at 0°C to minimise self-digestoin of cell organelles by the enzymes released from cell vesiceles in cell disruption.

quickly to avoid dust entering the microscope tube.

7. Replace the upper eyepiece lens, and return the eyepiece to the microscope. The eyepiece graticule is held in the plane of the primary image and therefore, is always in focus, whatever the magnification.
8. Using a prepared stained slide of unicellular animals such as *amoeba,* or *paramesium* measure the organism by mounting the slide on the microscope stage and focusing on the relevant part of the specimen. You may need to rotate the eyepiece so that the scale lies across the object.
9. Record the dimension of the organism in **arbitrary** units (a graticule has numbered divisions). Note the magnification.
10. Repeat this technique by taking measurements of the following:
    (a) the diameter of a parenchyma cell from the central pith of the stem;
    (b) the diameter of a nucleus (stained preparation);
    (c) the width of a capillary;
    (d) the length of an *amoeba* (stained preparation);
    (e) the diameter of the largest xylem vessel in the stem (TS);
    (f) the diameter of a red blood cell.

Calibration of the eyepiece graticule

1. Now the eyepiece graticule has to be calibrated. Hold up the stage micrometer slide in the light and observe the scale by means of a hand lens.
2. Most micrometer slides have a scale printed on them, e.g. 1cm with either 10 or 100 divisions. Each division is therefore equal to 10μm or 100μm (1μm = 0.001mm). Remember the scale on the micrometer slide can vary. *Check on the micrometer slide.*
3. Focus on the calibration scale and examine the micrometer slide under the microscope. Rotate the eyepiece until the graticule scale lies superimposed **Fig. 2.6.** Observe how many eyepiece divisions are equivalent to how many slide divisions. Do this at both medium and high-power magnification, for as the magnification is increased the eyepiece scale will cover a smaller area of the object, and each division measures a smaller length. Record the size of the divisions at each magnification.
4. List the eyepiece measurements (arbitrary units) of the objects you measured above, recording whether at medium or high power magnification. Multiply these measurements by the length calculated for the divisions at the magnification used.
   For example at low power, 60 eyepiece divisions are equivalent to 30-micrometer divisions.
   Therefore 60 eyepiece divisions = 3000μm

   $$1 \text{ eyepiece division} = \frac{3\,000}{60} = 50\ \mu m$$

5. Record the size of various unicellular organisms and cells.

Plant Histology

The microscopic study of tissue is called **histology**. You are required to study the histology of both plants and animals at a level of detail, which can be observed using the light microscope. At times, to provide greater clarification, it is appropriate to study electron micrographs produced with the electron transmission microscope, which is an extension of light microscopy, and can reveal details far beyond that of light microscopy.

Wherever possible, try and relate structure to function since function and structure are intimately interrelated. Bear in mind the three dimensional structures of cells and their relationship to each other.

Plant tissue can be divided into groups either based on types of cells or on ability to divide:

(1) Based on types of cells:

i. **simple plant tissues**-consisting of one type of cells;
ii. **compound plant tissues**-consisting of more than one type of cells.

(2) Based on ability to divide:

i. **meristematic tissue** e.g. root and shoot apex and cambium;
ii. **permanent tissue** such as ground tissue parenchyma, collenchyma and sclerenchyma; **vascular tissue** e.g. xylem and phloem.

Simple Plant Tissues

Parenchyma Fig. 12.11

All plant cells originate as parenchyma cells, which later specialise according to function.

Appearance: consists of living cells, which are roughly spherical, and may be elongated. The cells are unspecialised, with thin cellulose wall (which may contain pectin and hemicellulose) to allow expansion of turgid cells and for ease of diffusion of gases and dissolved solutes.

Usual colour when stained: light green or blue.

Location: parenchyma cells form bulk of various organs as 'packing' e.g. centre of stem (pith), periphery of stem (cortex), cortex of root, and occur among xylem and phloem, around midrib of leaves.

Function: metabolically active packing material, maintain turgidity, provide support, food storage (usually as starch) and transport of material through cells.

Collenchyma Fig. 12.12

Originate as parenchyma cells, but the cell walls become thicker with deposition of cellulose, especially at the corner of the cells.

Appearance: consists of living cells but modify to give support and mechanical strength. Cells appear very similar to parenchyma but is characterised by uneven deposition of extra cellulose at the corners of the cells, giving an angular shape to the cell. Cell wall consists of cellulose, pectin and hemicellulose, which allow extension of cells during cell growth.

Usual colour when stained: green.

Location: present in outer cortex of stem, vascular tissue in leaves, petioles, and midrib.

Function: give support and mechanical strength.

Sclerenchyma Fig. 12.13

Appearance: elongated and polygonal mature cells with tapering ends. The cells do not mature until elongation is complete, as the cells are dead at maturity and therefore incapable of elongation. Cell wall is mainly made up of lignin. Cellulose, pectin, and hemicellulose may also be present.

Usual colour when stained: red.

Location: present in outer regions of cortex, pericycle of stems, around xylem and phloem, supporting vascular tissue in some leaves.

Function: sole function is to provide mechanical strength and resistance to bending. Pits provide lateral transport between the cells.

Sclereids Fig. 12.13

Appearance: cells are dead, and roughly isodiametric.

Function: support and mechanical protection.

Location: scattered in groups or isolated through out the plant body e.g. gritty bits in pears, but most common in cortex, pith, phloem and seeds e.g. in shells of stony fruit endocarp, (the testa toughens e.g. almonds, plums).

Compound Plant Tissues

There are two types of conducting tissues in plants, namely the **xylem** and the **phloem**, both of which contain more than one type of cells. Together they constitute the **vascular tissue**, whose function is translocation. Xylem conducts mainly water and mineral salts from roots to all parts of the plant, while the phloem conducts organic food from the leaves to the rest of the plant. Both tissues increase in quantity as a result of **secondary growth**. Secondary xylem may become extensive to form **wood Fig. 12.5**.

Xylem Figs. 12.14–12.21

Appearance: in the stems of dicotyledons the xylem is arranged as peripheral rings, whereas in the monocotyledons they are scattered. In the root the distribution of xylem is central. It consists of four types of cells, **tracheids, vessel elements, parenchyma** and **fibres**.

Usual colour when stained: red.

Location: peripheral bundles in stem, central stele in roots, and in veins of leaves.

Function: plays two major roles, conduction and support.

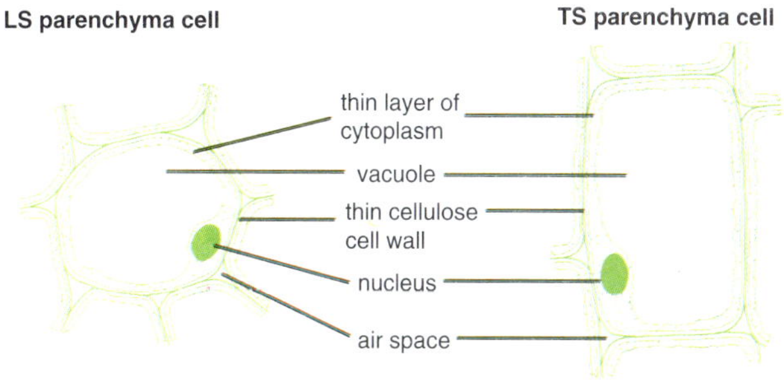

Fig. 12.11 Parenchyma Tissue

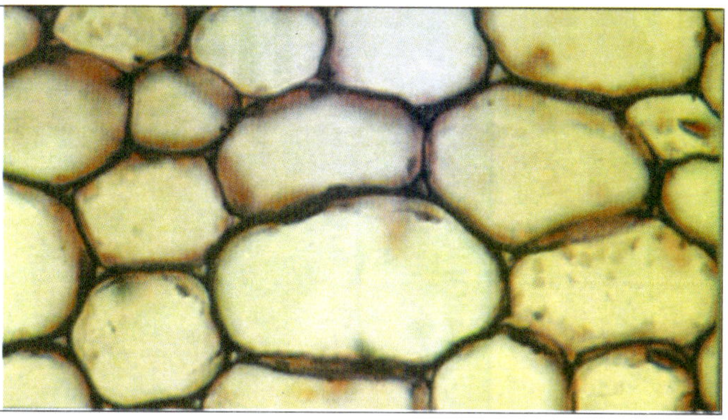

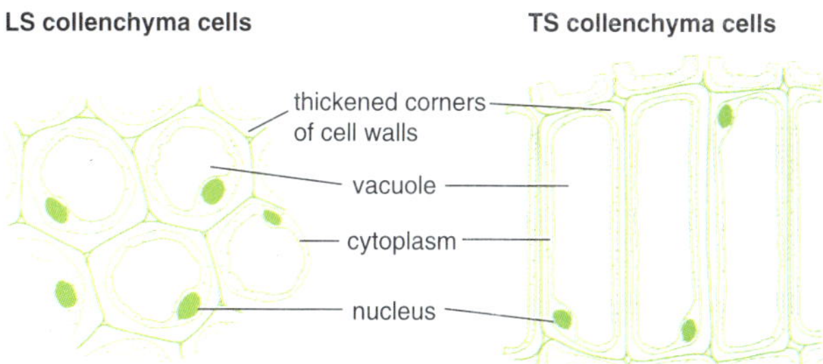

Fig. 12.12 Collenchyma Tissue

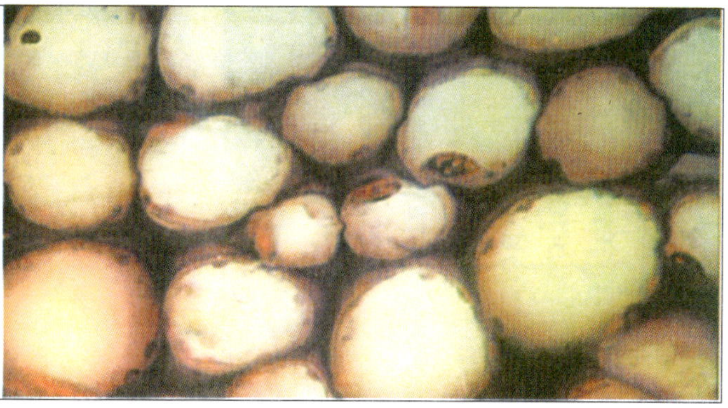

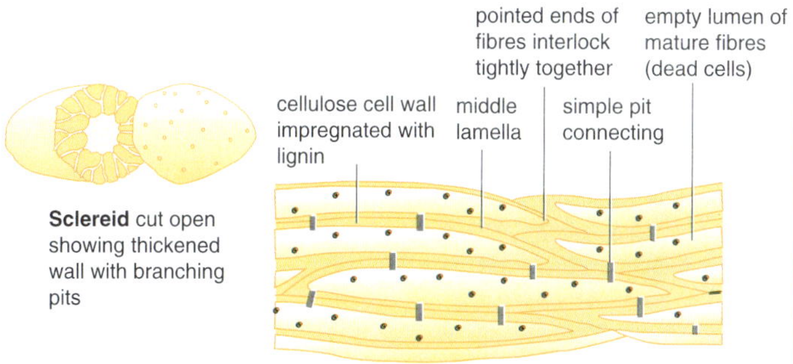

Fig. 12.13 Sclerenchyma Tissue LS Fibres

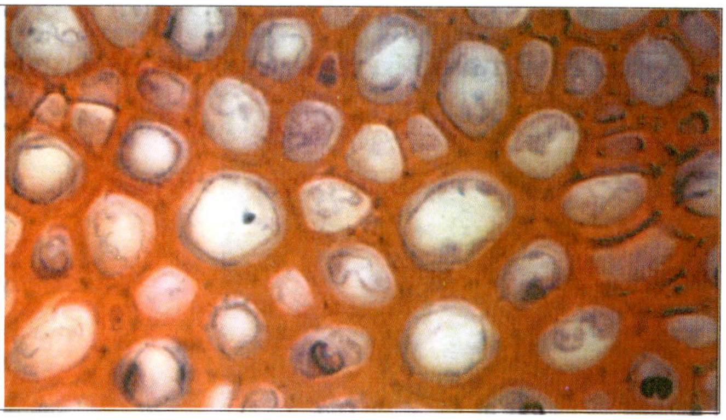

Tracheids Figs. 12.14–12.17, 12.21

Appearance: tracheids are single cells that are elongated and lignified. They have pointed end walls that overlap with adjacent tracheids. They are dead at maturity, therefore cytoplasm is absent and their walls are lignified in various patterns. These can be as annular rings, spiral, reticulated or simple pits. Water can pass from tracheid to tracheid through the pits via the 'pit membranes' or through unlignified portion of the cell wall.

Function: provides mechanical strength and support to the plant as well as transport of water and mineral salts.

Vessels Figs. 12.14–12.15

Appearance: they are long, tubular, cylindrical structures, formed by fusion of several cells placed end to end in rows. Each of the cells forming the xylem vessel is equivalent to a tracheid and is called a **vessel element**. However, vessel elements are shorter and wider than tracheids. The first xylem to appear in a plant is called the primary xylem and develops in the root and the

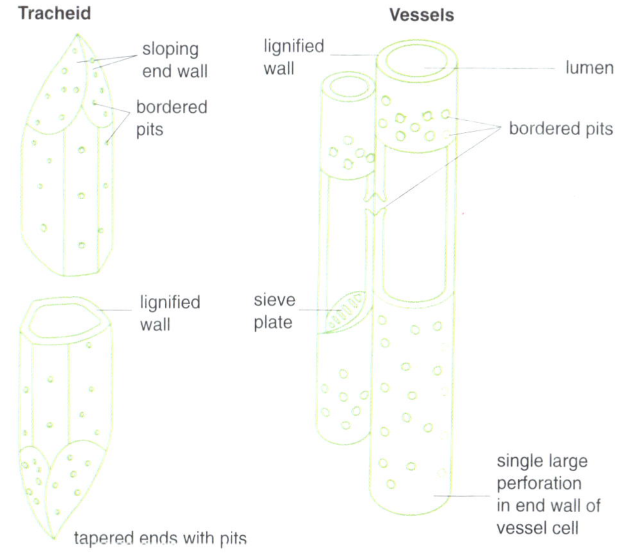

Fig. 12.14 Xylem Tissue – Tracheid and Vessels

Practical 5 – OBSERVING CELL STRUCTURE

Individual cells are extremely small and almost transparent, and are therefore difficult to observe unless treated with special stains. The various structures that are crammed into a theoretical diagram of a generalised cell are not all visible in any one cell. So to piece together the structure of a typical cell it is necessary to look at more than one type of cell. In light microscopy, it is common practice to add dyes or stains **(see page 20)** to introduce sufficient contrast, and observe different structures. Dyes and stains that are taken up by living cells are especially useful in this. The choice of stain is important since certain stains are specific to certain structures; for example actinocarmine stain is picked up by the nucleus and its contents, whereas iodine stains starch grains.

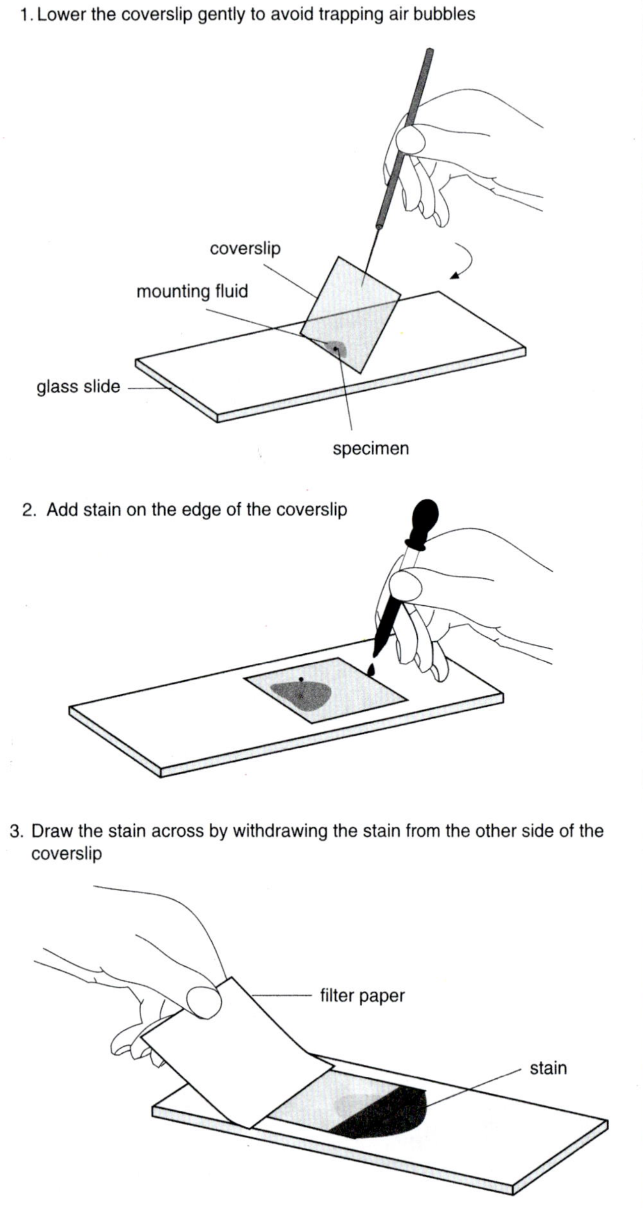

Fig. 3.7 Preparation of a Temporary Slide

Caution:

- *When working with dyes and stains, avoid contact with skin or clothing.*
- *Take care when using sharp dissection equipment.*

Observing human cheek cells

Caution:

Wash hands before you begin, and dispose of the slide in a beaker of disinfectant or absolute ethanol.

1. Gently wipe the inside lining of a your own cheek using a **fresh, clean** cotton bud or **sterilised** spatula.
2. Mount the scrapings in a drop of water on a clean microscope slide. Add a coverslip.
3. Observe first under low power, then under high power. Some of the cells will appear crumpled and irregular in outline because the cell membrane is extremely delicate and thin **Fig. 3.8.**

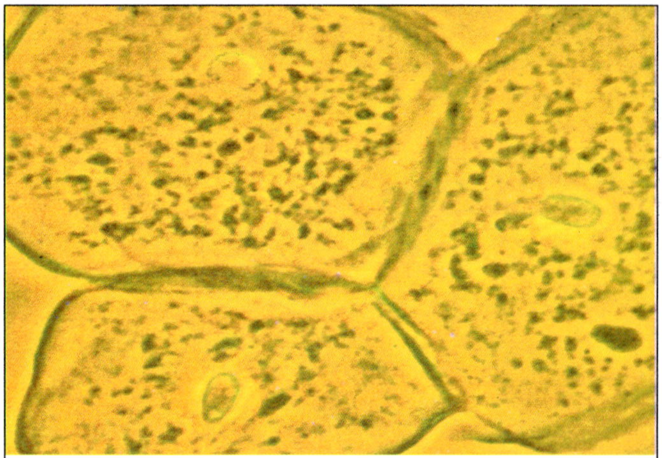

Fig. 3.8 Cells from Lining of Cheek Epithelium

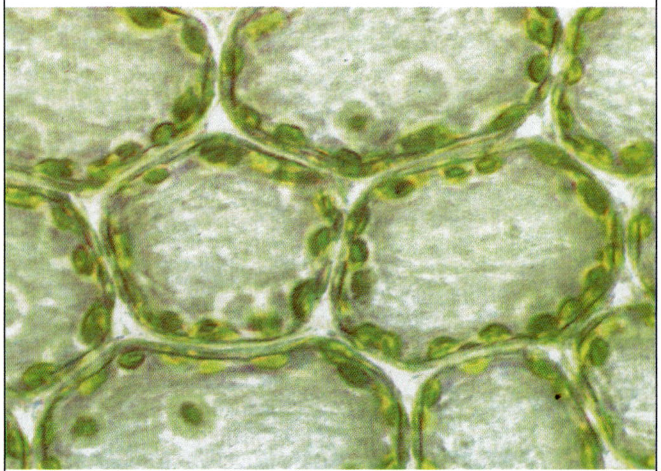

Fig. 3.9 Cells in a Moss Leaf

The Cell

Background Summary

A common characteristic shown by nearly all living things is that they all consist of cells. Cells were first described by Robert Hook in 1665 and are now known to be of universal occurrence in living organisms.

The **cell** is the functional unit of all tissues. It has the capacity to perform independently all life functions. Within the various tissues of the body, cells exhibit a wide range of specialisation, which are, merely amplifications of one or more of the cellular processes. Reflecting their particular functional specialization, mammalian cells have an extraordinary range of morphological forms, **Fig. 3.1** varying in size and shape, yet all cells conform to a basic model of cell structure. As viewed by the light microscope, all cells are seen to consist of **cytoplasm surrounded**

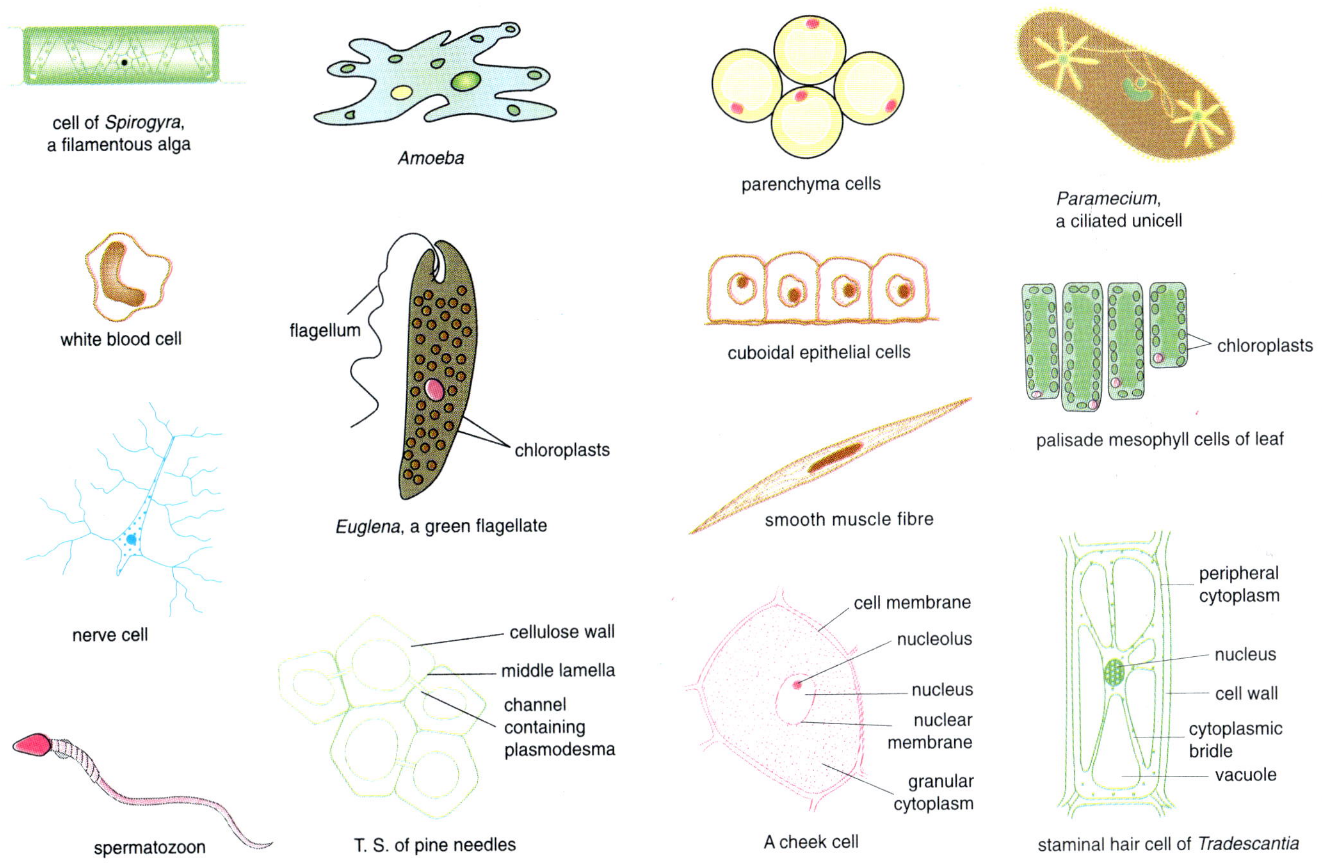

Fig. 3.1 A Variety of Different Cells (not to scale)
All cells are fundamentally similar, possessing a nucleus and cytoplasm with an array of organelles, enclosed within a membrane.

by a plasma membrane, and to contain a nucleus. As and when microscopic techniques advanced it became increasingly obvious that both the nucleus and the cytoplasm contain a number of subcellular elements, which are, called **organelles**. Typical plant cells differ from animal cells in lacking cillia or flagella and in possessing cellulose wall, chloroplasts, starch grains and permanent sap vacuole.

Most structures within cells are far too small to be resolved by light microscopy but can be observed with an electron microscope, see **Figs. 3.2–3.5**. The resolving power of the light microscope is limited to about 0.20µm (200 nm) and the study of the ultrastructure of the cell had to await the advent of the electron microscope, which at present permits the resolution of structures as small as 3.0nm (30 angstrom units).

Electron microscopy, together with the technique of **cell fractionation** i.e. disruption of cells to isolate the internal structures, **Fig. 2.5** has established a range of organelles. These cell organelles can be separated by **differentiation centrifugation** and are studied individually to ascertain their functions. The roles of the different organelles in the growth, behaviour and metabolism of cells are understood, at least in part.

Some organisms are unicellular whilst others are multicellular. Multicellular organisms show a great range of

***Phloem* Figs. 12.18–12.25**

Appearance: phloem resembles xylem in possessing tubular structure, modified for translocation. However, unlike the xylem, the cells are living and contain cytoplasm but play no role in mechanical strength. There are five types of cells present in the phloem namely, **sieve tube elements**, **companion cells**, **parenchyma**, **fibres**, and **sclerieds**.

Usual colour when stained: green or blue.

Sieve tubes are long tube-like structures that translocate solutions of organic solutes like sucrose throughout the plant. They are formed by the end-to-end fusion of cells called **sieve tube elements** or **sieve elements Fig. 12.24.** The end wall between adjacent cells, is called the **sieve plate**. It has characteristic pores, which are visible under the light microscope. Rows of these cells can be seen developing from the procambial strands of apical meristem where primary phloem develops, together with primary xylem in the vascular bundles.

The first phloem formed is called the **protophloem** and, like the protoxylem, it is produced in the zone of elongation of the growing root or stem. As growth proceeds, much of it collapses, and becomes non-functional, meanwhile more phloem continues to be produced, and the phloem that matures after elongation is called **metaphloem.**

Sieve tube elements have a very distinctive structure. Like parenchyma cells their walls are made of cellulose and pectin. Nuclei however, degenerate and are lost as the cells mature and the cytoplasm becomes confined to the edges of the cell. Though they lack a nucleus they remain living and are dependant on the adjacent companion cell, which has a dense active cytoplasm, that develops from the same original meristematic cell. The two cells together form a functional unit.

Function: play no role in mechanical strength and are modified for translocation.

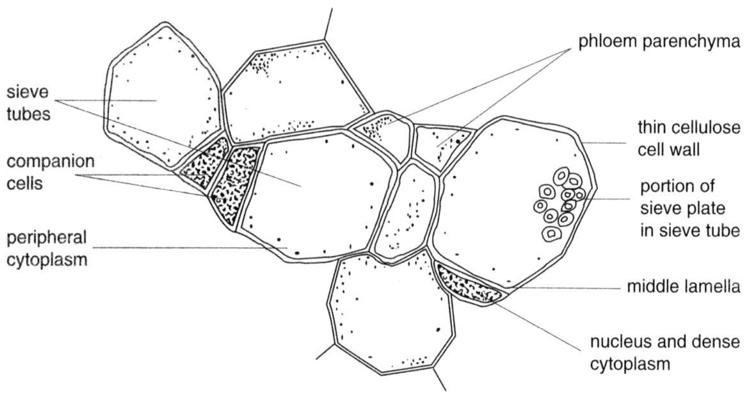

Fig. 12.22 TS Phloem from Marrow (*Cucurbita*) Stem

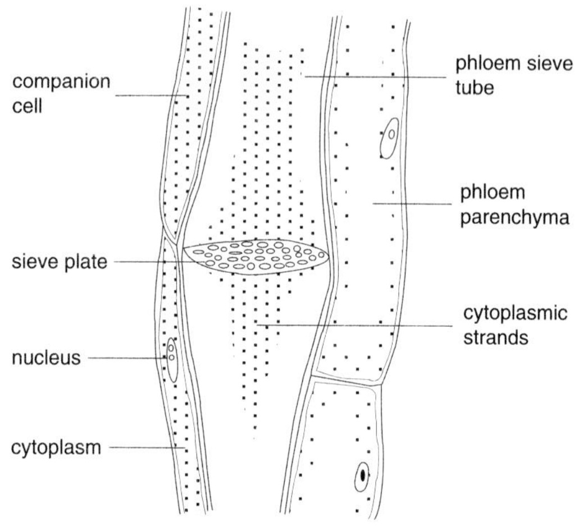

Fig. 12.23 LS Phloem from Marrow (*Cucurbita*) Stem

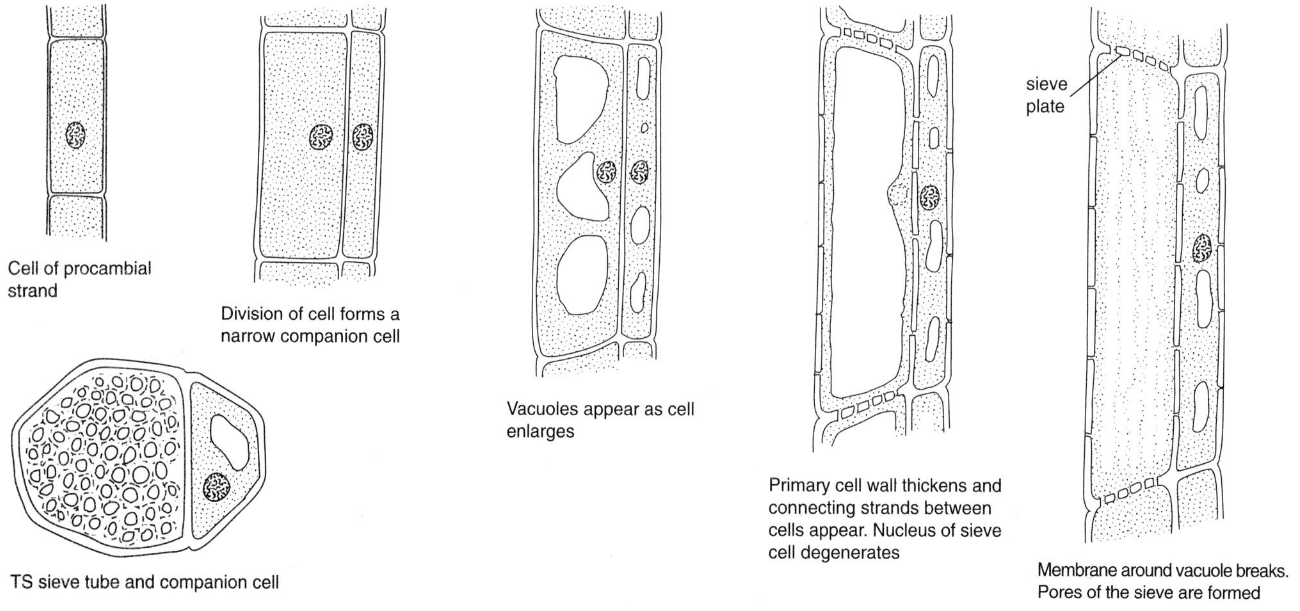

Fig. 12.24 Formation of Phloem Tissue (sieve tube and companion cell)

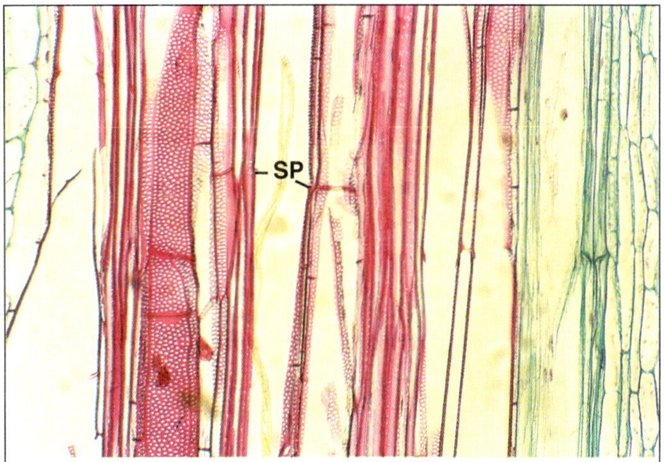

Fig. 12.25 Phloem Sunflower (*Helianthus*) LS Old Stem. Note the sieve plate within the sieve tube with adjacent companion cells.

Phloem parenchyma, fibres and sclereids

Are found in dicotyledons but not in monocotyledons. The structure of the cells resembles other similar cells.

Meristematic Tissue

Once the embryonic stage is passed, growth in plants is confined to certain localised regions called the **meristems Figs. 12.26–12.28**.

There are three types of meristems:

i. **Apical meristem**-occurs at tips of roots and shoots. Cells are small, and cuboidal with thin cellulose cell wall and dense cytoplasmic content.
The cell has few small vacuoles and contain undifferentiated plastids called **proplastids**.
The cells are packed tightly together, without any air spaces between the cells.
The cells are called **initials,** which divide by mitosis. One remains in the meristem, the other increases in size and differentiates to become the permanent plant tissue.

ii. **Lateral meristem (cambium)**-occurs as cylinders towards the outside of the stem, resulting in increase in girth annually, which is referred to as **secondary growth** in woody prennials such as trees and shrubs **Fig. 12.5**. Secondary growth takes place in the stem and the roots by mitotic cell division between the xylem and the phloem in the vascular bundles. These cells form the **cambium** and divide to form **secondary xylem** to the inside and **secondary phloem** to the outside. More xylem tissue is formed than the phloem tissue. In between adjacent vascular bundles **secondary parenchyma** is formed.
Increase in girth necessitates the epidermal layers of the plant tissue to undergo secondary growth also otherwise the epidermis would rupture. Just beneath the epidermis is a layer of cells called the **cork cambium**, which divides tangentially to form **secondary cortex** to the inside and **cork cells** to the outside. The walls of these cells become impregnated with **subrin**, which renders them impervious to water and gas. **Lenticles** are regions where cells are loosely packed, allowing gaseous exchange to take place between the inside and the outside of the stem.

iii. **Intercalary meristem**-occurs at nodes of grasses, allows growth in length in places other than the tip.

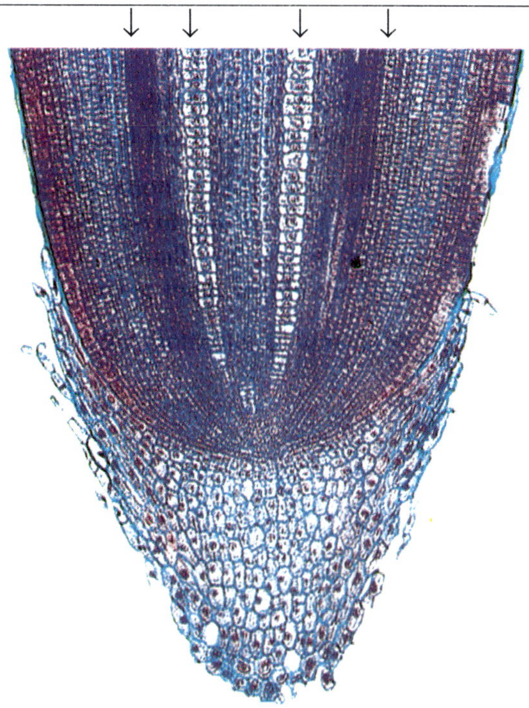

Fig. 12.26 Micrograph of Root Apical Meristem. The outer arrows mark the outer limit of the stele, the inner ones indicate the rows of cells differentiating as vessels.

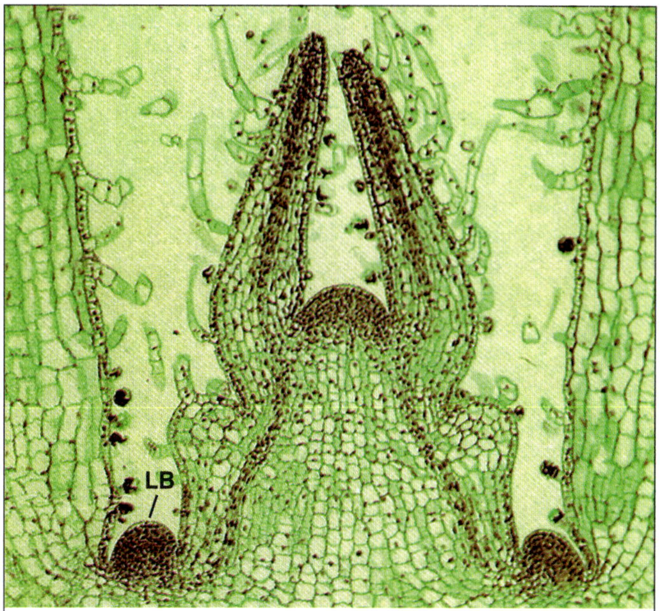

Fig. 12.27 Micrograph of Shoot Apical Meristem. The shoot apex appears as dome in the centre, flanked by young leaves. The darker rows of cells within the ground tissue are vascular bundles. Lateral buds are seen as dark tissue near the base of the micrograph.

Bacteria in Yoghurt

1. Pass a glass slide through the blue flame of a Bunsen burner using a pair of forceps, to remove grease.
2. Transfer a drop of sterilised distilled water on to the slide using a heat sterilised inoculating loop. Dip the sterilised cooled inoculating loop in the yoghurt. Mix about half a loopful of the yoghurt with the water on the slide.
3. Smear the resultant mixture in the centre of the slide **Fig. 3.13** using another glass slide.
4. Allow the **smear** to air dry. Then **heat-fix** the smear by quickly passing the slide through the blue flame of the Bunsen burner. The slide should not become too hot for comfort when touched against the back of your hand.
5. Using a dropper, flood the slide with crystal violet stain and leave for one minute.
6. Wash clear with a gentle flow of distilled water. Blot and allow to air dry.
7. Examine the stained smear directly (without a coverslip) first under high power, and then under immersion oil (**see page 18**). Bacteria are coloured red-violet.
8. Record your observations by drawing what you see.

Bacteria in Plaque (tooth scrapings)

1. Using a sterilised inoculating loop add two drops of sterilised distilled water to a clean microscope slid.
2. Using a sterile toothpick, scrape the surface and the crevices between your teeth and mix the scrapings with the distilled water on the slide.
3. Transfer a loopful of the mixture to another clean glass slide, add a drop of nigrosin, mix and prepare a smear using the end of another glass slide.
4. Air-dry the smear and dispose of other used slides in the sterilising fluid.
5. Observe and record your observations with annotated drawings under high power/oil-immersion without a coverslip. The bacteria appear colourless with an intense blue/black background (negative staining).
6. If time permits, use an eyepiece graticule and a stage micrometer slide to estimate the size and range of bacteria present (**see page 20**).

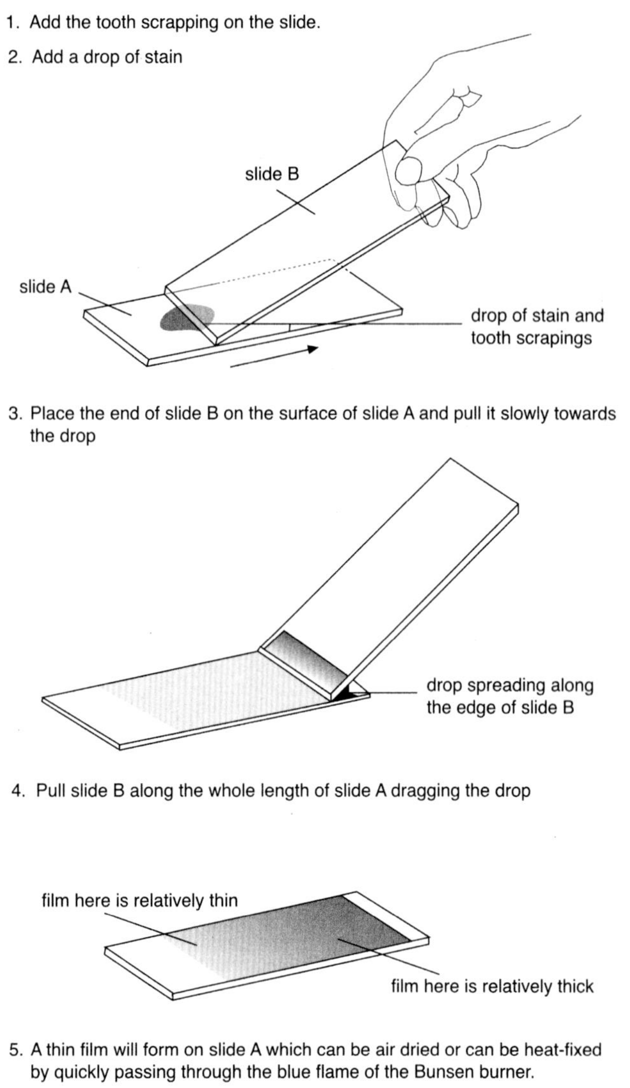

Fig. 3.13 Preparation of a Smear

For consideration

(a) Compare and contrast bacterial cells with other cells you have observed in previous investigations.

(b) What are the sources of danger from bacteria when you are working with materials such as yoghurt and tooth scrapings?

4. Find a single intact cell and draw your observations. Label nucleus, nuclear membrane, nucleoplasm, chromatin granules, nucleolus, granular cytoplasm and cell membrane.
5. Prepare another cheek cell slide as before.
6. Add a drop of methylene blue dye to the edge of the coverslip and remove the bulk of the dye, by withdrawing it with a piece of filter paper from the other edge **Fig. 3.7.** Examine some of the individual cells present under medium and high power magnification.
7. Observe and record your observations with annotated drawings. When drawing cells remember that each cell has its own separate cell wall, connecting to the adjacent cell with the middle lamella **Fig. 3.10**. Look for nucleus, cell membrane, and the granular cytoplasm. Pay special consideration to how the cells join with adjacent cells and the shape of cells.
8. Work out the total magnification of your drawings.
9. Now using prepared slides examine as many different plant and animal cell types as possible.

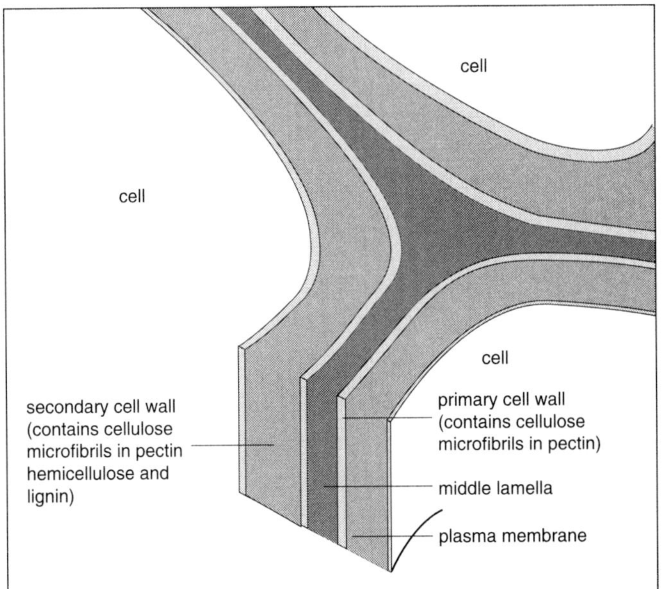

Fig. 3.10 Diagram of Cell Walls of three Connected Plant Cells

Observing chloroplasts

1. The leaf of the moss plant *(Mnium sp.)* is typically one cell thick. Place a single leaf from a moss plant, mount it on a microscope slide in a drop of glycerol, and carefully add a coverslip. Avoid trapping air bubbles.
2. Then examine individual cells under low and high power of your microscope **Fig. 3.9**.
3. Make labelled drawings of your observations.

For consideration

(a) What is the green colour of the chloroplasts caused by?

(b) What other structures (if any) of these plant cells are visible?

(c) When cells were first observed why do you think it was easier to observe plant cells than animal cells?

Observing onion (Alluim cepa) epidermis cells

1. Slice an onion bulb into half, and cut into pieces about 0.5 cm long. With a fine forceps peel off the epidermis from the inner, curved surface of one of these pieces.
2. Place this film of tissue on a microscope slide in a drop of iodine solution (I_2/KI) and carefully place a coverslip on top, making sure the tissue layer is flat and not folded. Avoid trapping air bubbles **Fig. 3.7.**
3. Leave this **temporary mount** for one or two minutes whilst the iodine penetrates the cell membrane.
4. Examine and make a labelled drawing of the cells under medium and high power magnification.
5. Notice that the iodine solution stains the living contents a light yellow colour, but the nucleus takes up the stain more strongly than the cytoplasm. The bulk of these cells are filled by a vacuole which remains unstained.
6. Observe the nucleus, nucleoli, and chromatin granules inside the nucleus, the distribution of granular cytoplasm surrounding the vacuole and the cellulose cell wall.
7. Record your observations by drawing.

For consideration

(a) Why do you think onion tissue was chosen for this exercise?

(b) What can you say about the 3-dimensional shape of the cells?

(c) The onion is a plant organ but why does it not contain chloroplasts?

(d) The leaf bases of the onion bulb are concerned with food storage, but the onion does not store carbohydrate as starch. Why do you think this is fortunate for this investigation?

(e) Make a table of the cell structures observed and relate them to their functions. Also record how each responded to the stains used.

(f) What value, if any, is there in the concept of 'the generalised plant or animal cell'?

(g) Examine some electron micrographs of plant and animal cells, identifying as many structures as possible with reference to **Figs. 3.3, 3.5.**

(h) Work out and record the size of the cell and of each organelle you have observed from the scale given on the electron micrograph.

(i) Compare the structure of plant and animal cells observed.

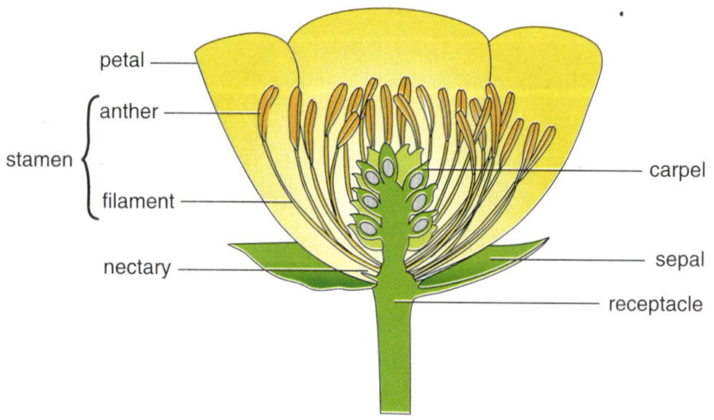

Fig. 12.31 Section of a Buttercup Flower showing Radial Symmetry

Gynaecium–collection of **carpels/pistil**. Each carpel consists of **stigma**, **style** and **ovary**. The stigma receives the pollen during pollination; the style carries the stigma and supplies nourishment to the pollen tube and the pollen nucleus as it grows through it. The ovary is a swollen hollow base of the carpel, which contains one or more **ovules**.

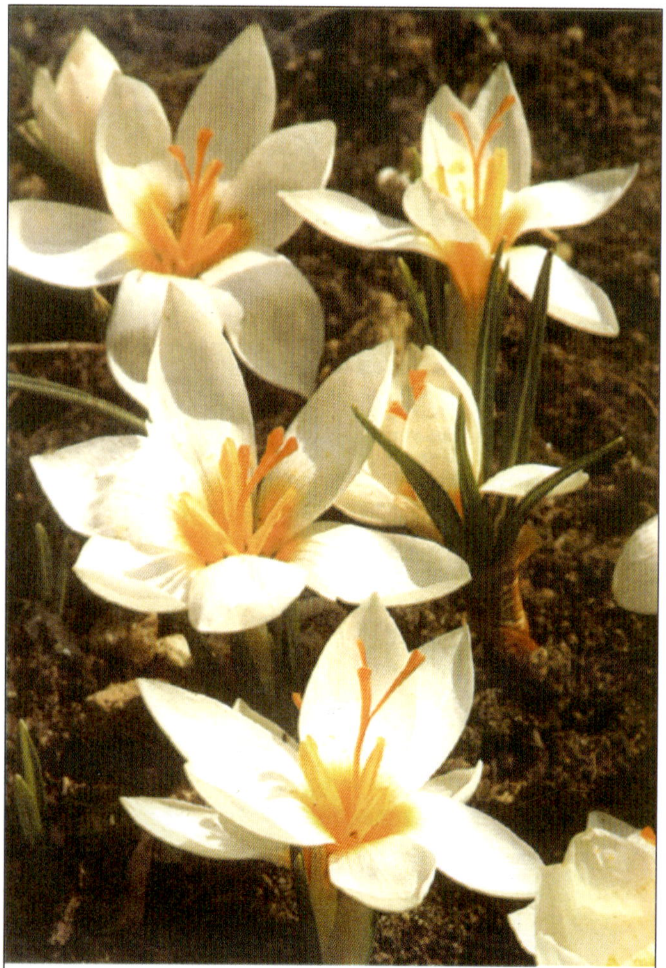

Fig. 12.32 Crocus sieberi 'Bowles' White'

At the base of the ovary are the **nectaries**. These are glandular structures, which secrete nectar, a sweet sticky substance that attracts insects and birds.

All the floral parts are arranged on a flattened tip of the pedicel called the thalamus or the receptacle. The pedicel, calyx, corolla and the thalamus are **vegetative parts** of the flower. The androecium and the gynaecium are the **reproductive parts.**

8. Now look at a **Compositae** flower such as the dandelion (*Taraxacum*) kakronda, daisy (*Bellis*), or the sunflower (*Helianthus*) suraj mokhi **Figs. 12.33** and **12.34**. This is a specialised form where the thalamus is expanded and flattened and bears numerous small flowers (each petal of the flower is in fact a complete flower). This type of inflorescence is called **capitulum**.

   If the flower parts are arranged in radial symmetry around the recepticle (i.e. can be cut in two equal halves in any direction) the flower is said to be a regular or **actinomorphic** flower e.g. buttercup. If the flower is bilaterally symmetrical (can be cut in two equal halves in one plane only) it is said to be an irregular or **zygomorphic** e.g. sweet pea (*Lathyrus odoratus*) muttery **Fig. 12.35**.
9. Take a regular flower such as petunia (*Solanaceae*) or buttercup (*Ranunculus*) make labelled drawing of the whole flower and then carefully cut it in half. Make a labelled drawing of the half flower **Fig. 12.31**.
10. Now examine as many different flowers as possible. Determine if they are actinomorphic or zygomorphic. Identify all the structures within them.
11. Examine an irregular zygomorphic flower such as the sweet pea (*Lathyrus odoratus*) **Fig. 12.35**. Note that there is a large odd petal outermost. This is called the **standard** or **vexillum**. The two petals below the standard are called the **wings**. The last two petals are tightly packed together to form a **keel** or **carina** enclosing the stamens and the carpels. All ten stamen filaments are fused to form a tube. The fruit is a **legume**, which splits at both ends.
12. Take other irregular flowers such as lupine or salvia, observe their structure and record your observations by means of drawing. Cut the flowers in two equal halves and make annotated diagrams of your observation.
13. Observe and draw flowers from any species of grass **Fig. 12.36**.

Variations in Flower Structure

Numerous variations in size, scent, colour, shape and structure have evolved over the 130 million years of angiosperm history. Much of this diversity represents adaptation of flowers to different pollinators.

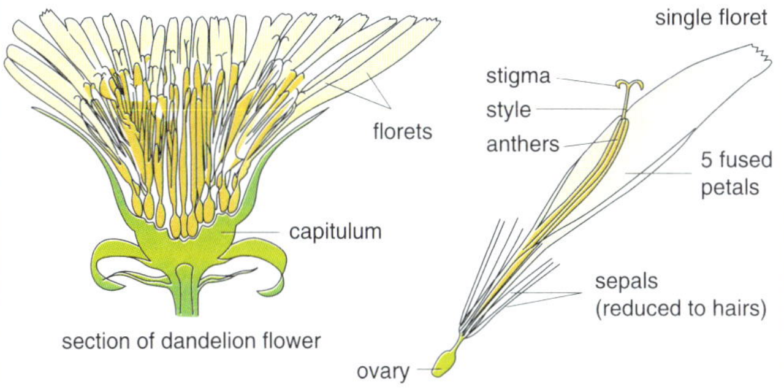

The flower head consists of flattened, disc-shaped stem called the capitulum, which carries a large number of flowers called florets.

Fig. 12.33 Structure of the Dandelion, (*Taraxacum officinale*) Capitulum

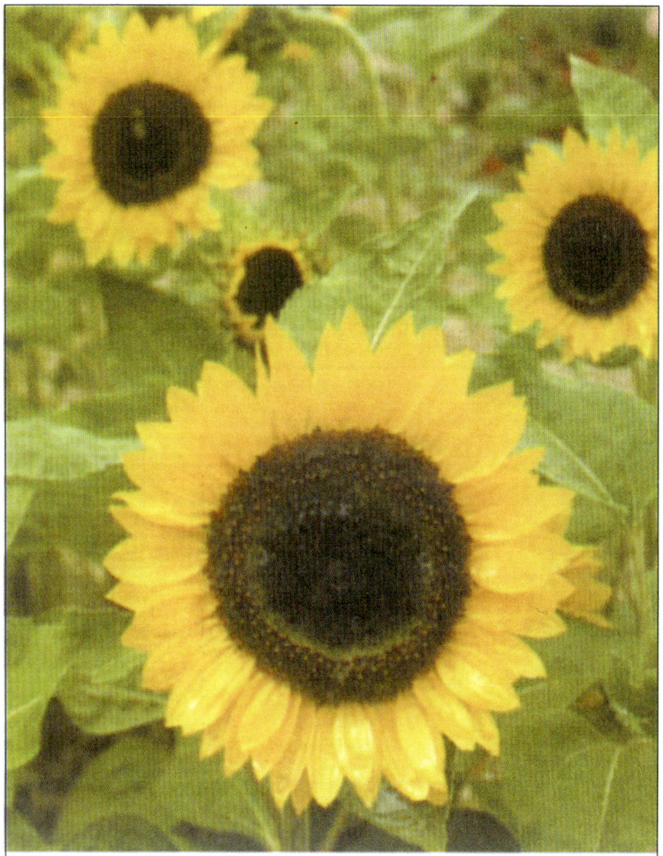

Fig. 12.34 Sunflower (*Helianthus*) Suraj Mukhi

Sepals–number variable; show varying degrees of fusion; may be absent altogether; may be green and leaf-like, or coloured and petal-like (**petaloid**) e.g. Bougainvillea (*Nyctaginaceae*).

Petals–number variable; like sepals, show varying degrees of fusion, in some cases forming tube (corolla tube) e.g. petunia, foxglove (*digitalis*). Sepals and petals may be fused or indistinguishable from one another, in which case they together form the **perianth**.

Nectaries–may be absent; scent varies widely.

Stamens–number may be large and variable or small and fixed; anthers vary in size.

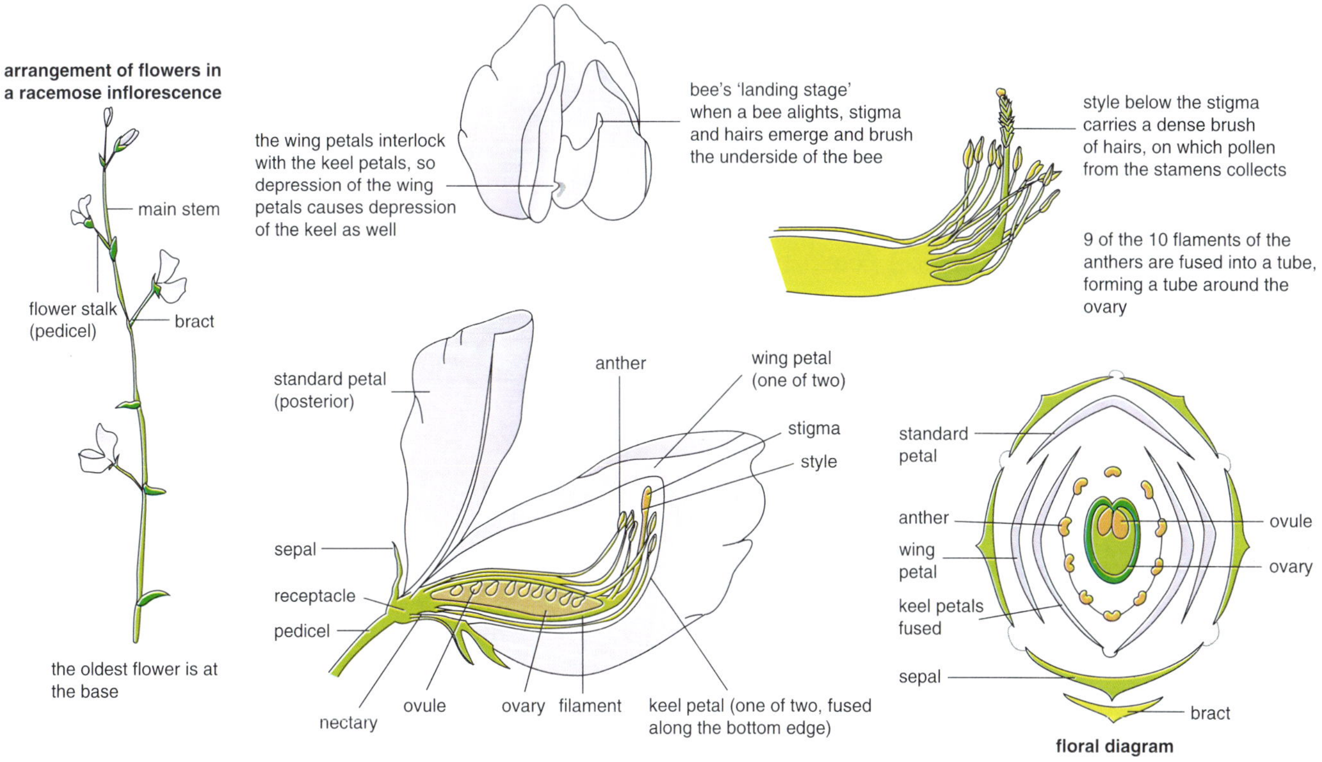

Fig. 12.35 The Flower Sweet pea (*Lathyrus odoratus*) muttery

Osmosis

Osmosis is the one-way net diffusion of solvent (particularly water) across a **selectively permeable membrane**. It plays a vital role in cell homeostasis. Cell water relations are determined by osmotic concentration of the cell sap (**solute potential**) and the **pressure potential** of the cell (pressure due to the cell wall or the turgidity of the cell).

The osmotic movement of water can be expressed in terms of **osmotic pressure**. This is the tendency of a solution to take in water across a selectively permeable membrane.

An animal cell immersed in a **hypotonic** (external solution more dilute than the cell) solution swells and may burst unless it has means of disposing of the water that enters by osmosis. In a **hypertonic** solution the cell shrinks and the cell membrane crinkles. Whereas a plant cell immersed in water or a hypotonic solution becomes **turgid**. If immersed in a hypertonic solution the protoplast shrinks and **plasmolysis** occurs. (The protoplast membrane is selectively permeable but the cellulose wall is fully permeable.)

As a way of expressing water movement, osmotic pressure is increasingly being replaced by the **water potential** concept. For practical purposes, water potential is the capacity of a system to give out water, and it is given a negative sign. The component of the water potential, which is caused by the presence of solutes, is called the **osmotic potential**. The symbol for water potential and related energy potentials is the Greek letter psi (ψ).

The water relations of a plant cell can be summarised as follows:

$$\psi_{cell} = \psi_s + \psi_p$$

Where:

ψ_{cell} is the water potential of the cell (usually negative),

ψ_s is the osmotic potential of the sap (negative),

ψ_p is the **pressure potential** – that is the inward pressure exerted by the cell wall against the protoplast (zero or positive).

The water potential of a plant tissue can be determined by balancing it with an external solution, which produces no mass or volume change in the tissue. The osmotic potential can be determined by balancing it with an external solution that produces incipient plasmolysis.

Active transport is a highly selective process in which the movement of particles is against a concentration gradient. It is an energy requiring process involving the use of protein carriers in the cell membrane.

Bulk transport of substances in the cells takes place by invagination of the cell membrane to form vesicles, generally referred to as **endocytosis.** There are three types of endocytosis, **phagocytosis** ('cellular eating'), **pinocytosis** ('cellular drinking') and **receptor-mediated endocytosis**. The reverse process is known as **exocytosis** (expulsion out of cells). Basically the cell wraps pseudopodia around the substance to be engulfed, forming a membrane-enclosed vacuole. The package is digested after the vacuole is fused with a lysosome containing hydrolytic enzyme. The receptor-mediated endocytosis is very specific. The extracellular substance binds to the receptor (called **ligand**) located in the cell membrane, forming a pit and the substance is transferred inside this pit. Endocytosis and exocytosis provides a means by which liquids and macromolecules may be brought in and out of cells.

4 Transfer of Substances through the Cell

Transfer of Substances through the Cell

Cells and Osmosis

Red Blood Cells

Plant Epidermis

Filamentous Algae

Effect of Temperature on Cell Membrane

Movement of Ions through the Cell Membrane

The Water Potential of Cells of an Inflorescence Stalk

Osmotic Fragility of Red Blood Cells

Water Potential of Plant Cells

Practical 48 – MICROSCOPIC STRUCTURE OF STAMEN AND CARPEL

In a flower, the stamens and carpels contain pollen grains and egg cells respectively. The pollen-containing part of the stamen is the anther. The egg-containing part of the carpel is the ovule: the ovary contains one or more ovules, each of which contains an embryo sac with an egg cell inside **Fig. 12.39**.

Anther

1. Examine a transverse section of a flower bud of a lily (*Lilium*) and identify the anthers **Fig. 12.37**.
2. Examine an anther under high power. Note the four pollen sacs and examine their contents. The contents depend on the state of maturity of the anther:
   i. If immature, the pollen sacs will be full of closely packed pollen mother cells.
   ii. If more mature, they will contain pairs or tetrads of cells (pollen tetrads) resulting from meiotic division of the pollen mother cells. Chromosomes may be observed, telling you at what stage of meiosis the cells have been fixed.
   iii. If completely mature they will contain fully formed pollen grains
3. Observe the wall of the pollen sac, noting the inner **tapetal** layer, which nourishes the developing pollen grains, and the middle and fibrous layers. Drying out of the cells of the fibrous layer creates tension which causes the anther to split open at the **stomium**, a line of weakness running longitudinally along each side of the anther from top to bottom.
4. Observe and compare pollen grains from different flowers **Fig. 12.38**.

Ovary

5. Locate the ovary in the centre of the flower bud, carefully cut it in half and examine under high power. With reference to **Fig. 12.39** record your observations by drawing.

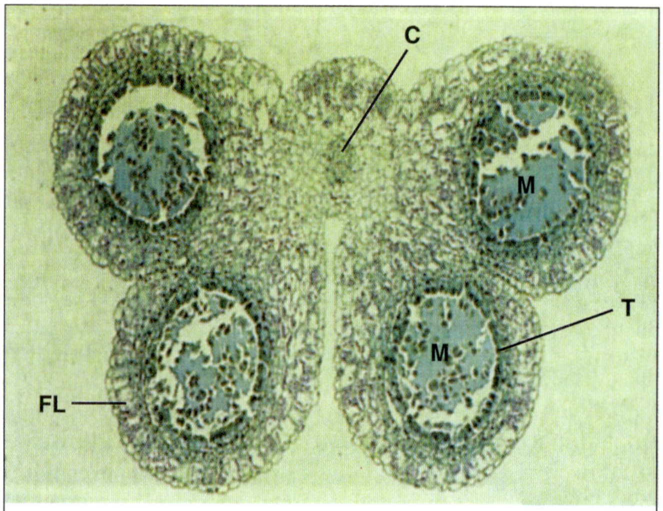

Fig. 12.37 TS of a young undehised anther of Lilum.
Note the connective **C**, fibrous layers **FL**, tapetum **T**, microsystem mother cells inside the microsporanguin **M**.

The embryo sac has a single **haploid** nucleus, which is formed by meiosis from an embryo sac mother cell. It undergoes successive mitotic divisions to give eight nuclei, two of which (the **polar nuclei**) will fuse to form a central fusion nucleus. Each of the seven resulting nuclei becomes surrounded by membranes. The **antipodal cells** at the **chalazal** end of the embryo sac are thought to provide nourishment for the **embryo sac**, the **synergids** at the **micropyle** end are non-functional eggs and degenerate. In the act of fertilisation, the egg cell (**ovum**) fuses with one male nucleus to give the **zygote**. The diploid **fusion nucleus** fuses with the other male nucleus to form the triploid **primary endosperm nucleus**, this latter gives rise to the endosperm tissue, which envelops and nourishes the embryo.

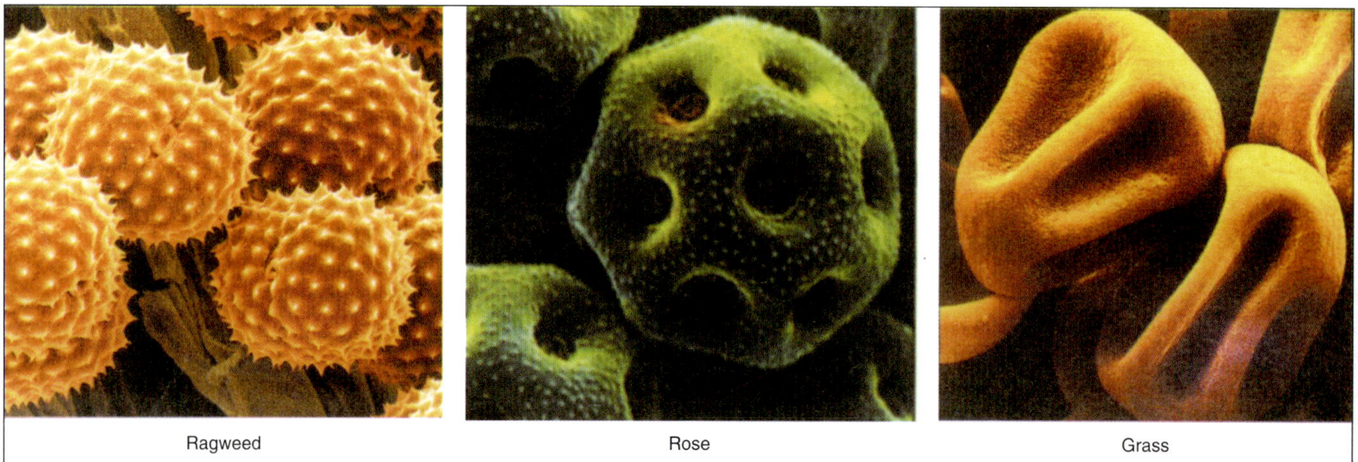

Fig. 12.38 Pollen Grains

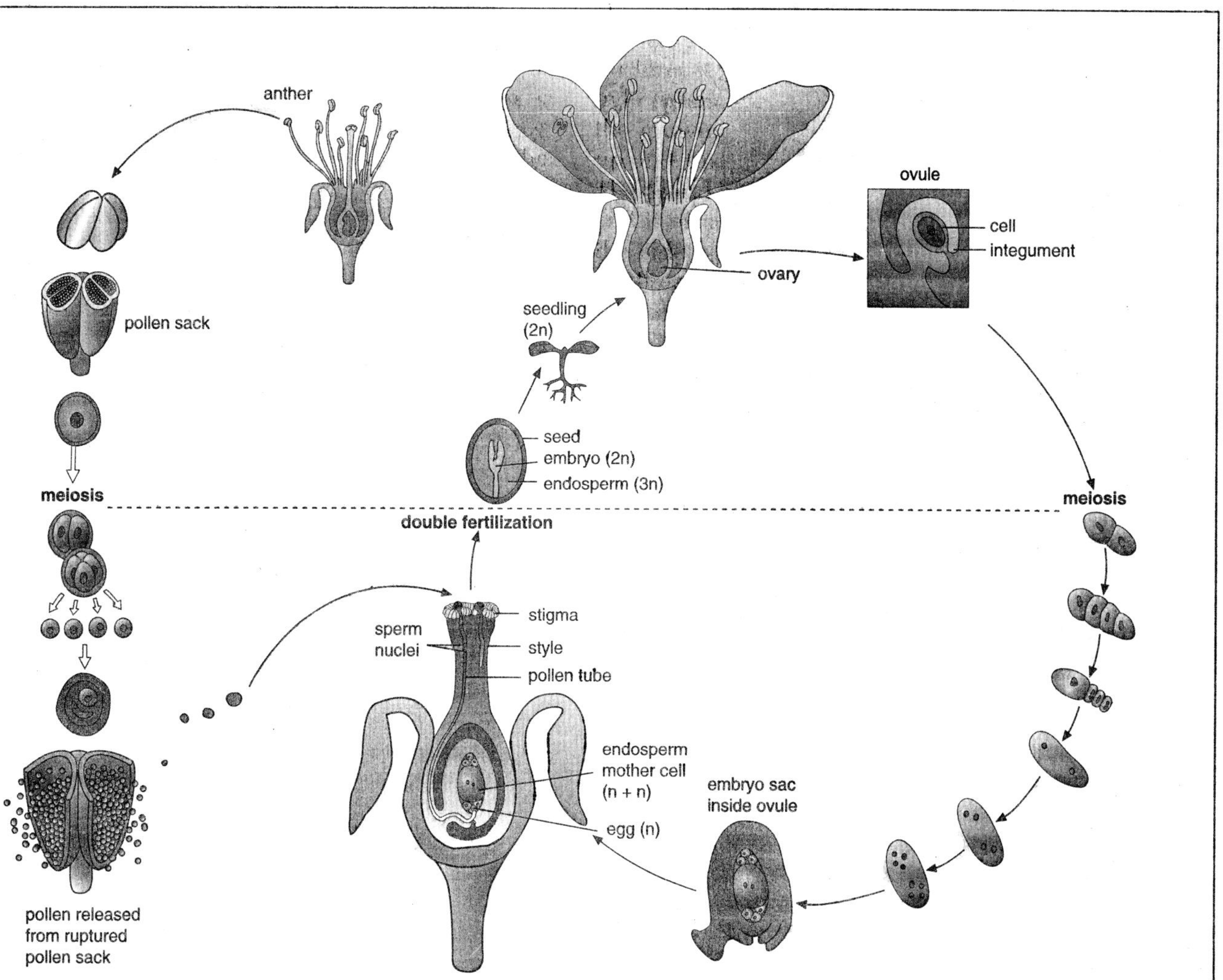

Fig. 12.39 Pollination and Fertilization

For consideration

(a) Where and when does meiosis take place in a flowering plant?

(b) Compare the gametes and the way they develop in the flowering plant and mammal.

(c) Consider each of the flowers that you have examined and try to decide how efficient it is at securing cross-pollination and preventing self-pollination.

(d) Although cross is genetically desirable, it is not necessary that it should happen invariably. For this reason the various mechanisms listed above are by no means foolproof. Indeed, some plants have mechanisms which specially encourage self-pollination. Can you suggest what these mechanisms might be?

Practical 49 – GERMINATION

A seed in itself is a life support package. Inside is the embryonic plant, containing a store of food and all the necessary ingredients to develop into a new plant. The stored food either is packed around the embryo as **endosperm** (e.g. maize) in the monocotyledons or is stored in special seed leaves called the **cotyledons** (e.g. broad bean) in the dicotyledons **Figs. 12.40–12.42.** This is required to keep the embryo alive and for energy during the process of germination. The seed may remain inactive (dormant) for months, years or even centuries. When the conditions are right the seed suddenly comes alive and begins to grow. It absorbs water, cell division begins to take place, the seed coat or the **testa** ruptures, and a root or **radicle** emerges and grows downward (**geotropism**). A shoot or **plumule** begins to grow pushing its way through the soil upward towards the light (**phototropism**). It is usually bent double to protect the growing tip, but once above ground it straightens up and from this the stem and leaves appear.

The apical meristem is at the tip of the growing shoot and if nipped off further growth has to take place from the side buds. Once the true leaves are produced the seedling begins to photosynthesise and no longer relies on the stored food supply, which by now is depleted

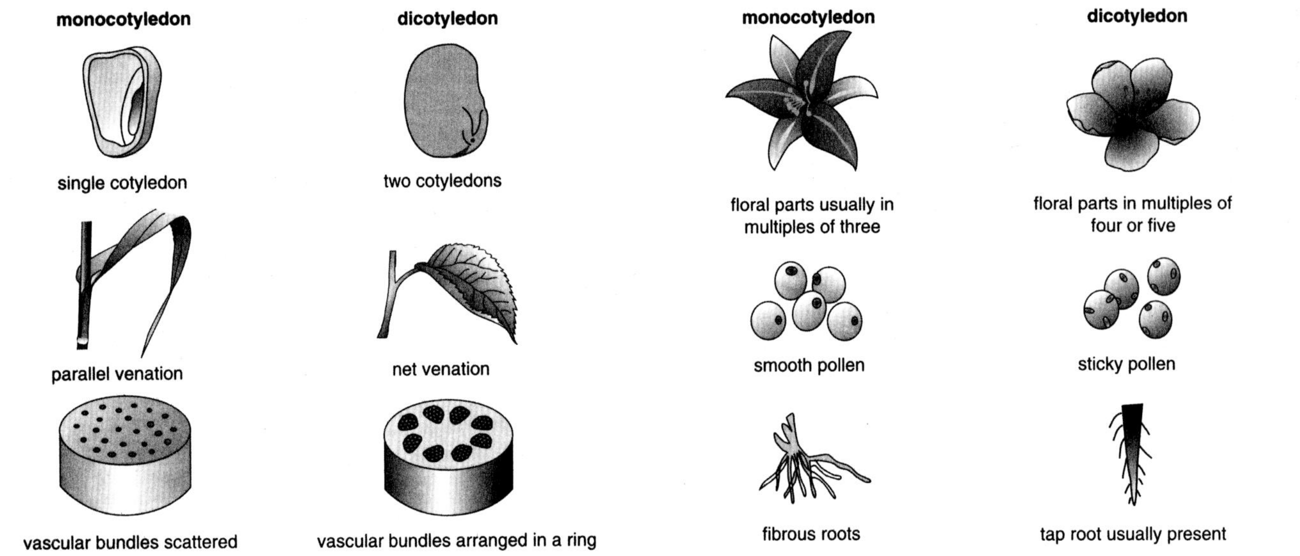

Fig. 12.40 Comparison of Monocotyledon and Dicotyledon Plants

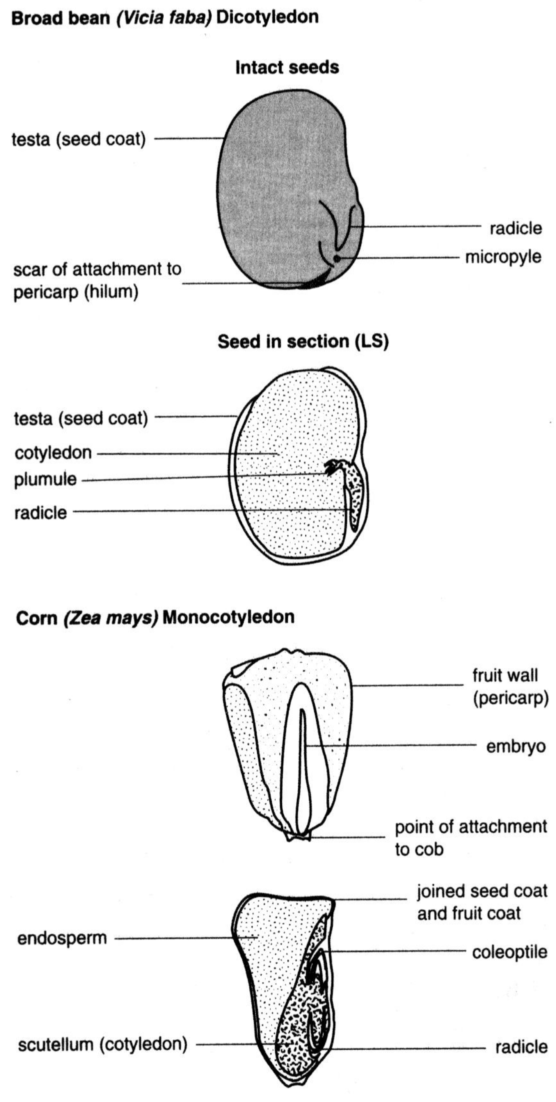

Fig. 12.41 Structure of Seeds

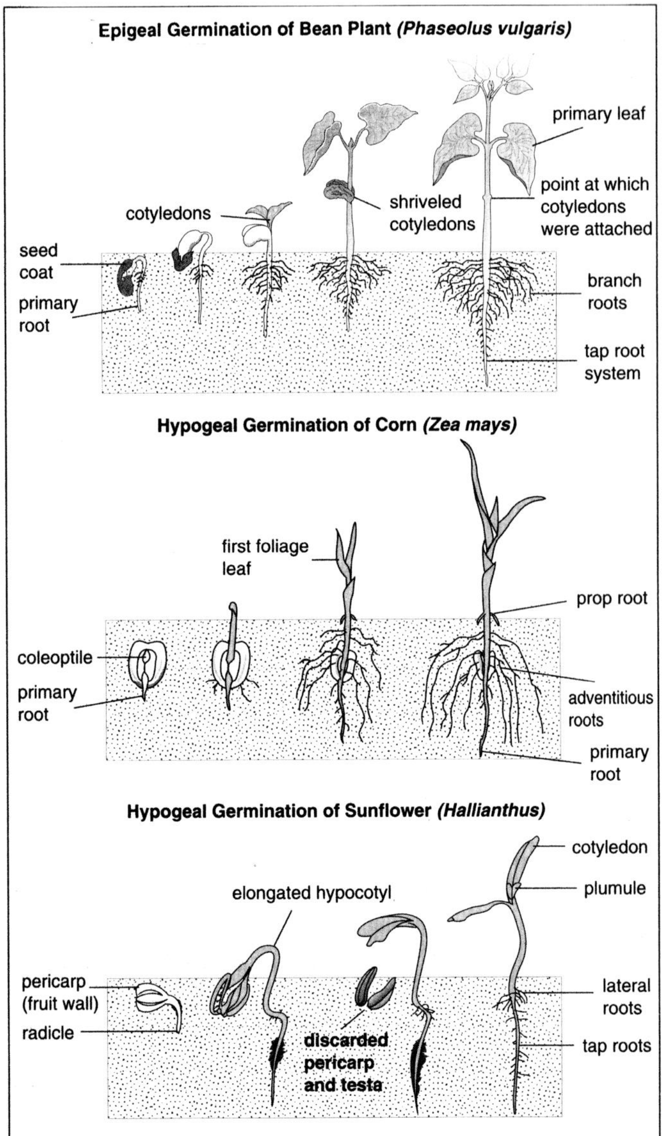

Fig. 12.42 Germination

and the shrivelled remains of the seed fall off.

Flowering plants are divided into monocotyledons (having only one cotyledon) and dicotyledons (having two cotyledons). Monocots have a single seed. The young shoot grows upwards protected by a tube called the **coleoptile**. The growing point or the apical meristem is at the base of the plant at ground level so even when the tip is removed as is the case in pasture, the plant continues to grow.

Procedure

1. Examine dry and soaked broad beans, caster oil seeds, sunflower seeds and maize seeds. Notice the seed coat (**testa**), **micropyle** and the **hilum Fig. 12.41**. Make drawings of your observations.
2. From the broad bean carefully remove the testa and split open the two cotyledons and notice the plumule, radicle and the absence of the endosperm tissue.
3. In the caster oil seed note the **caruncle**, which covers the helium and the micropyle. The caruncle plays a part in the imbibition of water. Using a sharp blade slice the seed horizontally down the flattened side and observe the radicle and the plumule and the endosperm. Record your observations with careful drawings.
4. Test the seeds for the presence of carbohydrates, protein and fats.
5. Observe the germinating broad bean **Fig. 12.42**. This type of germination is referred to as **hypogeal** germination in which, the **epicotyle** elongates and the cotyledons remain below the ground.
6. In the **epigeal** germination of the sunflower seeds, the **hypocotyl** elongates with the result that the delicate cotyledon remain protected by the ruptured seed coat. They turn green and begin to photosynthesise and eventually fall off after the true leaves have emerged.
7. Examine and make annotated drawings of the germinating seeds of broad bean, and the sunflower.

For considerations

(a) What are the ideal conditions for seed germination?

(b) Why is it necessary to have ideal conditions before the seed germinates?

Practical 50 – RATE OF TRANSLOCATION OF SUCROSE IN A STOLON OF POTATO

Food manufactured in the leaves by photosynthesis is distributed to the whole plant and excess is stored in the storage organs. This transport of the organic food material is called **translocation** and takes place in the **phloem** of the plant. In the potato plant *Solamum tuberosum* in early summer, sucrose is translocated from the leaves to the developing tubers - the 'new potatoes'. Each tuber develops at the end of a stolon, which grows out from the base of the main stem.

In this investigation you will determine:

i. The volume of sucrose, which enters the tuber in a given period of time.

ii. The cross-sectional area occupied by sieve tubes in the stolon.

From these two values, you can calculate the rate of translocation of sucrose in the stolon.

In summer before the growing season for potatoes has ended, extract a potato from the soil with its living stem still attached. Find out when the seed potato from which the tuber has developed was planted.

Procedure

Determination of the volume of sucrose entering the tuber per unit time

All the starch in the tuber is derived from sucrose transported down the phloem into the tuber. Some of the sucrose which enters the tuber, however, will not be stored but will be used in cellular respiration. This provides ATP for growth of cellulose cell wall, for storage cells etc.

1. Clean the potato, by wiping with cotton wool and weigh the potato on an accurate balance.
2. Keeping in mind the above assumptions calculate:
   i. The dry mass of the potato.
   ii. The mass of the starch in your tuber.
   iii. The length of time for which the tuber has been accumulating starch. The figure for the mass of starch accumulated by the potato tuber each hour is an estimate of the mass of sucrose, which entered the tuber each hour.
   iv. The amount of starch accumulated per day, per hour.
   v. Recalculate the mass of sucrose reaching the tuber per hour. This new estimate will be higher than the previous one.
   vi. The volume of sucrose that must have travelled down to the tuber per hour.

To determine the volume of sucrose entering the tuber per unit time following assumptions have to be made:

- That 80 % of the mass of the potato is water and that 20 % of the dry mass is starch.
- That the tuber arises at the end of an underground stem about thirty days after planting.
- 25 % of the sucrose entering the tuber has been used for cellular respiration, growth of new cell walls etc.
- Sucrose in the tuber is a 2% sucrose solution.

Determination of the cross-sectional area occupied by sieve tubes in the stolon.

1. Using a sharp razor cut thin cross-sections from your tuber.

2. Place them on a microscope slide, add a few drops of phloroglucinol and hydrochloric acid (**corrosive**), stains lignin pink. Add a coverslip.
3. Calibrate an eyepiece graticule under the high power of the microscope, using a stage micrometer slide **(see page 20)**.
4. Observe and draw plan diagram of the tuber section under low power of the microscope. Notice that the bundles of xylem and phloem are arranged in a ring, as in a stem, instead of in the centre, as in a root **(see page 126)**.
5. Observe a vascular bundle under high power. Measure the distance across the phloem area in two directions at right angles. Average the two estimates. Assuming that the area covered by the phloem is rectangular, calculate the cross-sectional area of the phloem in this bundle.
6. Experimental evidence suggests that only a fifth of this cross-sectional area consist of the sieve tube elements. Divide your estimate of the cross-sectional area of the phloem in one bundle by five. The result represents the area of sieve tube elements in a bundle. Multiply by the number of bundles in the cross-section.

Calculation of the Rate of Translocation of Sucrose in the Stolon

You now know the volume of sucrose transported and the cross-sectional area of the phloem sieve tubes (volume = length x area).

To calculate the length of phloem sieve tube, which empties per hour, divide the volume of sucrose, which enters the tuber per hour by the cross-sectional area through which it has travelled. This is the rate of phloem transport, i.e. the rate at which sucrose is translocated in the stolon.

For consideration

(a) Compare your estimate of the rate of translocation with those in the table below.
(b) Do your results compare with those of the table? If not, suggest possible reasons.
(c) Of what practical use might these estimations be?
(d) Suggest possible factors, which might determine the rate at which a tuber fills up with starch, and its eventual size.

Plant and organ	Translocation rate (cm h^{-1})	Experimenters
Potato tuber stem	225	Dixon & ball
Potato tuber stem	105	Crafts
Yam tuber stem	220	Mason & Lewin
Bean (*Phaseolus*) petiole	28	Birch-Hirchfield

Measured rates of transport in plant organs. Based on the solute in the translocated solution to be 2% sucrose. Adapted from M.J. Canny, Biological Reviews, Vol. 35, 1966.

Practical 51 – STRUCTURE OF LEAVES

Leaves are of many shapes and sizes varying from the six foot long leaves of some tropical palms to the pinhead-sized leaves of *Wolffia*, one of the duckweeds. Some are slender smooth and elegant while others are stubby, thick and prickly. They may be pointed, rounded or blunt ended. The variation is endless. The arrangement of the leaves on the stem is in just as many multitude of differing ways. Taxonomists use the leaf shapes to distinguish species and hence an elaborate terminology has evolved to define leaf characteristics. Some of the leaf shapes are illustrated in **Fig. 12.43**.

The leaf is the plant's specialised organ of photosynthesis. Since structure and function are related, it is logical that the basic leaf structure be thin and flat for maximum exposure to the light. The leaf attachment to the stem is such that there is a minimum of overlap allowing maximum light exposure. The thin **lamina** is attached to the plant by a short stalk called the **petiole**. Through transpiration and osmotic pressure within the cell, the leaf literally sucks water, dissolved minerals and ions from the soil.

With the help of radiant energy from the sun it manufactures nutrients required by the plant (sugars, proteins, fats etc.) through photosynthesis. As would be expected the photosynthetic tissue is located in a position to secure maximum illumination of the chloroplasts. The leaf must obviously be in functional connection with the rest of the plant, in order to transport water and mineral salts to the photosynthetic tissues and to distribute the products of photosynthesis to the rest of the plant. Leaf structure and functions are highly adapted to satisfy these conditions and are closely linked with **midrib**, **veins** and **veinlets**.

In some plants, such as the xerophytes the leaves become a disadvantage because of water loss. Elaborate modifications in structures have taken place to conserve water. The leaves are either succulent to store excess water **Fig. 12.56** or are reduced to spines and other organs of the plant such as the stem take on the function of the leaves **Fig. 12.55, 12.56**.

Procedure

External structure

1. Observe:
   (i) Evergreen leaves, which stay on the tree for most of the year such as young leaves of Peepul (*Ficus religiosa*), Eucalyptus (*Myrtaceae*) Safada.
   (ii) Mulberry (*Moracae*) shehtoot, Buddelia (*Loganiaceae*) Din-ka-Raja, dahlia or any other deciduous leaves which are lost in the winter.

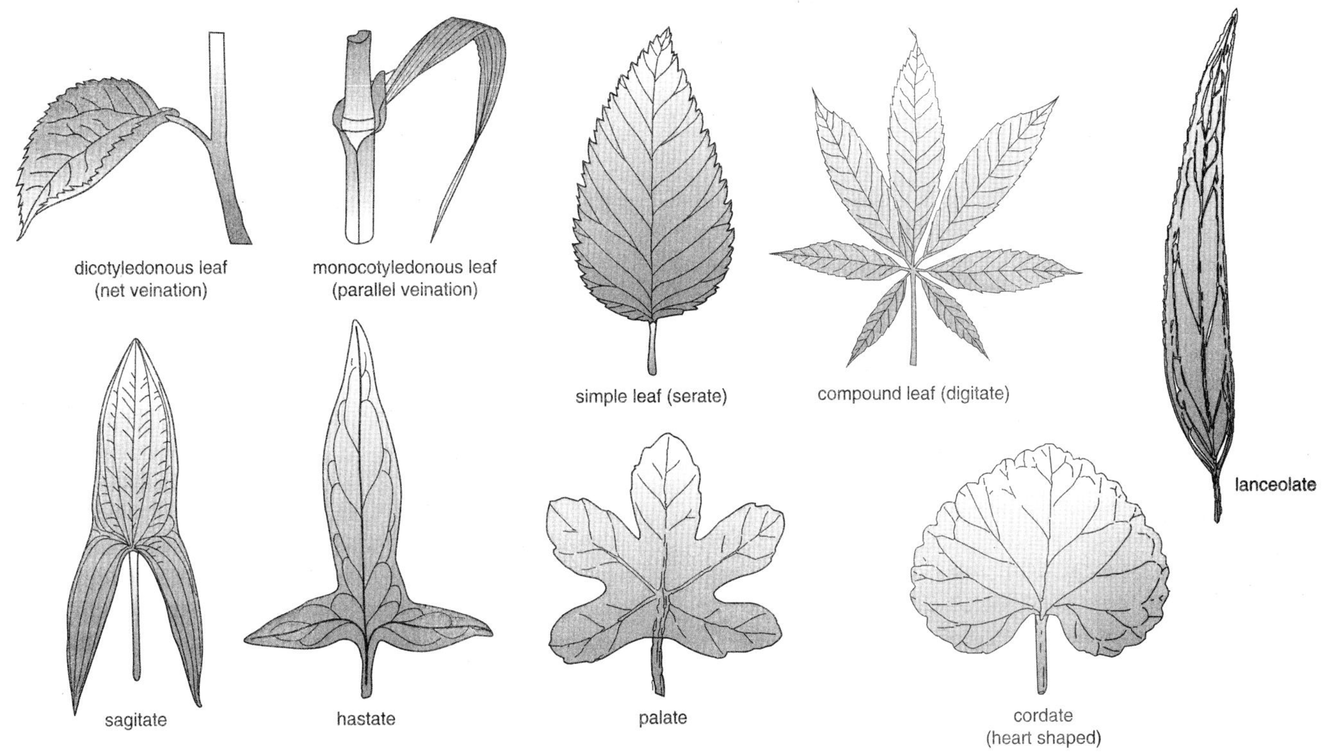

Fig. 12.43 Structure of Leaves

(iii) Monocotyledon leaf, e.g. Spiderwort (*Tradescantia pallida*), grasses (*Poaceae*), lily (*Lilium*), iris (*Iridaceae*), and record the similarities and the differences in a table.

2. Study and record your observation by drawing the external features of a leaf of a dicotyledon and monocotyledon.
3. Note that the dicotyledons generally display a network of veins whereas monocotyledons have parallel veins. The upper surface of the leaf is darker green and shiny as compared to the lower surface.
4. Observe the location of the midrib and the network of veins in as many leaves as are available.
5. With some leaves such as *Tradescantia* and *Buddelia* (Din-ka-Raja) and *Bryophyllum* (pather chat) it is possible to strip the upper and the lower leaf surfaces. Tear an edge and pull the two edges in the opposite directions pulling at an angle. After some practice you will be able to separate some of the thin, almost transparent upper and lower epidermis. You only require a tiny piece, about 2-3mm is sufficient for observation under the microscope.
6. Float it in a watch glass of water. Transfer it with a small soft brush onto a clean glass slide, making sure to keep the section flat. Add a few drops of water to prevent the specimen from getting dry. Gently place a cover slip on top.
7. Observe first under low power then under high power of the microscope, noting epidermal cells in surface view, stomata and guard cells. Make labelled drawings of your observations **Figs. 12.49, 12.50.**

Internal Structure

1. Cut transverse sections of a dicotyledonous leaf, by inserting it in the centre of a slit made in a piece of potato or carrot tuber or elder pith, **Fig. 12.2.**
2. Hold the tuber in one hand, cut rapidly and smoothly thin section almost gilding over the surface using a sharp razor blade. Float the sections in a dish of water.
3. Using a fine brush transfer one or two of the thinnest sections, including at least one that is cut through the midrib, and mount them in water on a glass slide. Observe first under low power, then under high power. Note all the structures you can identify in **Figs. 12.44–12.46.**
4. Examine and draw the plan of the leaf lamina under low and high power. Note the following:
   Upper epidermis–one or more layers of rectangular cells, generally with thick waxy cuticle of cutin to reduce water loss by evaporation. Transparent to allow light through to the photosynthetic mesophyll layers. No air spaces between cells to reduce penetration by pathogen. Few, if any, stomata. No chloroplasts. Some plants have epidermal hairs to reduce pathogen attacks.

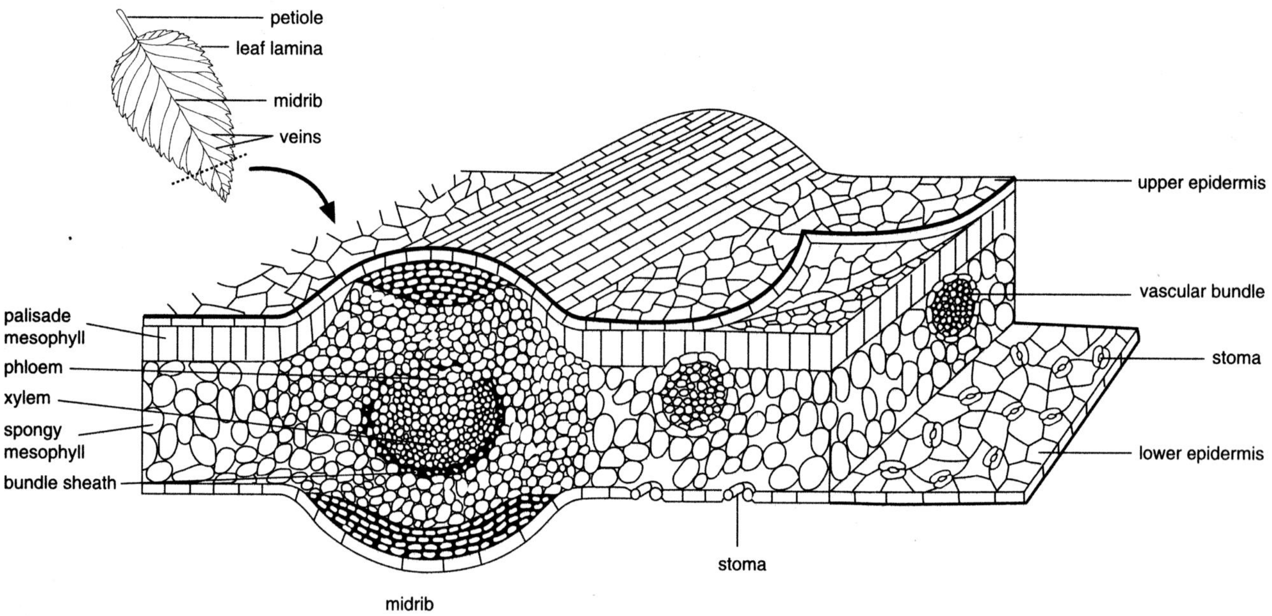

Fig. 12.44 Schematic Representation of Internal Structure of the Leaf

Palisade mesophyll–one to three cells thick rectangular cells elongated at right angles to leaf surface to allow maximum surface area for light absorption; narrow intercellular air spaces appear as dark lines flanking many of the cells. Large vacuole provides support and turgidity. Thin cellulose walls to allow diffusion of gases and solutes. Main sites of photosynthesis hence is dense green due to presence of numerous chloroplasts.

Spongy mesophyll–irregular shaped cells, fitting loosely together to leave large air spaces as main respiratory surface of plant. Increased surface area for gaseous exchange provided by spherical or sausage-shaped cells. Transpiration from sub-stomatal chamber keeps cell moist to allow gases to dissolve. Fewer chloroplasts so some photosynthesis can take place.

The palisade and spongy mesophyll together make up the photosynthetic tissue (**chlorenchyma**) in the leaf.

Lower epidermis–single layer of cells with a very thin layer of cuticle, with many stomata. Main sites of gas exchange via the stomata **Figs. 12.49, 12.50.** Also a site for water loss through evaporation regulated by guard cells. Generally, guard cells are only present in the lower epidermis. They are the only cells in the lower epidermis to have chloroplasts, so are quite obvious. They appear a little sunken below the surface of the epidermis.

5. Examine the **vascular bundles** in the leaf lamina (not the midrib). The vascular bundles may have been cut through transversely or obliquely. The upper part consists of water-conducting **xylem tissue Fig. 12.18;** the lower part consists of food-conducting **phloem** tissue. Thick-walled **sclerenchyma** fibres may be seen immediately beneath the phloem. If the bundle is cut obliquely, spirally thickened xylem elements may be seen.
6. Find a section of the midrib and observe and compare the vascular tissue with that of the leaf lamina, note:
   Vascular tissue–large circular/oval vascular bundle (s) in centre; phloem is usually to the underside of the xylem but in some plant species it may surround the xylem.
   Strengthening tissue–variable amount of **parenchyma** tissue surrounds vascular area, usually as packing material; **collenchyma** immediately below the lower epidermis, **sclerenchyma** close to the phloem.
7. Add a drop of iodine solution to the edge of the cover slip, you may need to draw the iodine solution under the coverslip by touching the other edge of the coverslip with filter paper.
8. Observe under high power. All lignified walls will be stained yellow and any starch present will be stained dark blue.
9. Mount a section in Sudan III. This stains fat and will stain the cuticle.
10. Stain another section with FABIL. This is a good stain to show various structures, xylem elements will stain brown, sclerenchyma pink, cellulose pale blue, cytoplasm and nuclei dark blue, starch black.
11. Observe and draw different types of cells and tissues paying special attention to detail of cell shapes and size under high power **Figs. 12.11–12.13.**

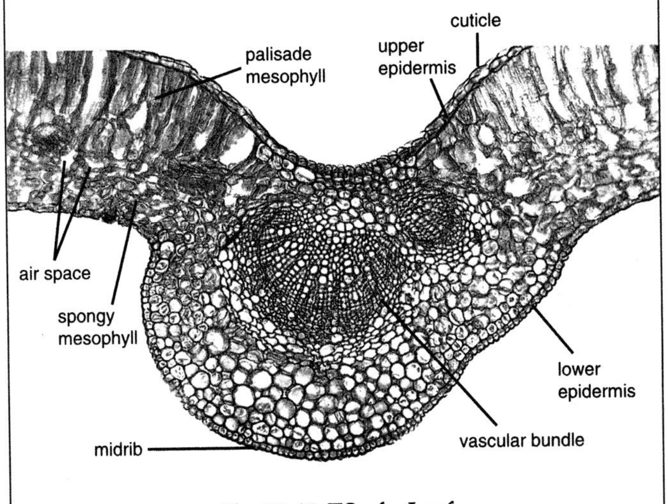

Fig. 12.45 TS of a Leaf

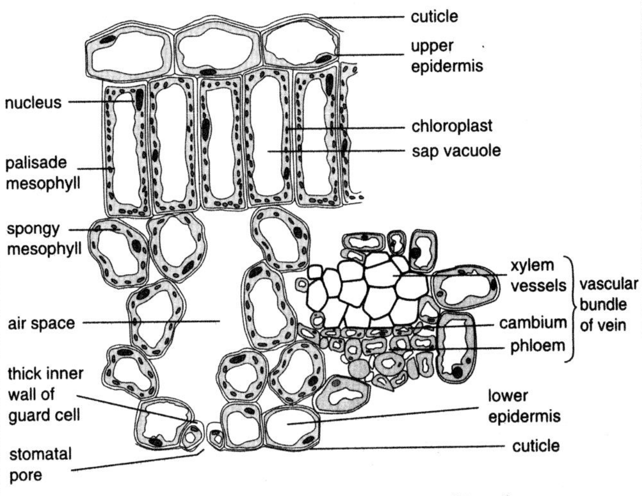

Fig. 12.46 Internal Structure of Leaf

Structure of the Chloroplasts

1. Observe chloroplasts in your section, these are very prominent in moss leaves (**see page 28**). Compare with electron micrographs and diagrams in textbooks.
2. With reference to **Fig. 12.47** identify the various structures in the micrograph. Notice in particular the **thylakoid membranes** (the photosynthetic pigments are located in the thylakoid membranes), **grana** and **stroma** and relate structure to functions.

Further Investigations

1. Observe the differences between the internal structure of leaves in the shade and those in bright sunlight. A shade leaf can absorb light available at low light intensity. If exposed to high light most of the light passes through. Observe leaves from the exposed top of the tree and from the bottom which is in shade.
2. Cut transverse sections of a monocotyledon leaf, e.g. grasses, lily, iris. Observe and draw under the high power of the microscope.
3. Compare the internal leaf structure of mesophytes, hydrophytes and xerophytes **Fig. 12.52–12.59**.

For consideration

(a) What is the function of the midrib and veins in the leaf?
(b) Why is the upper surface darker and shinier than the lower surface in most leaves?
(c) What would be the difference in the structure of leaves growing in differing habitat?
(d) How does the internal structure of the monocotyledonous leaf differ from that of the dicotyledon leaf? Explain the differences.
(e) Construct a three-dimensional diagram of the dicotyledonous leaf. Include the vascular bundle and strengthening tissues as well as the photosynthetic tissue.
(f) How is the structure of the mesophyll tissue adapted for its function of photosynthesis?

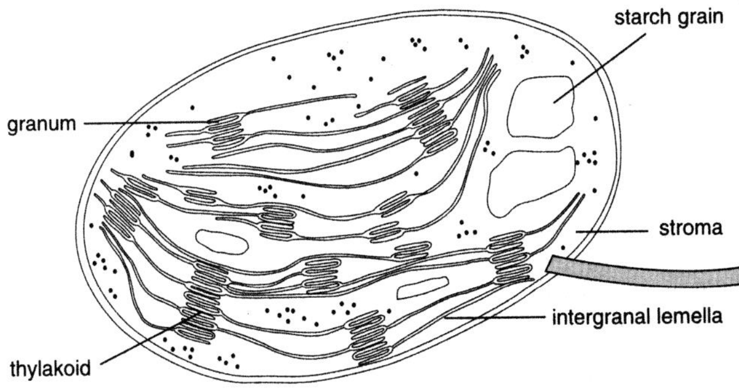

Fig. 12.47 Drawing from Electron Micrograph of a Chloroplast

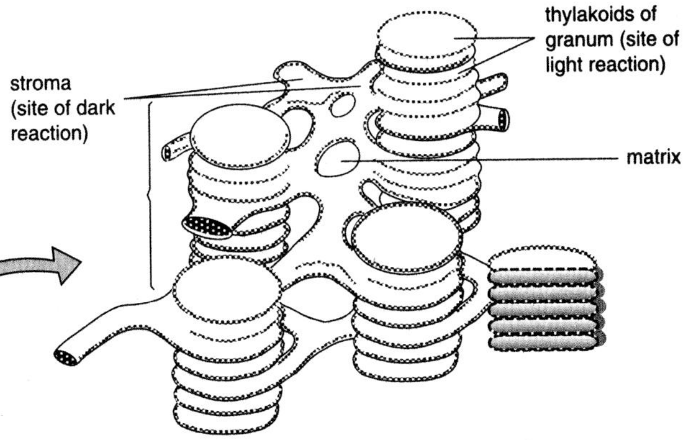

Thylakoids of Grana and Stroma

(g) How does the structure of the leaf permit gases exchange to take place readily between the outside air and the photosynthetic cells?
(h) To what extent do the stomata resemble the generalised diagram in **Fig. 12.49**.
(i) The stomata are distributed mainly in the lower surface, why?
(j) Guard cells are the only cells in the lower epidermis with chloroplast, what is the functional significance of this?
(k) If no starch is present in the vascular tissue what is the explanation?
(l) Make sure you know the structure and function of all the **bold words** in this investivation.

Reference: UCLES, Question 2, 4th Nov. 1998.

Practical 52 – INTERNAL STRUCTURE OF THE LEAF

In the previous investigation a traditional method to study the internal structure of a leaf was described. Another simple method is described below.

Caution: ***Super glue (Elfi) is a very strong adhesive, which will stick anything, including your skin. Use gloves and be very careful with it.***

Procedure

1. From a **young** (*Ficus religiosa*) peepul or dahlia leaf blade (lamina) cut two squares approximately 10 x 10mm, avoiding the midrib and the main veins.
2. Label two clean glass sides **U** (upper), and **L** (lower).
3. Stick the squares of leaf blades on the glass slides using a drop of 'super glue' (Elfi), different surfaces uppermost on the appropriate slide **Fig. 12.48.** Alternatively, wide Scotch tape or a transparent adhesive covering used to cover books with a 'peel' off backing can be used.
4. Peel off the squares, and examine the glue surface for the impression left by the leaf cells, under the microscope.
5. Count the number of stomatal impressions visible under low power, in one field of view for both slides.
6. Repeat the procedure for the upper and lower epidermis of other leaves; use leaves from plants that have leaves all year round e.g. *Ficus religiosa* (Peepul) and from plants that produce leaves in summer only e.g. Mulberry (*Moracae nigra*) shehtoot; as well as monocotyledonous leaves such as lily and grasses.

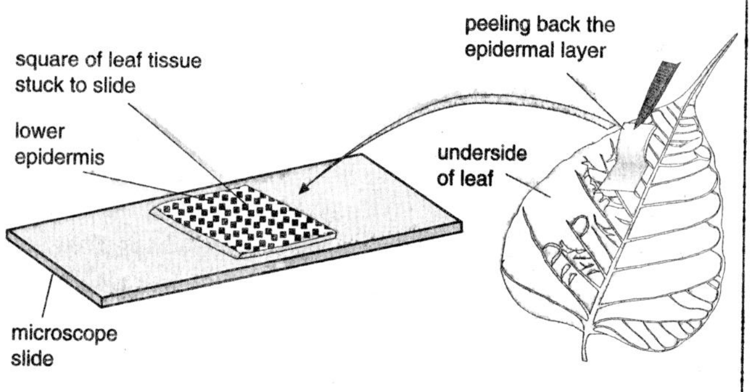

Fig. 12.48 Examination of Leaf Tissue

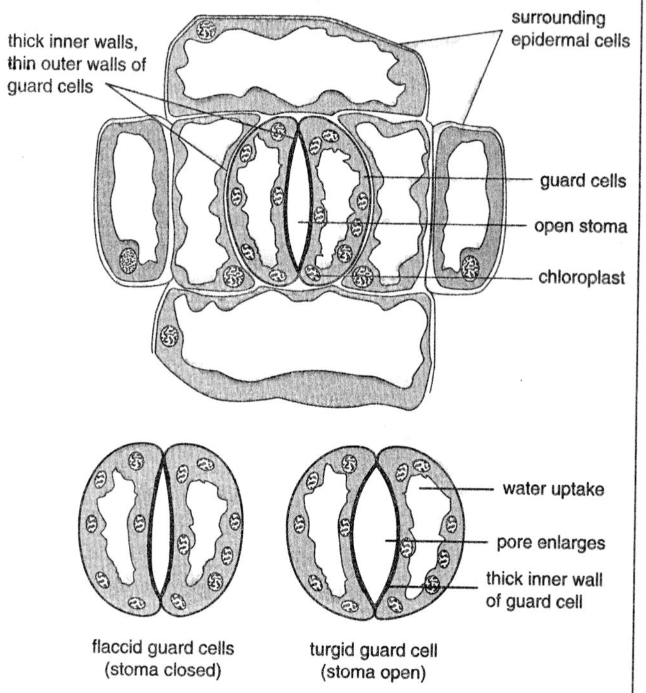

Fig. 12.49 Lower epidermis of a Leaf Showing a Stoma

Examination of the leaf mesophyll cells

8. Stick another leaf lamina on a glass slide, with the upper epidermis facing the slide, cut at an angle with a sharp blade so as to expose as much of the internal structure of the leaf as possible.
9. Examine the internal structure under high power without a coverslip.

Examination of the lower epidermis of the leaf

10. Peel off the lower epidermis either with a pointed scalpel or by tearing the edge of the leaf and then pulling the torn edge at an angle in the opposite direction.
11. Transfer the transparent epidermal layer into a drop of water on a microscope slide, making sure to keep it flat.
12. Remove the water with some filter paper.
13. Add a drop of toludine blue stain. Remove the stain with the filter paper, and mount in water.

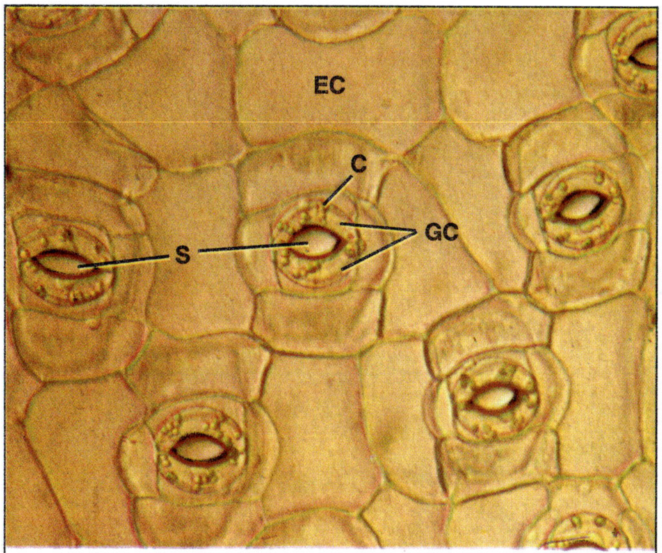

Fig. 12.50 Lower Epidermis of Leaf, showing epidermal cells **EC**, guard cells **GC**, and stomata **S**; note the presence of chloroplasts **C** in the guard cells.

14. Observe and draw some guard cells and surrounding subsidiary cells under high power.
15. Compare stomatal distribution in two different leaves.
16. Compare your preparation with prepared slides and with **Figs. 12.49, 12.50.**

For consideration

(a) Relate the difference in stomatal distribution in the two leaves you have studied to the function of the leaves.

(b) Relate the leaf structure you observed to the function of photosynthesis.

(c) Did you manage to observe all the structures in the textbook diagrams? If not explain why?

(d) What advantages are there in looking at the arrangement of cells in a fresh, living tissue than in a dehydrated, stained and mounted section?

Reference: UCLES, Question 2, 4th Nov. 1998.

Practical 53 – DISTRIBUTION OF WATER IN THE BROAD BEAN PLANT

Water, the most abundant constituent of organisms is a fundamental requirement for life because it is the medium for all chemical reactions. Water lost through transpiration is continually replaced by uptake from the vascular bundles of the stem. Water is brought to the leaf (from where most water loss occurs about 90%) by the xylem of the vascular bundles, which spreads to form a fine branching network throughout the leaf. The branches end in one or a few of the tracheids, from where the water can escape through their cellulose walls to mesophyll cells that they supply. It then travels through the apoplast (through cell walls), the symplast (cytoplasm and plasmodesmata), and from vacuole to vacuole. The quantity of water loss through transpiration is very large. A herbaceous plant such as sunflower or cotton can loose between 1-2 dm^3 of water per day, and a large oak tree can lose as much as 600 dm^3 of water per day. In this investigation you will observe the network of the vascular bundles in the stem, petiole and the leaves of a broad bean plant *Vicia feba.*

Procedure

1. Fill a large beaker with water and two test tubes almost to the brim with the stain provided (0.1% aqueous rose Bengal).
2. Select two healthy shoots from a broad bean plant, cut them at root level and immediately immerse them in a beaker of water.
3. Obliquely cut the ends of each shoot in turn, under water, to within 5cm of the lowest petiole and immediately transfer it to the test tube of stain. Make sure the whole shoot is fully immersed in stain.
4. Leave the shoots in the stain, for about 30 minutes, well ventilated and illuminated near the window.
5. Cut transverse sections from the bottom end of the shoot and examine a section under low and high power of the microscope. Make labelled drawings of your observations.
6. Repeat steps 4 and 5 with the leaf petiole and the midrib.
7. Use a blunt razor and gently scrape the surface on one of the angles of the stem just below a fully expanded leaf, until you can see the stained vascular bundle.
8. Continue to scrape and dissect out the stained xylem as far as possible into the stem, petiole and the leaf. Try and follow the path of the xylem from the bottom end of the stem right into the leaf. Make annotated drawings of your findings.
9. Cut thin sections of the stem and observe under the microscope.

For consideration

(a) Explain with reference to the internal structure of the plant stem why the water movement is restricted to the vascular bundles.

(b) Speculate on the factors which determine the formation and arrangement of vascular bundles during the plants' development.

(c) How does water reach individual cells from the xylem vessels?

Variation in Leaves

Photosynthesis is the process by which plants manufacture food using energy from sunlight and simple raw material such as water and carbon dioxide. The most important single factor controlling the rate of photosynthesis is light and plants exhibit a wide variety of adaptations for acquiring maximum illumination. Other limiting factors are carbon dioxide, and suitable temperature. Water availability and chlorophyll concentration are not normally limiting factors in photosynthesis. Plants have adapted to the most adverse conditions by altering their external and internal structure to conform to their environment.

Mesophytes

These are plants, which normally grow in temperate climate with no storage of water. Most angiosperms around you are regarded as typical plants for this comparison. The general leaf structure of mesophytes is described on **pages 136–141**, and **Fig. 12.52**.

Hydrophytes

These are aquatic plants and have adaptation for buoyancy and oxygen storage e.g. Water lily (*Nymphaea*) kanwal and *Victoria amazonica*. They have very little mechanical tissue, as the surrounding water supports them **Fig. 12.51**.

Hydrophyte leaf adaptations

1. Stomata on upper epidermis allows gas exchange (lower surface is submerged); hardly any epidermis.
2. Very large air spaces **Figs. 12.53, 12.54** in the mesophyll for buoyancy and for storage of oxygen, as less is available in the water.
3. Veins contain few xylem, as water can be obtained directly through the leaf surface.
4. Star shaped sclereides (modifies sclerenchyma cells) in the mesophyll tissues provide some mechanical support although most come from the water.
5. There are numerous small veins in the midrib sections as the leaf is thick.

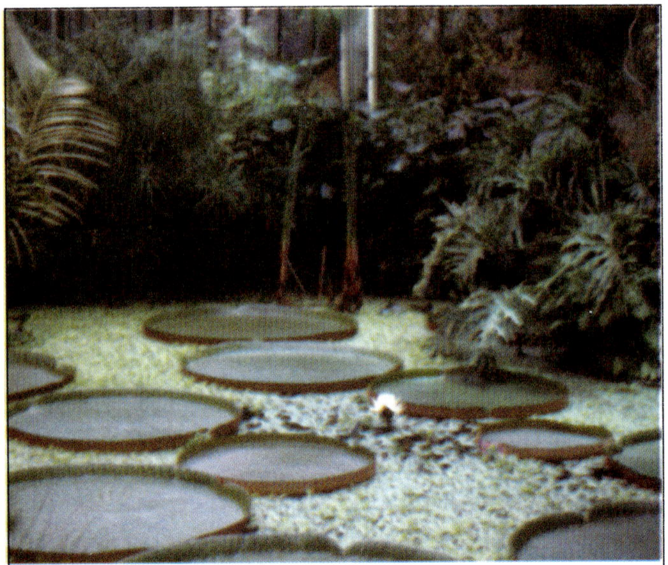

Fig. 12.51 *Victoria amazonica*

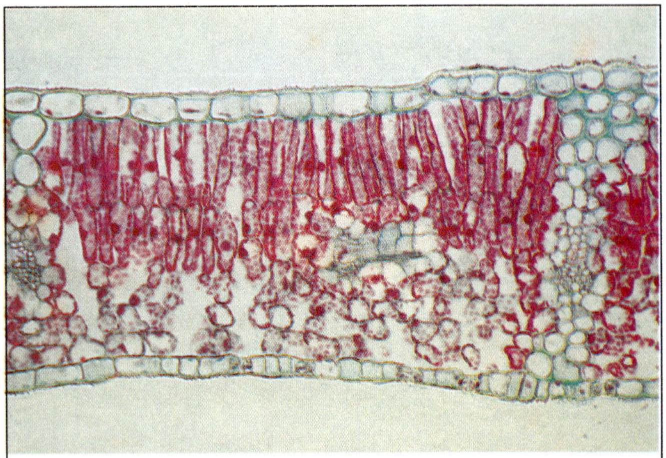

Fig. 12.52 Internal Structure of a Mesophyte TS

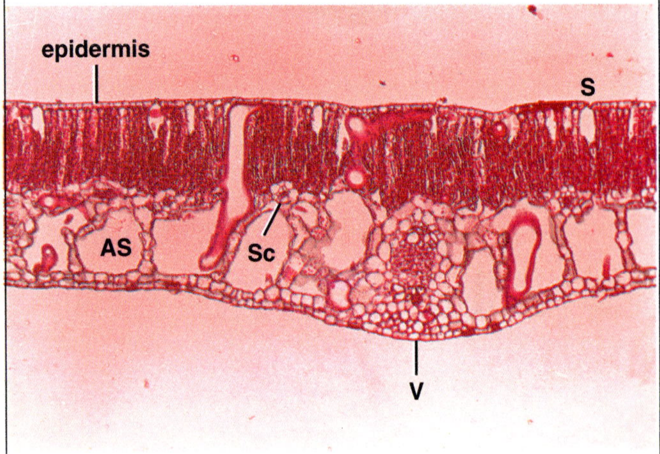

Fig. 12.53 Internal Structure of a Hydrophyte TS. Note the stoma (**S**) in thin upper epidermis, large air spaces **AS**, and star shaped sclereids **Sc**.

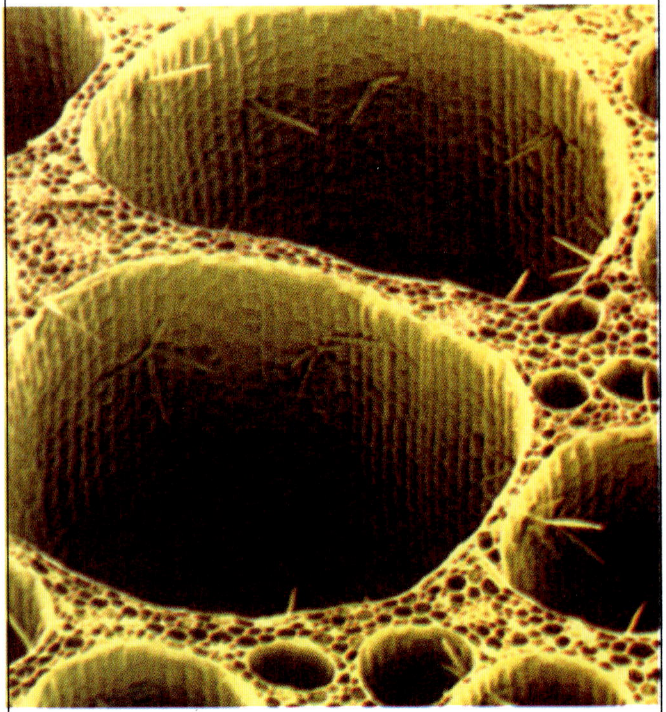

Fig. 12.54 SEM of Air Spaces in Hydrophyte Stem.

Xerophytes

These are plants, living where water is scarce such as deserts or where water may be frozen. They have adapted to conserve water by reducing transpiration. Succulents have ideal leaf form for dry regions as the thick small leaves allows maximum water storage capacity with reduced surface area. The cactus such as the prickly pear *(Opuntia)* naag phun and torch cactus have these characteristics where the leaves are reduced to spines and the function of photosynthesis is taken over by the stem **Fig. 12.55**.

Xerophyte leaf adaptation

1. Thick waxy cuticle on both upper and lower epidermis to reduce transpiration.
2. Two layers of palisade mesophyll.
3. Thickened epidermal layer to provide barrier to water loss.
4. Layers of hair on epidermis to reduce cuticular transpiration.
5. Main vein is deep within the midrib to reduce loss of water from vascular tissue.

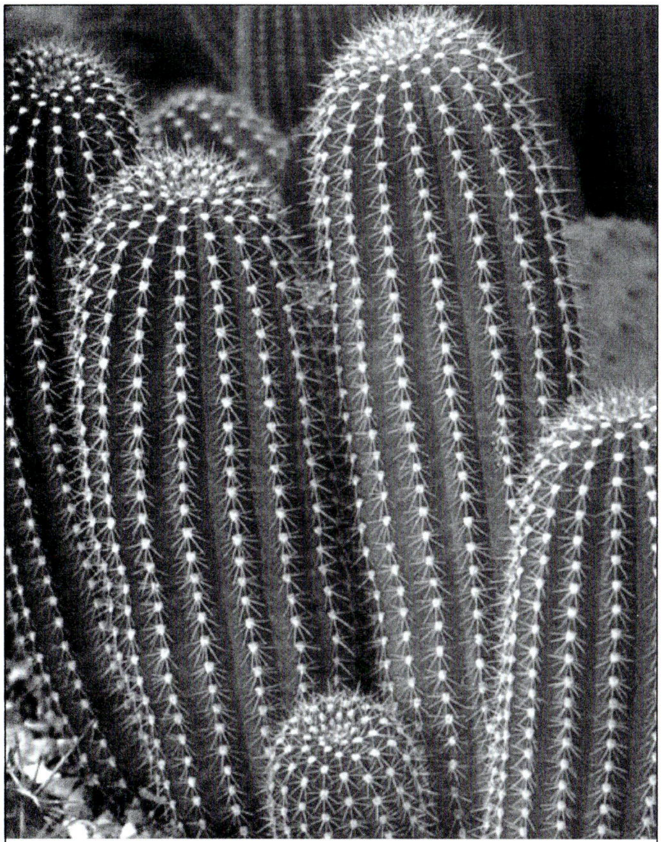

Fig. 12.55 Torch Cactus (*Trichocereus Spachianus*).
The leaves are reduced to spines.

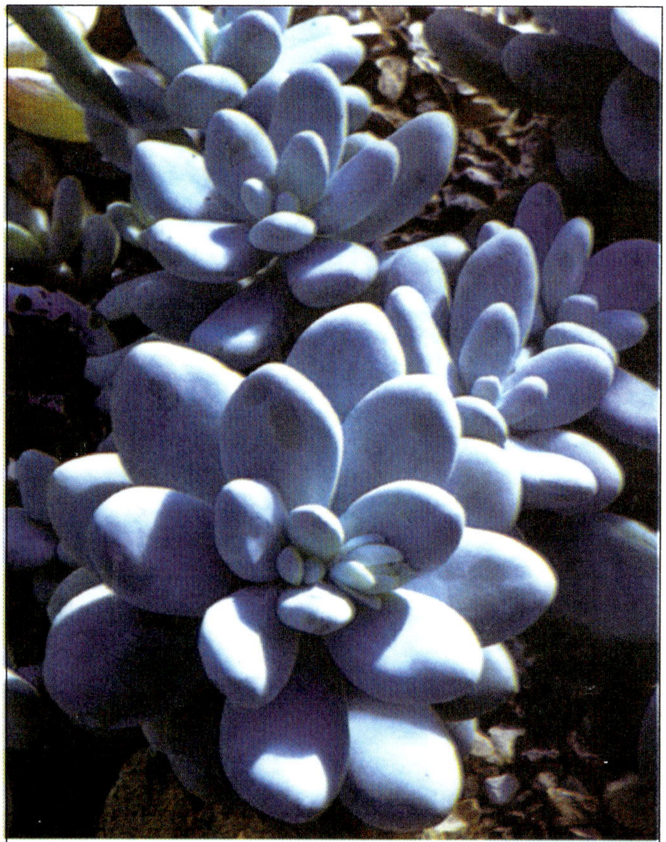

Fig. 12.56 Moonstones – Sugar Almond Plum (*Pachphytun*).
Thick small leaves which reduce evaporation and store water.

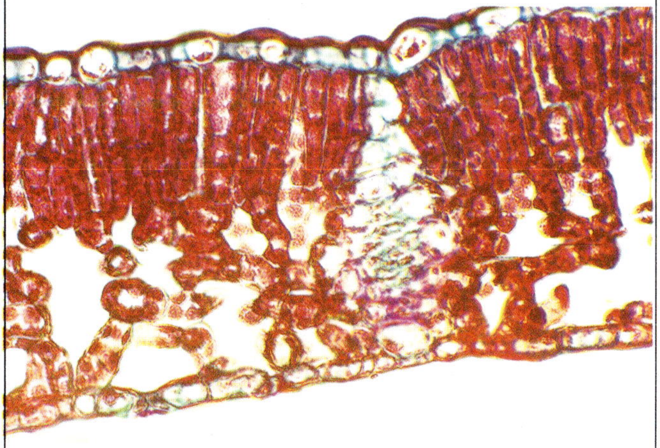

Fig. 12.57 Sun leaf.
Thick layer of palisade mesophyll often 2-3 layers deep.

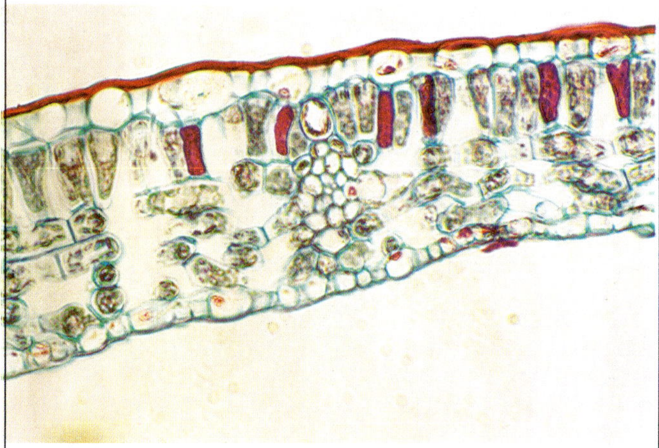

Fig. 12.58 Shade leaf.
Single layer of palisade mesophyll.

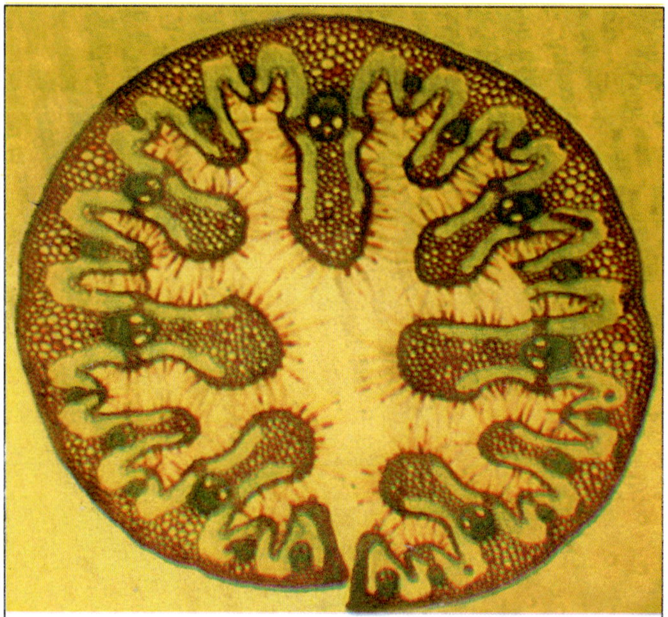

Fig. 12.59 TS of Marram Grass Leaf.

6. Stomata are often in sunken chambers with hairs to trap moist air (less likely to be moved away from the leaf surface by air current).
7. Leaves are rolled up to reduce surface area over which water can be lost **Fig. 12.59**. At times leaves are reduced to spines, or are absent altogether.
8. Survive periods of drought by storage of water in leaves or stem (succulents).
9. Also in CAM (crassulacean acid metabolism) stomata close during the day and open at night, but photosynthesis proceeds unhindered.
10. Leaves are massed into rosettes at ground level.

Reference: UCLES, Question 3, 3rd Nov. 1997.

Practical 54 – DISTRIBUTION OF STOMATA IN A LEAF

In general the greater the number of stomata the greater the transpiration rate. However, the distribution and location of stomata is also very important. For example, dicotyledonous leaves are held horizontally and there are more stomata in the lower epidermis than in the upper epidermis. In monocotyledons, the stomata are distributed evenly in both the upper and the lower surfaces of the leaves and the leaves are held vertically. The number of stomata is very low in leaves of plants growing in dry conditions and some plants have modified their structure to suit the environment e.g. deeply embedded stomata in marram grass (*Ammophil*), stomata on the upper epidermis in hydrophytes.

A very simple method of observing the stomata is to peel off the upper and the lower epidermis and examine under the microscope. This is not always possible with certain leaves, in which case a replica of the epidermis can be made by coating the epidermis with a layer of clear nail varnish, allowing it to dry and then carefully peeling off the layer for microscopic examination.

Procedure

1. Select a variety of leaves such as monocotyledonous, dicotyledonous, shade plants, light plants etc. Also select leaves from the top of a plant and leaves deeply embedded at the bottom of the same plant, leaves from plants that loose their leaves in winter, and those that do not, and from succulents (xerophytes) and hydrophytes.
2. Apply clear nail varnish on the lower surface of the leaf, allow to dry and repeat two or three times. When dry peel off the replica with a pair of fine forceps and place it on a microscope slide under a drop of water. Add a coverslip.
3. Count and record the number of stomata in the field of view and repeat this several times in different areas of the leaf.
4. Measure the field of view of the microscope using a stage micrometer slide or a transparent ruler and using the formula πr^2, where r = radius and $\pi = 3.142$, estimate the number of stomata per square centimetre.

For consideration

(a) Relate the stomatal distribution of different leaves in relation to their habitat and species.

Practical 55 – WATER LOSS FROM LEAVES OF A PLANT

The rate of transpiration from the leaves of a plant depends on characteristics of the leaves and its habitat. In general, the greater the number of stomata the greater the transpiration rate.

In this investigation, you will observe the correlation between the mass of water lost from the leaves of a plant and the stomatal frequency and distribution. Evergreen deciduous plants such as Eucalyptus (*Myrtaceae*), Silver Oak (*Grevillia robusta*) are recommended.

Water loss can be determined, by weighing a bunch of leaves with an electrical top-pan balance. Alternatively, to weigh a single leaf a sensitive microbalance can be used.

Estimation of Water Loss by Weighing (work in pairs)

1. Pick leaves from two different species of evergreen shrubs with their stalks (petioles) attached. Estimate the stomatal distribution of each species as instructed in **practical 54**.
2. Tie about 10g of the leaves from each of the two species with their petioles on a piece of thread at about 5cm intervals along the thread.
3. Record the exact weight as accurately as possible for each species.
4. Suspend the strings between two stands like a washing line **Fig. 12.60**. Note the time.
5. Repeat this procedure with a similar bundle of leaves of the same species. On this occasion suspend the bundle on a 'washing line' under a fan.
6. Create four more bundles of leaves, two from each species. Smear Vaseline or silicone grease thinly on the upper surfaces of the two groups of leaves and on the lower surfaces of the other two. Place a tissue paper on the balance first to avoid getting Vaseline on it. Weigh each group separately, and hang them up to dry. (Deduct the weight of the tissue paper from the weight of the leaves.)
7. If you have enough time and leaves, subject several bundles to each treatment. The results can then be analysed statistically to see if the water loss differs significantly between contrasting treatments.
8. If a microbalance is available, these procedures can be carried out using single leaves. Trace the outline of the leaf on graph paper before the initial weighing and estimate the surface area. Water loss can then be related to the unit area of the leaf.
9. Re-weigh each bundle of leaves (or if a microbalance is used, re-weigh each individual leaf) at least three times, at intervals of about 10 minutes. Record and analyse your results.

Estimation of Water Loss with Cobalt Paper

1. Whilst the leaves are drying, apply a strip of anhydrous cobalt chloride or cobalt thiocyanate paper to the upper and lower surfaces of a leaf of each species on an intact leafy shoot **Fig. 12.61**. Hold the paper in place with two glass slides held firmly together with elastic bands or paper clips. Note the time.
2. Anhydrous cobalt paper is blue, but in the hydrated state it turns pink. When the leaf surface loses water, the paper will change colour from blue to pink. Note the time taken for the paper to turn pink.
3. Tabulate your results.

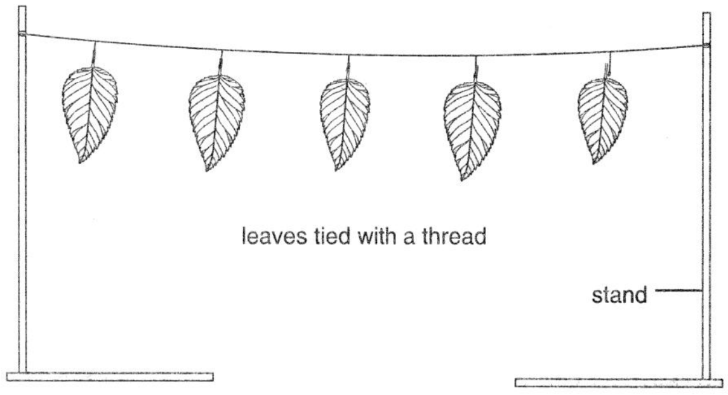

Fig. 12.60 Water loss from Leaves of a Plant

4. Calculate the percentage decrease in mass at each interval, from the formula:

$$\% \text{ decrease in mass} = \frac{a - b}{a} \times 100$$

where
a = initial mass and
b = new mass

5. Estimate the time taken for the cobalt paper to change colour on the upper and lower surfaces of the leaves.

Comparison of these plants can also be made with xerophytes such as Yucca (*Sansevieria trifasciata*) Mother-in law's tongue, Spurge or Milkweed (*Euphorbia*).

(For very large leaves such as Yucca or mother-in-law's tongue, cut the leaves in one inch pieces, pierce a hole in it and pass a thread through the hole to hang on the line.)

For consideration

(a) Why does the water loss from the upper surface of the leaves differ from that of the lower surface? Explain in relation to the structural features of the leaves.

(b) What other structural features of the plant might affect the rate of transpiration?

(c) What effect did the altered conditions have on the rates of transpiration?

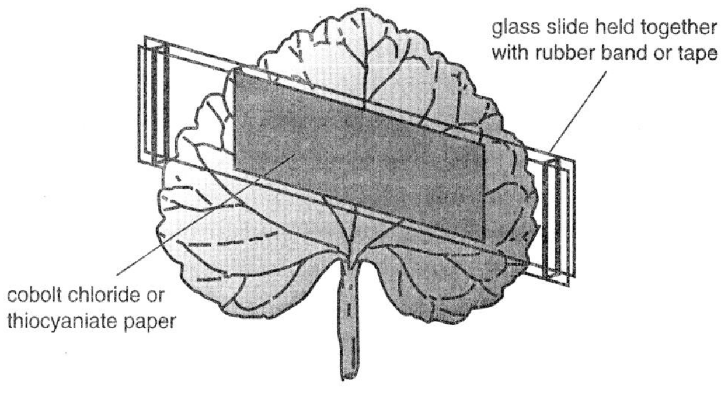

Fig. 12.61 Estimation of Water loss with Cobalt Paper

(d) Explain the rate of water loss in relation to the stomatal distribution of the two species.
(e) Why would the rate of uptake of water not be the same as the rate of transpiration?
(f) How could your results be used to estimate the rate of transpiration of the whole plant from which the shoot was taken?
(g) Why would the rate of transpiration of a cut shoot not reflect the rate of transpiration of a similar shoot which is still intact on the plant in similar conditions?
(h) How could you modify this investigation so that you can measure the rate of transpiration of an intact whole plant under similar conditions?
(i) Was there a difference in time taken for the cobalt paper to change colour on the upper and lower surfaces of the leaf? If so, explain why?

Practical 56 – FACTORS AFFECTING THE RATE OF TRANSPIRATION

Water normally leaves the plant as vapour, from three sites:

i. **Stomata**-by evaporation from cells and stomata found in the lower epidermis of leaves and stem (about 90%).
ii. **Cuticle**–by evaporation from the epidermal cells through the cuticle on the epidermis of leaves and stems (about 10%).
iii. **Lenticels**–evaporation through lenticles (minute amounts >1%), is the main source of water loss in deciduous trees after leaf fall.

All the water that evaporates ends up in the air spaces (sub-stomatal chambers) in the spongy mesophyll of the leaves and escapes through to the atmosphere via the stomata. The rate at which water enters a plant depends on the rate at which it evaporates from the leaves, into the surrounding atmosphere. Various environmental conditions affect the rate of transpiration.

In this investigation you will use a **potometer** to investigate the effect of various external conditions on the rate at which water enters a leafy shoot.

The potometer is designed to measure the rate of water uptake by a cut shoot. It does not measure the rate of transpiration but since most of the water loss is through transpiration the two processes are closely related.

The potometer consists of a length of a graduated capillary tubing, which can be attached to the cut end of the shoot. The capillary tube is filled with water, which is continuous with the water columns in the xylem elements in the shoot. The rate at which water traverses the capillary tube is then measured and the rate of water uptake is calculated.

This is a difficult set up but if you follow the instructions carefully, you will succeed.

Various types of potometers are illustrated in **Fig. 12.62.** In all cases, water uptake is measured by timing the rate at which an air bubble moves along the graduated capillary tube.

Procedure

Setting up the Potometer

1. Select a plant with leafy shoots. Cut a shoot with lots of leaves with an end thick enough to fit firmly in the hole in the rubber stopper in the potometer. Immediately immerse it in water, keeping the cut end under water, cut off about 2-3 cm obliquely. Keep the shoot immersed in the water to minimise the risk of air entering the xylem vessels.
2. Completely fill the potometer with water by immersing it into a large container of water.
3. Keeping the potometer and the shoot under water attach the shoot to the potometer as shown in **Fig. 12.62.**
4. Once the shoot is attached to the apparatus and there are no air bubbles in the capillary tube take the set-up out of the water and set it up in a fixed position, as shown in **Fig. 12.62** keeping the end of the capillary tube in a beaker of water.
5. If you encounter problems and have to start again cut off obliquely a few centimeters again, to ensure that air has not entered the xylem vessels, and that the water column is continuos with the capillary tube.
6. It may be necessary to smear Vaseline or plaster of Paris on the joints in the apparatus to ensure there are no leaks.
7. Expel any air bubbles in the capillary tube by letting in water from the reservoir (type 1) or squeezing the rubber tubing (type 2), and pushing the syringe plunger (type 3).

Using the Potometer

1. Perform a trial run with the plant in normal room conditions. Introduce an air bubble in the capillary tube and again put the end of the capillary tube back in water.
2. Once the plant settles down to a steady rate, record the distance moved by the air bubble in a certain interval of time.
3. Return the bubble to the beginning and repeat the procedure.
4. In the case of type 1 the air bubble can be returned by carefully letting in water from the reservoir; the same air bubble can then be used again. In type 2 it is necessary to expel the air bubble into the beaker by pressing the rubber tubing; a new one may then be introduced. In type 3, the air bubble can be moved to starting position by pushing the syringe plunger.

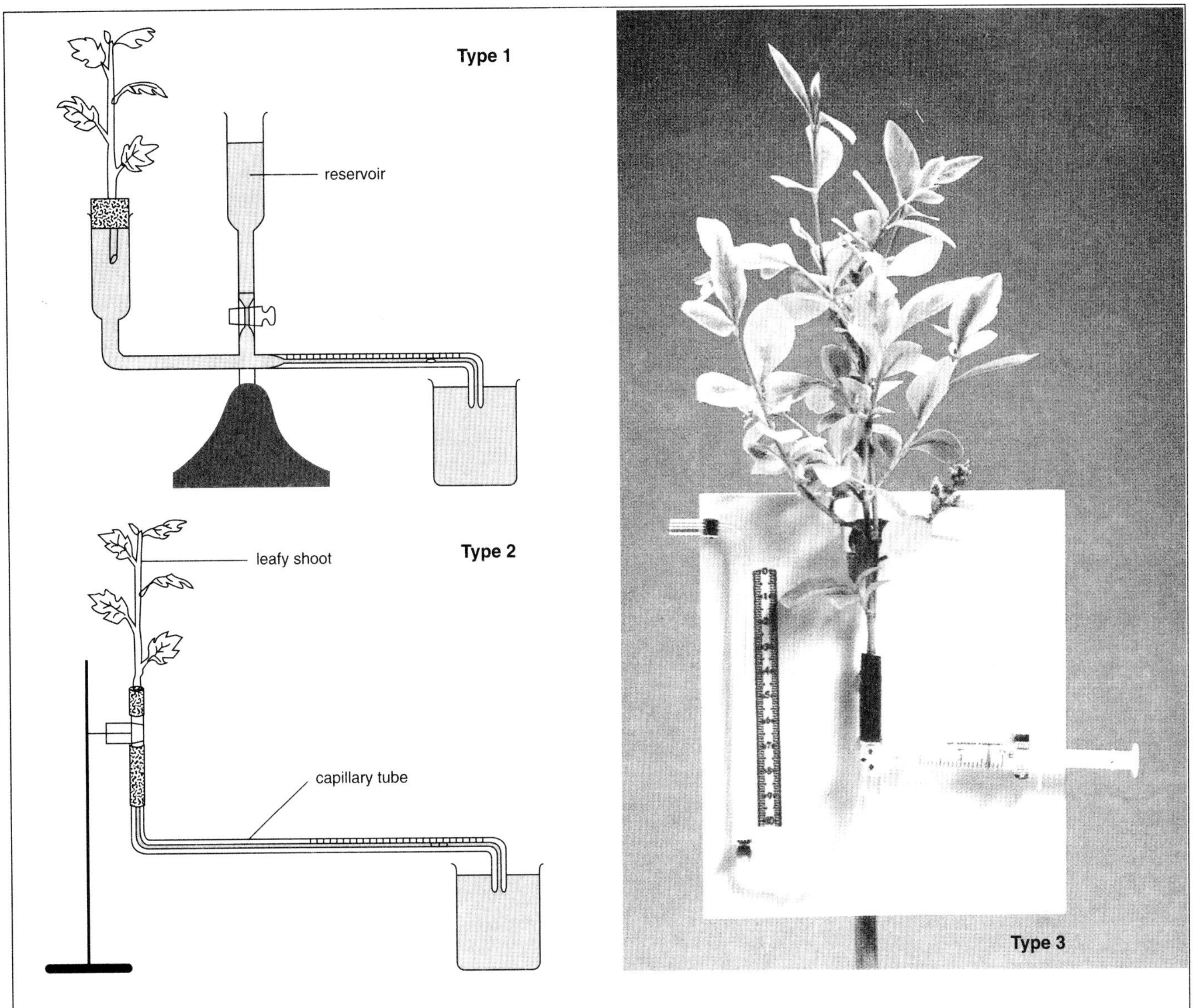

Fig. 12.62 Potometers

In Order to Investigate the Effect on the Rate of Transpiration with Change of Conditions, try the following:

1. Place the plant/potometer set up under an electric fan in a current of air.
2. Cover the plant with a clear plastic bag to create a humid environment.
3. Place the plant close to a heat source such as a lamp or outside in the sun to increase the temperature.
4. Enclose the plant in a black bag to exclude light.
5. Smear Vaseline or silicone grease on the lower and/or upper surface of the leaves to block the stomata.
6. Remove half or all of the leaves from the plant.
7. When you are investigating the effect of **one** condition, try and keep all other conditions constant.
8. Express the rate of water uptake as distance moved by the air bubble per minute (mm min^{-1}).
9. If you know the radius of the capillary tube you can convert these results to volume of water taken up per unit time (e.g. mm^3min^{-1}), volume = $\pi r^2 d$ where d is the distance travelled by the bubble and $\pi = 3.142$.
10. Estimate the total leaf area of your plant. Remove the leaves and lay them flat on graph paper. Draw around each leaf and count the squares. Express the water uptake in volume per unit time per leaf area (e.g. $mm^3\ m^{-2}\ h^{-1}$).

For consideration

(a) Discuss the effect of change of each condition on your results.

(b) Will evaporation alone account for the movement of

water through a plant? What other factors might be involved?

(c) What effect might the absence of roots have on the flow of water through the plant?

(d) When you altered one condition were you able to keep all other conditions constant? If not what effect might the difference in conditions have on your results? How would you overcome them if you were to repeat the experiment?

(e) If you have failed to obtain the desired results explain why and how you could overcome the problems.

13 Tissues, Organs and Systems

Animal Histology

All multicellular organisms are made up of groups of cells of common structure and function, assembled together to form **tissues** e.g. muscle and nervous tissues. The microscopic study of tissue is called **histology**. A group of different tissues together form an **organ** e.g. stomach, heart, liver, kidney etc. In higher animals, organs group together to form an even larger functional unit known as the **system** e.g. respiratory, digestive, nervous etc.
The cells of a tissue may all be of the same type, e.g. cuboidal epithelium in animals. Alternatively, the tissue may contain a mixture of different types of cells, e.g. the connective tissues or the pancreas in animals. Generally the cells of the tissue share a common embryological origin.

Animal tissue are generally divided into four groups:

i. Epithelial
ii. Connective
iii. Muscle
iv. Nervous

Preparation of sections for observation under the microscope is a very skilled and tedious task. The most convenient method of studying this section is to obtain commercially prepared slides and using the information provided here, observe under low and high power of the microscope and make detailed drawings of your observation (**see page 5**). List of suitable slides is on **page 222**.

Epithelial Tissue

The epithelia are a diverse range of tissues, which line all body surfaces, cavities and tubes in a single layer (**simple**) or multilayered (**compound**-more than one cell thick), with a very few exceptions. The epithelia thus function as interface between biological compartments and are involved in a wide range of activities such as protection, secretion, and absorption. Epithelium tissue is not supplied by blood vessels and relies on the lymph system for supply of nutrients and diffusion of oxygen. All epithelial tissue is supported by a basement membrane of varying thickness, which separates the epithelia from the underlying connective tissues.
Epithelia are classified into various types according to the number of cell layers, shape of individual cells, and the presence of surface specialisation features such as cilia and keratin.

Simple epithelia

Surface epithelia, consisting of a single layer of cells, are almost always found on absorptive and secretory surfaces and never on surfaces subjected to stress and abrasion as they provide little mechanical protection.
The cells can range from flat thin, to tall columnar depending on the function and location. They provide little resistance to passive diffusion and are therefore found in alveoli, the lining of blood vessels and renal tubules.
Highly active epithelial cells such as those lining the small intestine are 'tall' to accommodate the large number of organelles. Simple epithelia may exhibit a variety of surface specialisation such as microvilli and cilia, which facilitate their specific surface functions. They can range from **simple squamous**, sometimes called **pavement epithelium** (blood vessels), **simple cuboidal** (collecting ducts in kidney), to **simple columnar** (lining of gall bladder) and **simple columnar cilliated** (lining of oviduct).

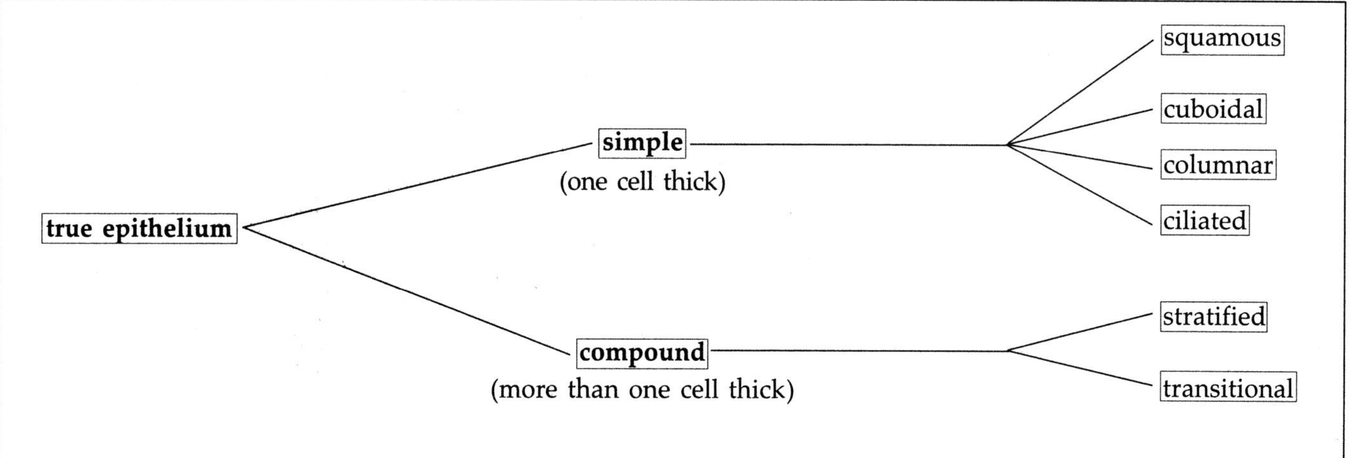

Classification of Epithelia

Simple Epithelia

Cuboidal epithelium

Appearance: least specialised of all epithelia, cells are cube-shaped, possess a prominent central spherical nucleus. Viewed from the surface, appear pentagonal or hexagonal in outline. May have microvilli to increase surface area.

Location: part of gut lining, respiratory tract lining, and many duct lining e.g. salivary, pancreatic and collecting ducts of kidney where they are non-secretary. Also found in secretary glands such as salivary, mucus, thyroid and sweat glands.

Function: secretion, absorption, provides protective yet permeable surface.

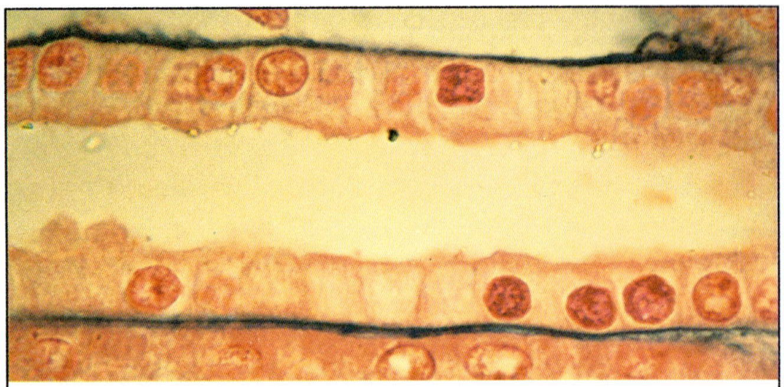

Simple Cuboidal Epithelium in Rat Kidney (VS).
The cells appear square in the VS but in surface view appear polygonal in shape. Boundaries between cells are indistinct but nucleus is prominent. Basement membrane (stained blue).

Columnar epithelium

Appearance: tall narrow cells, with nucleus placed at basal end. May have microvilli at its free surface.

Location: lines the stomach, intestine, where mucus secreted by goblet cells protects the stomach lining from acid and from digestion by enzymes and lubricates passage of food. Lines kidney ducts, thyroid gland and gall bladder

Function: secretion, absorption, allows passage of material.

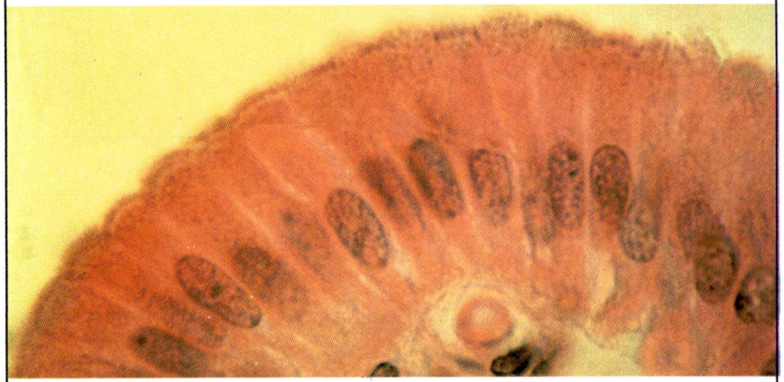

Simple Columnar Epithelium in Gall Bladder (VS).
It is similar to cuboidal epithelium except that the cells are taller. Height of cells varies according to location and function. Nuclei are elongated and located at the base of the cell.

Squamous or pavement epithelium

Appearance: cells are thin and flat, contain little cytoplasm, enclosing a disc shaped centrally placed nucleus which appears to bulge into the vessel. The margins are irregular in surface view.

Location: in Bowman's capsule, alveolar lining of lung and walls of blood vessels where it is known as endothelium, as well as chambers of the heart.

Function: thinness of cells allows ease of diffusion, and friction-free passage of fluids.

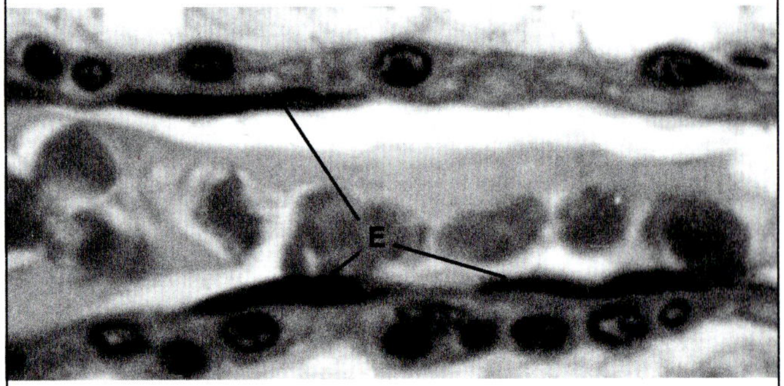

Simple Squamous Epithelium (SSE).
The epithelium lining cells **E**, (called endothelial cells in the circulatory system) are thin and flat with bulging nuclei.

Ciliated epithelium

Appearance: columnar in shape, with numerous cilia at the free surfaces. Always associated with mucus-secreting goblet cells producing fluids in which the cilia set up currents.

Location: lines oviducts, ventricles of the brain, spinal canal and respiratory tract.

Function: moves material from one place to another.

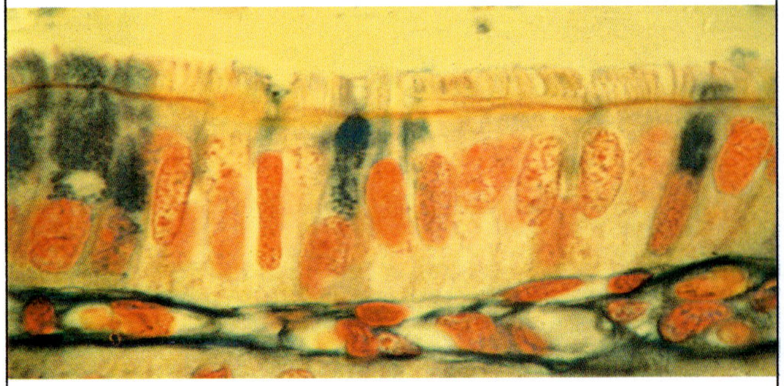

Simple Ciliated Columnar Epithelium in Oviduct (VS).
The cilia propel fluids or minute particles over epithelial surface.

Cubiodal Epithelium

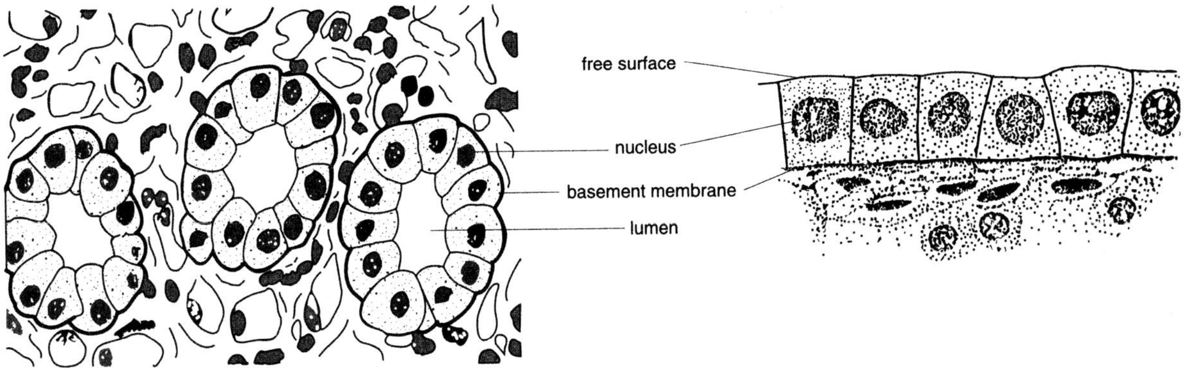

Columnar Epithelium

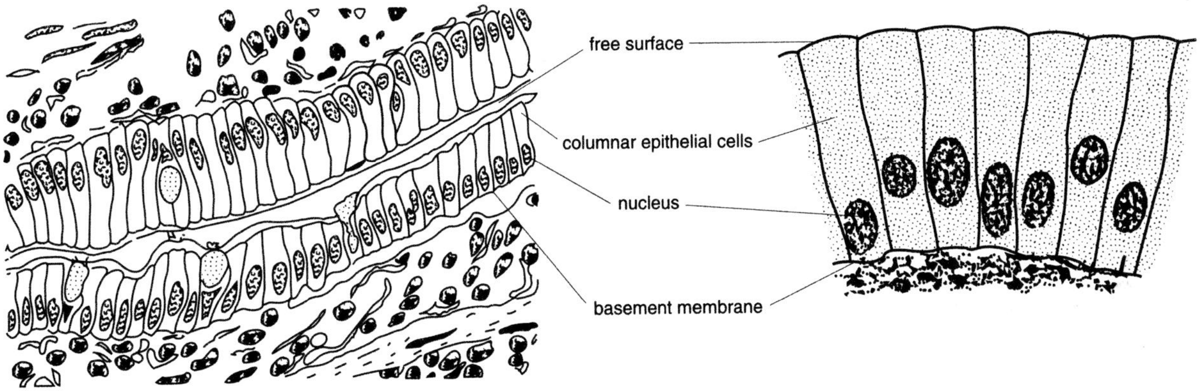

Squamous (or pavement) Epithelium

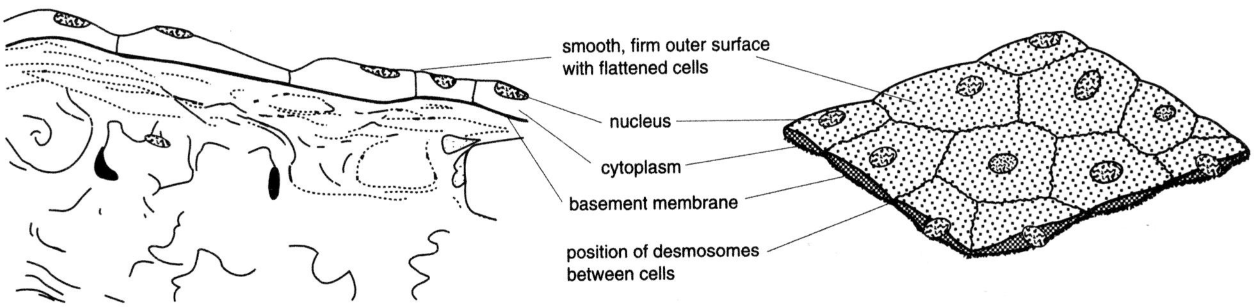

Simple Epithelial Tissue

Compound Epithelia

Stratified epithelia consist of more than one layer of cells. They have a protective function and the degree of stratification depends on location and the kind of physical stresses to which it is exposed. Classification of the stratified epithelium is usually based upon the surface structural layer since cells of the basal layer are generally cuboidal in shape.

Range from stratified squamous (vagina), stratified squamous keratinising (skin), stratified cuboidal (large excretory ducts of exocrine glands such as salivary glands) to transitional epithelium.

Stratified squamous epithelium

Appearance: comprises of a number of layers of cells. The first formed cells are cuboidal, but nearer the free surfaces of tissue are flattened, and are called **squamous**. May be uncornified as in oesophagus.

May become dead, horny layer of **keratin**, which ultimately flakes away. In this condition it is said to be **cornified**.

Location: lining of buccal cavity, vagina, skin, oesophagus, bladder, and mammary glands.

Function: protection against abrasion, invasion by pathogens and water.

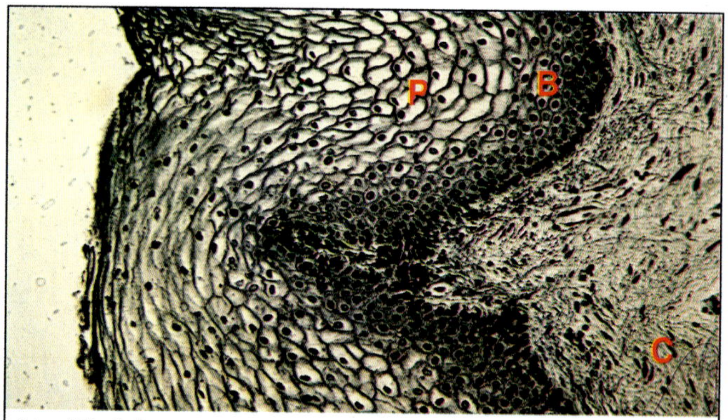

Stratified Squamous Epithelium in Vagina (VS).
Note the highly cellular basal layer **B** and the transformation through the large polygonal cells **P** of intermediate layer to squamous cells. Connective tissue **C** is highly irregular.

Transitional epithelium

Appearance: surface cells are usually large and pale-stained and appear to have scalloped surface outline. Nuclei of surface cells are large and rounded, and may be binucleate. The shape and size of intermediate and basal cells vary depending on degree of distension.

Location: almost inclusively confine to urinary tract in mammal.

Function: withstand great degree of stretch and toxity to urine.

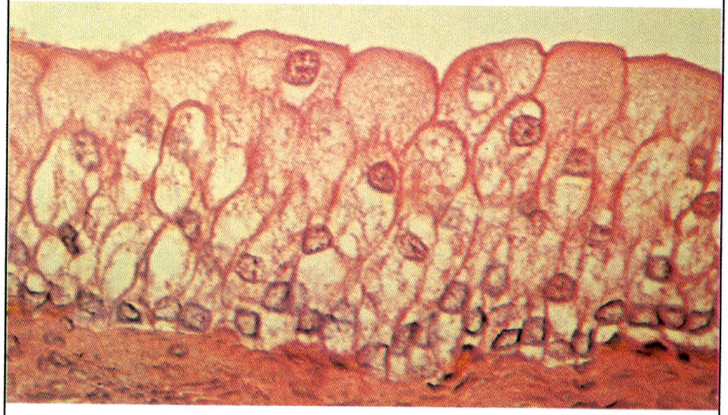

Relaxed Transitional Epithelium (TE) in Bladder (VS).
TE is a form of stratified epithelium almost confined to urinary tract to withstand great deal of stretch and toxity of urine. Is four to five layers deep.

Glandular epithelium

Glandular epithelium is involved in secretion, and is often arranged in structures called glands, which are invagination of the epithelial surfaces. Those glands, which maintain their continuity with the epithelial surface via a duct, are called **exocrine glands** and secrete into the free surface.

In some cases the ducts degenerate during development to leave isolated glands. These glands are referred to as **endocrine glands;** their secretions are passed directly to the bloodstream, and are termed ductless glands.

Appearance: folded epithelium with specialised secretary cells, may be individual glandular cells, such as the goblet cells, or aggregates of glandular cells forming multicellular gland.

Location: pancreas, mammary glands, sebaceous glands, and sweat glands.

Function: secretion, protection.

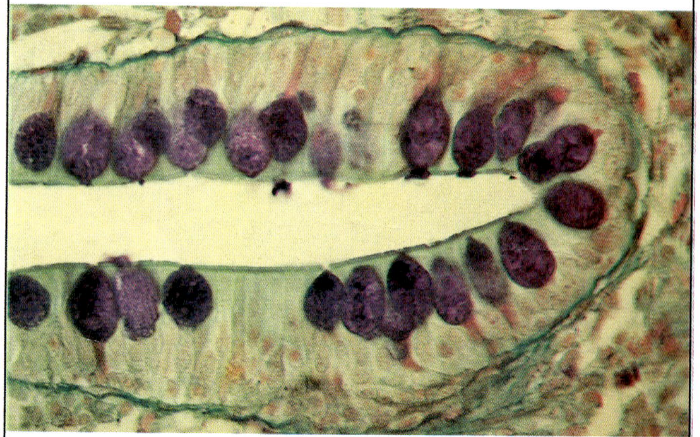

Goblet Cells (GC) Mammal (VS).
GC are modified columnar epithelial cells which secrete mucous. Dense aggregation of mucigen granules are visible in the cytoplasm.

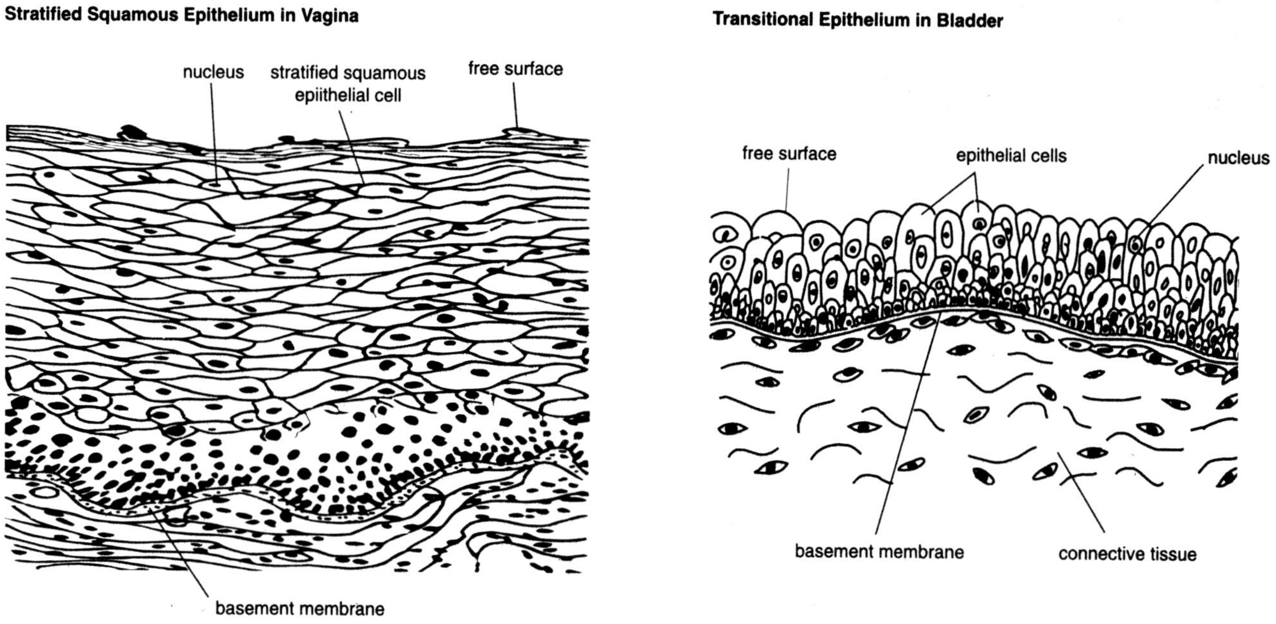

Compound Epithelia

Connective Tissue

The overall function of connective tissue is to bind other tissue types together, which provides structural and metabolic support to tissues and organs. It is the major supporting tissue of the body, which includes skeletal tissue, bone, and cartilage.

Connective tissue carries blood vessels and mediates the exchange of nutrients, metabolites and waste products between tissues and the circulatory system.

It occurs in many different forms with diverse properties. All connective tissues have two major constituents, cells and extra cellular material. Extra cellular material consists of a matrix of organic material, non-cellular component collagen and elastic fibres, but each type of connective tissue has its own characteristics, cells and fibres.

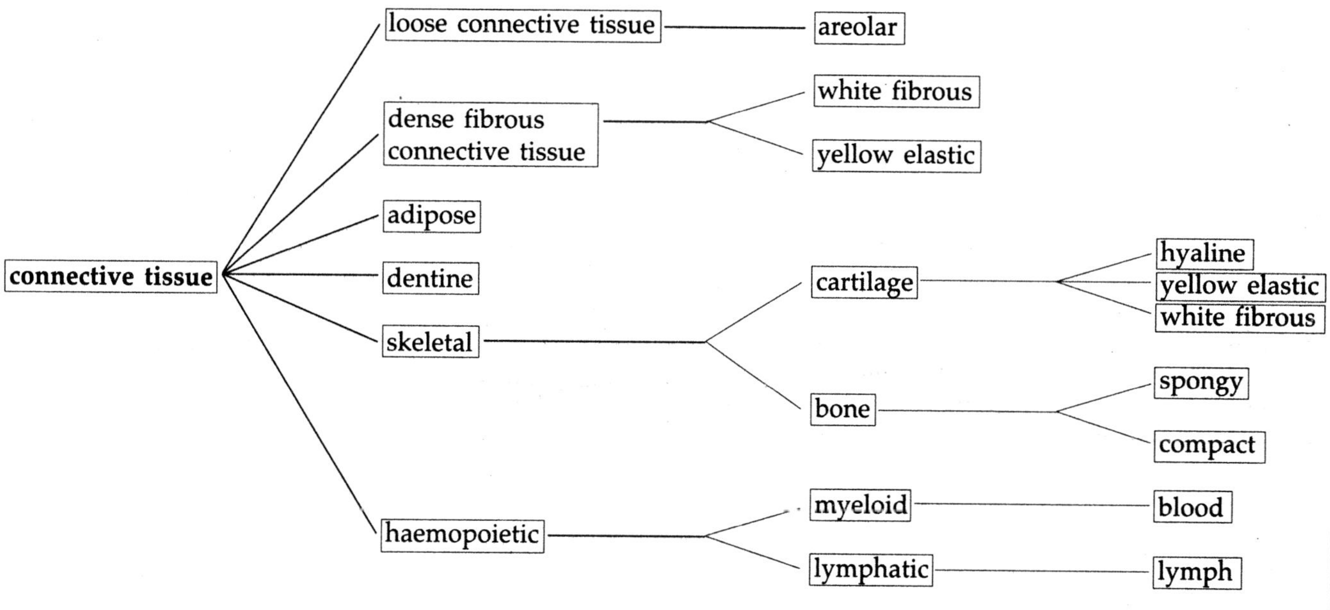

Classification of Connective Tissue

Connective Tissue

Appearance and location: forms sheaths around organs of body, its composite structure is made of a variety of cells, with several types of fibres which are non-living products of cells, and a fluid or semi-fluid intercellular matrix consisting of hyaluronic acid, chondroitin, chondroitin sulphate and keratin sulphate. Cells are wide spread, with extensive vascular network, but this is concerned with supplying other structures such as the epithelium rather than the connective tissue itself.

Function: packing, binding structures together, protection against damage by bacterial invasion (skin), insulation (adipose), and support (cartilage and bone) production of blood (haemopoietic tissue).

Location: around organs of body, blood vessels and nerves, mesenteries, skin etc.

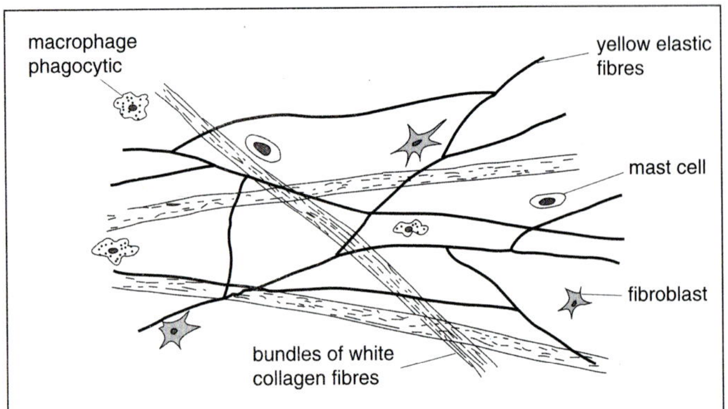

Loose Connective Tissue

Loose connective tissue

This tissue contains cells widely dispersed in intercellular material and has fibres loosely woven in a random manner.

Areolar tissue

Appearance and location: transparent semi-fluid matrix containing mixture of **mucin, hyaluronic acid** and **chondroitin sulphate**. With scattered bundles of wavy **collagen fibres** and straight fibres of **elastin**. Fine thread-like **reticular fibres are also present**. Located around blood vessels and nerves, and forms connective tissue covering around muscle fibres. Interspersed around matrix are variety of different types of cells, such as fibroblasts, macrophages, mast cells, plasma cells, chromatophores, fat and mesenchyma cells.

Fibroblasts, which produce the fibres are flattened, spindle shaped cells containing flattened nucleus. These lie close to the fibres they synthesise and around wounds to seal off injured areas.

Macrophages (histocytes) are amoeboid cells, which engulf foreign particles. Together with lymphatic system they comprise the **reticulo-endothelial system** of the body.

Mast cells are oval, small, containing granular cytoplasm, and are found around blood vessels.

Plasma cells are rare, **chromatophores** present in specialised areas such as skin, eye. The cells are branched and densely packed with melanin granules.

Fat cells, containing large lipid droplets, which fills bulk of the cell. The cytoplasm and nucleus are confined to margins. Areolar tissue is found around all organs of body. It connects skin to structures below and binds sheets of epithelia to form mesenteries. Also forms sheaths around blood vessels and nerves where they enter or leave the organ. Its functions are to mediate exchange of nutrients, metabolites and waste products between tissues and circulatory system and provide support.

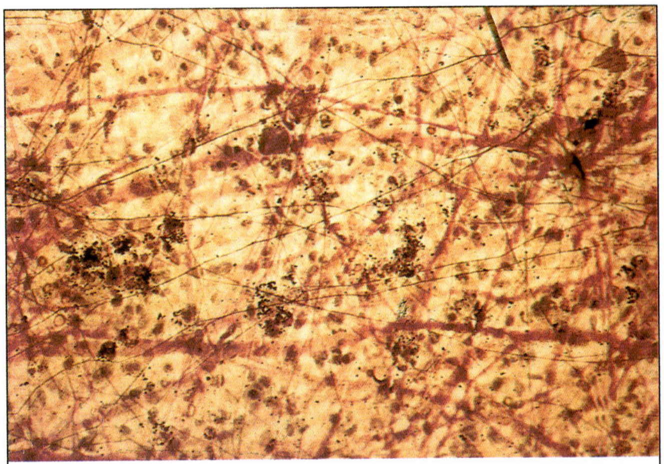

Areolar Tissue (spread rabbit).
The elastin fibres are (stained black) collagen fibres (stained pink) and nuclei (stained blue).

Dense (compact) fibrous connective tissue

Has more fibres in matrix than cells. Fibres may be irregularly arranged or regular.

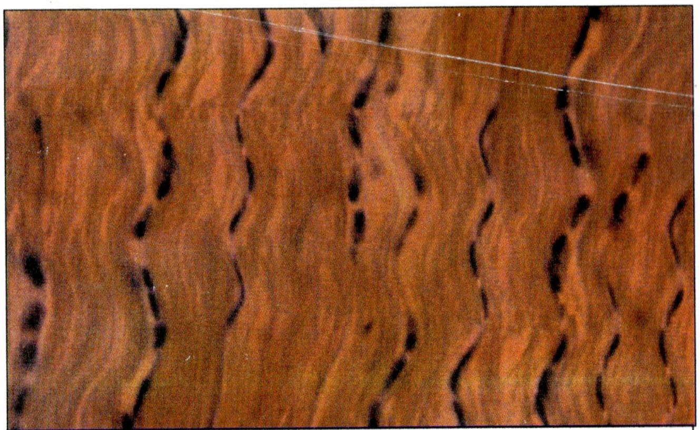

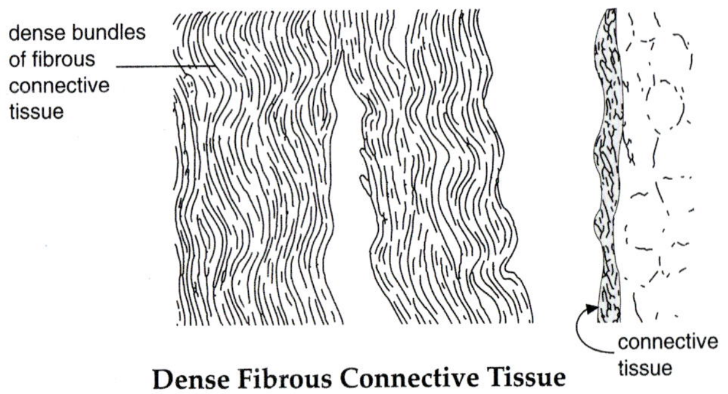

Dense Fibrous Connective Tissue

White fibrous

Appearance: tough shiny tissue, composed of highly organised bundles of collagen fibres, closely packed, lying parallel to each other. Rows of fibroblasts interspersed among the collagen run alongside the bundles. Each bundle is bound to its neighbour by areolar tissue.
Location: in tendons, ligaments, eye-sclerotic and cornea, kidney capsule, bone and cartilage.
Function: tensile strength with flexibility.

Yellow elastic

Appearance: unlike white fibrous tissue, possess loose network of irregularly arranged-branched yellow elastic fibres. Scattered fibroblasts throughout the matrix.
Location: ligaments, walls of arteries, lung and associated air passages, and in the great cords of the neck.
Function: strength with flexibility.

Adipose tissue

Appearance: has no specific matrix, and is areolar tissue containing large number of cells arranged into lobules. Each cell is filled with central fat drop, with cytoplasm and nucleus pushed to periphery.
Location: dermis of skin mesenteries around kidney, heart.
Function: energy reserve, shock absorber and insulation.

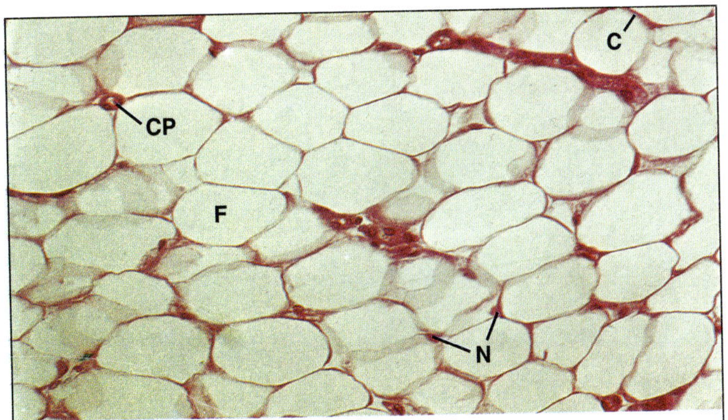

White Adipose Tissue (TS).
The nucleus **N** is compressed and pushed to one side by the stored fat droplet **F**. Cytoplasm **C** is reduced to a thin rim around the periphery. Capillaries **CP** are also visible.

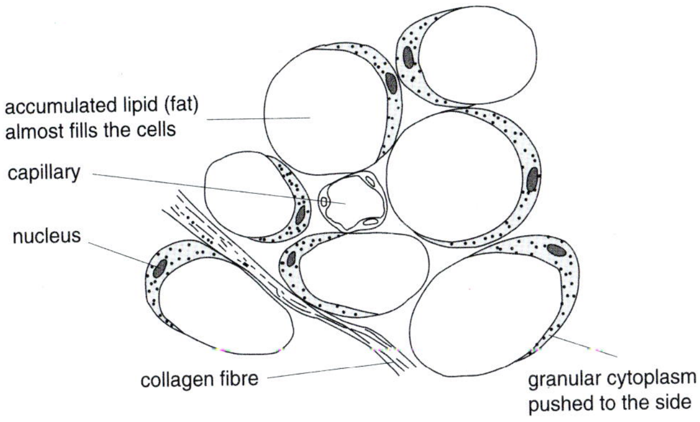

Adipose Tissue

Skeletal Tissues

The skeletal system is composed of a variety of specialised forms of connective tissue. **Bone** provides a rigid framework for most of the soft tissues of the body, whereas **cartilage** provides semi-rigid support in limited sites such as the respiratory tract, nose and the external ear.
The functional difference between the various tissues of the skeletal system relates principally to the difference of the ground substance and fibrous elements of the extra cellular matrix. The cells of all the skeletal tissue, like the cells of the connective tissue in general have close structural and functional relationship. The skeletal tissue is able to provide strength with flexibility and is able to absorb mechanical shocks.
The matrix is deposited by cells called **chondroblasts** and possesses many fine collagen fibrils. Chondroblast becomes enclosed in space called **lacunae,** and are then called **chondrocytes.** Dense layer of cells encloses the margin of cartilage and fibrils called **perichondrium.**

Cartilage

Cartilage is a semi-rigid form of connective tissue, characteristics of which generally stems from the nature of the predominance of ground substance in the extracellular matrix tissue. Within the ground substance are embedded various amounts of **collagen** and **elastic fibres** giving rise to three main types of cartilage: **hyaline cartilage, fibro-cartilage** and **elastic cartilage.**

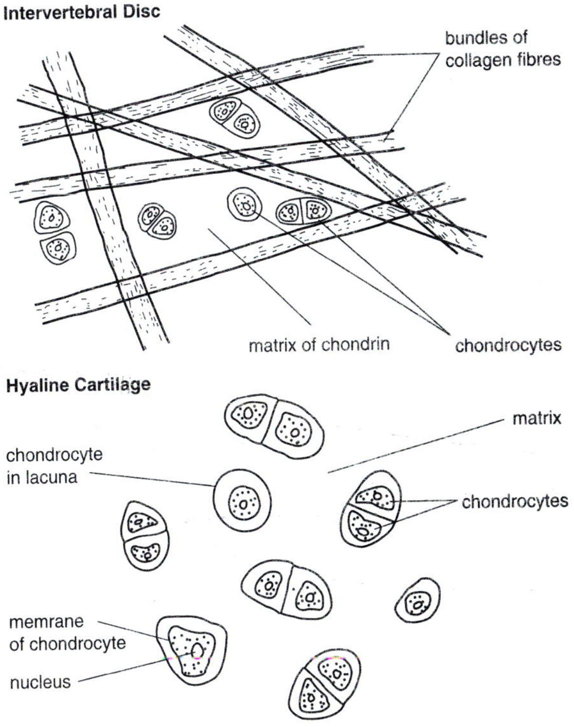

Cartilage

Hyaline cartilage

The matrix is semi transparent consisting of **chondroitin sulphate** and **fine collagen fibrils**. Peripheral chondrocytes are flattened, internally situated and are angular. Each chondrocytes is contained within a lacuna. Each lucuna may enclose from one to eight chondrocytes. No blood vessels are found. All exchange between chondrocytes and lacunae takes place by diffusion.

Function: structural with flexibility.

Location: ends of bones, nose, air passage of respiratory system, ear, and forms embryonic skeleton.

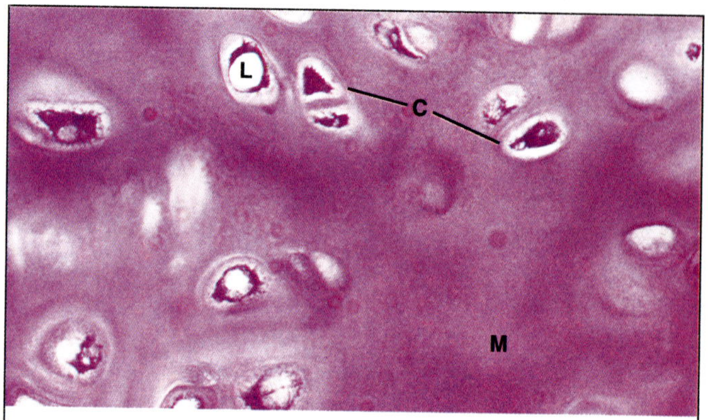

Hyaline Cartilage in Human Trachcea (TS).
Most common type of cartilage found in articular surfaces. Characterised by small aggregation of chondrocytes **C** embeded in amorphous matrix of ground substance **M**. Mature **C** characterised by small nuclei with dispersed chromatin and basophilic granular cytoplasm. Lipid droplets **L** prominent feature of **C**.

Yellow elastic cartilage

It has semi-opaque matrix which contains network of yellow elastic fibres.

Function: considerably more strength and flexibility than hyaline cartilage.

Location: external ears, Eustachian tube, the epiglottis, and cartilage of pharynx.

White fibrous cartilage

It has large numbers of bundles of densely packed white fibrous collagen fibres in the matrix.

Function: provides great tensile strength as well as small degree of flexibility and cushioning

Location: as discs between adjacent vertebrae (intervertebral discs) between pubic bones of pelvis and ligamentous capsules of joints.

Bone

Bone is the most abundant of all animal skeletal tissues, providing support and protection to soft tissues and

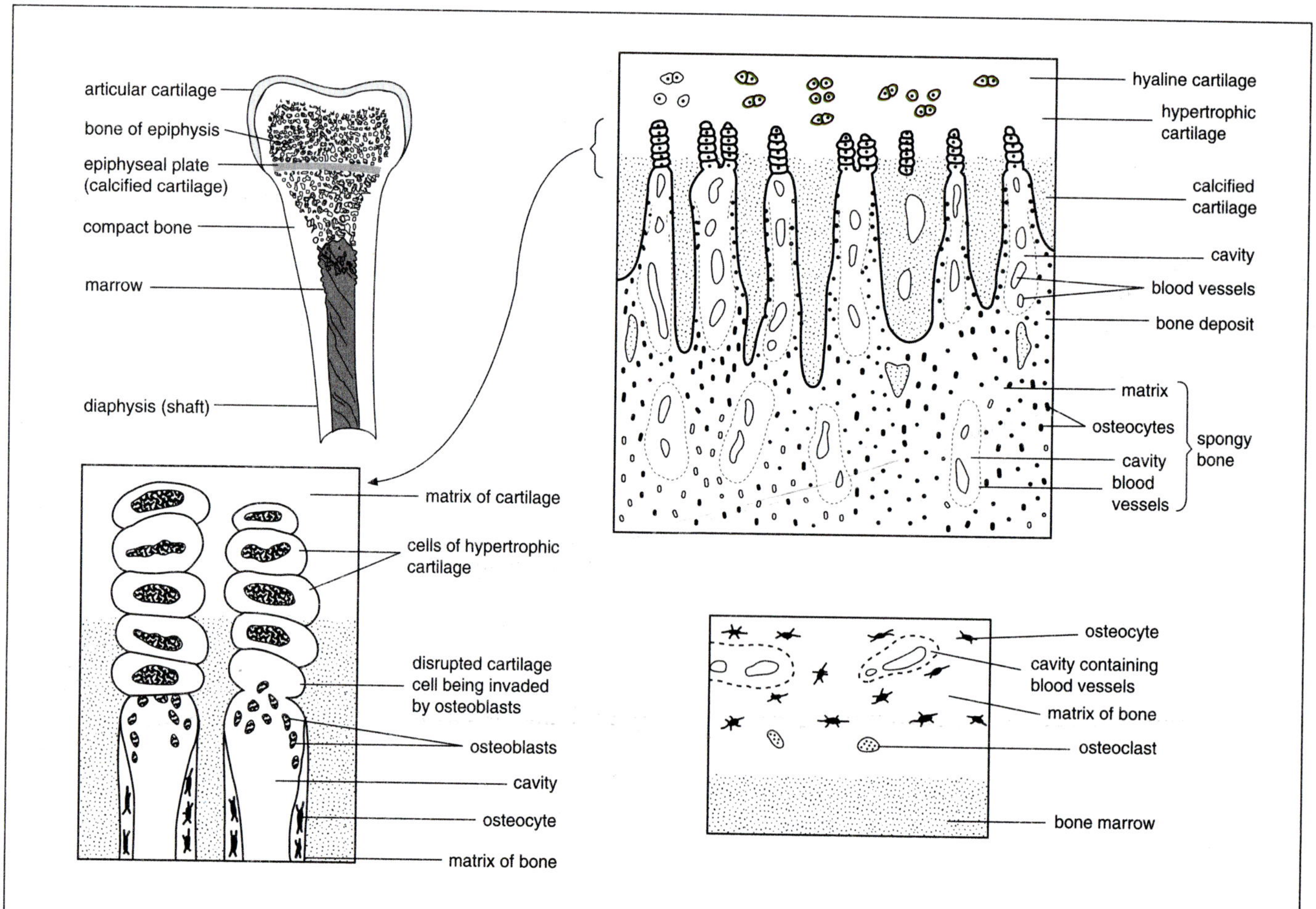

Growth of Long Bone

organs. It is a specialised form of connective tissue in which the extracellular components are mineralised. Thirty per cent of the matrix is composed of organic material, consisting mainly of collagen fibrils, and seventy per cent inorganic bone salts. In addition, bone constitutes a variable store of calcium phosphate (85%), calcium carbonate (10%) and other inorganic ions, and actively participates in the maintenance of calcium homeostasis in the body as a whole. To accommodate changing mechanical stresses and demands of calcium homeostasis, all the bones in the body are in a dynamic state of growth and resorption throughout life. The structure of individual bones provides the maximum resistance to mechanical stress whilst maintaining the least bony mass (approximately 15% of the body mass of adult mammals).

Like other connective tissues, bone is composed of cells and an organic extracellular matrix containing **glycoprotein ground substance** and **collagen fibres**. The cells found in bone are of three types:

(i) **Osteoblasts** are immature bone cells responsible for the synthesis and secretion of the organic components of the extracellular matrix of bone, a substance known as **osteoid**; osteoid rapidly undergoes mineralisation to form bone.

(ii) **Osteocytes** are osteoblasts which become trapped within bone and are then responsible for maintenance of the bone matrix.

(iii) **Osteoclasts** are multinucleate cells that are actively involved in resorptive processes associated with continuos remodelling of bone.

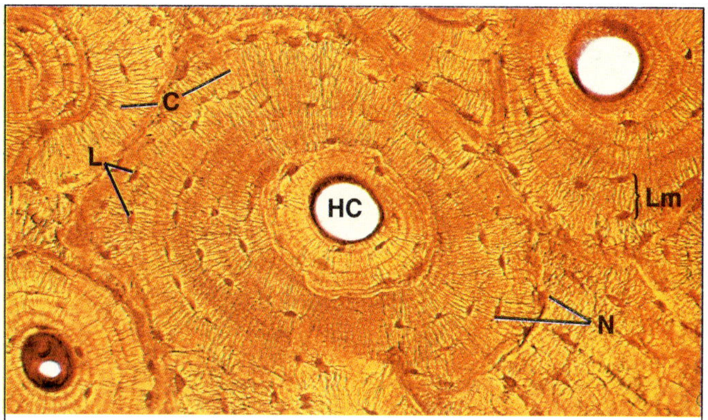

Compact bone (TS).
Compact bone is made up of parallel bony columns. Each column is made up of concentric bony layers or lamellae **Lm** around central canals (Haversian canals) **HC** containing blood vessels lymphatic vessels and nerves. Note the canalaculi **C** and lacuna **L**.

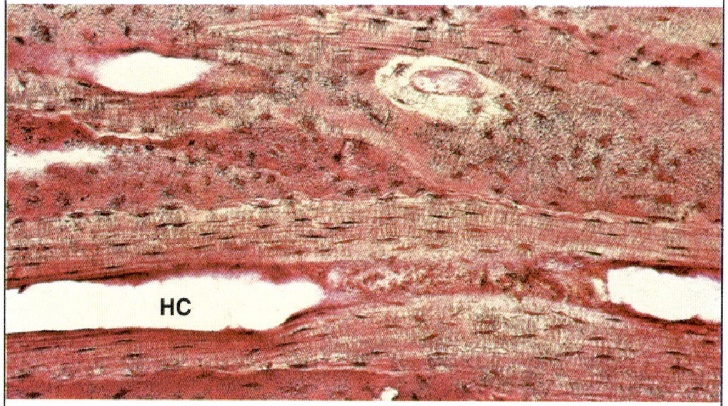

Compact Bone (LS).
Haversian canal **HC**, lacunae appear as elongated spaces arrange in concentric layers around **HC**.

Spongy bone

Spongy bone occurs in embryo, growing organisms, and epiphysis of long bone. It consists of meshwork of interconnecting bony struts called **trabeculae**. The spaces between the trabeculae are filled with soft **marrow tissue**. If the marrow is red as at the ends of femur, cells are predominantly red blood cells, if the marrow is yellow, as in the diaphyses of long bones, the cells are primarily fat cells.

As in the compact bone, three different types of cells are present in the spongy bone, the **osteoblasts** that synthesise spongy bone, **osteocytes** that are resting osteoblasts, and **osteoclasts**, which can resorb calcified matrix. Trabeculae are orientated in the direction in which the bone is stressed.

Compact dense bone

Compact bone consists of numerous cylinders of concentric bony **lamellae** each surrounding central neurovascular channels called the **Haversian canal**. One such cylinder plus its canal is called **Haversian system** or **osteon**. Each cylinder consists of concentric rings of osteocytes and the calcified matrix. An artery and a vein as well as a lymph vessel and nerve fibre run through each Haversian canal and capillary branches pass via **canaliculi** to the osteocytes in spaces called **lacunae Fig. 13 (a)**.

Bone is too tough and brittle to be cut for histological sections. Consequently, it is decalcified in acid solutions prior to sectioning and staining and the blood vessels etc. are therefore not present in such sections.

Transverse Haversian canals communicate with marrow cavity and interconnect with longitudinal Haversian canals. The outer and inner surfaces of the bone lamellae are not in the form of concentric cylinders but are orientated circumferentially over it. The **canal of Volkman** separates these areas. The canals contain blood vessels, which pass through them to link with those in Haversian canals. A dense connective tissue called **Periosteum** covers the bone.

For consideration

(a) How is the structure of the bone suited to bear heavy loads?

(b) Why are pregnant women advised to drink plenty of milk and asked to get their teeth checked after the birth of the baby?

(c) The occurrence of osteoporosis (brittle bone disease) is higher in females than in males. Why do you think this is so?

(d) Compare the structure of the bone, cartilage and tendons in relation to their task.

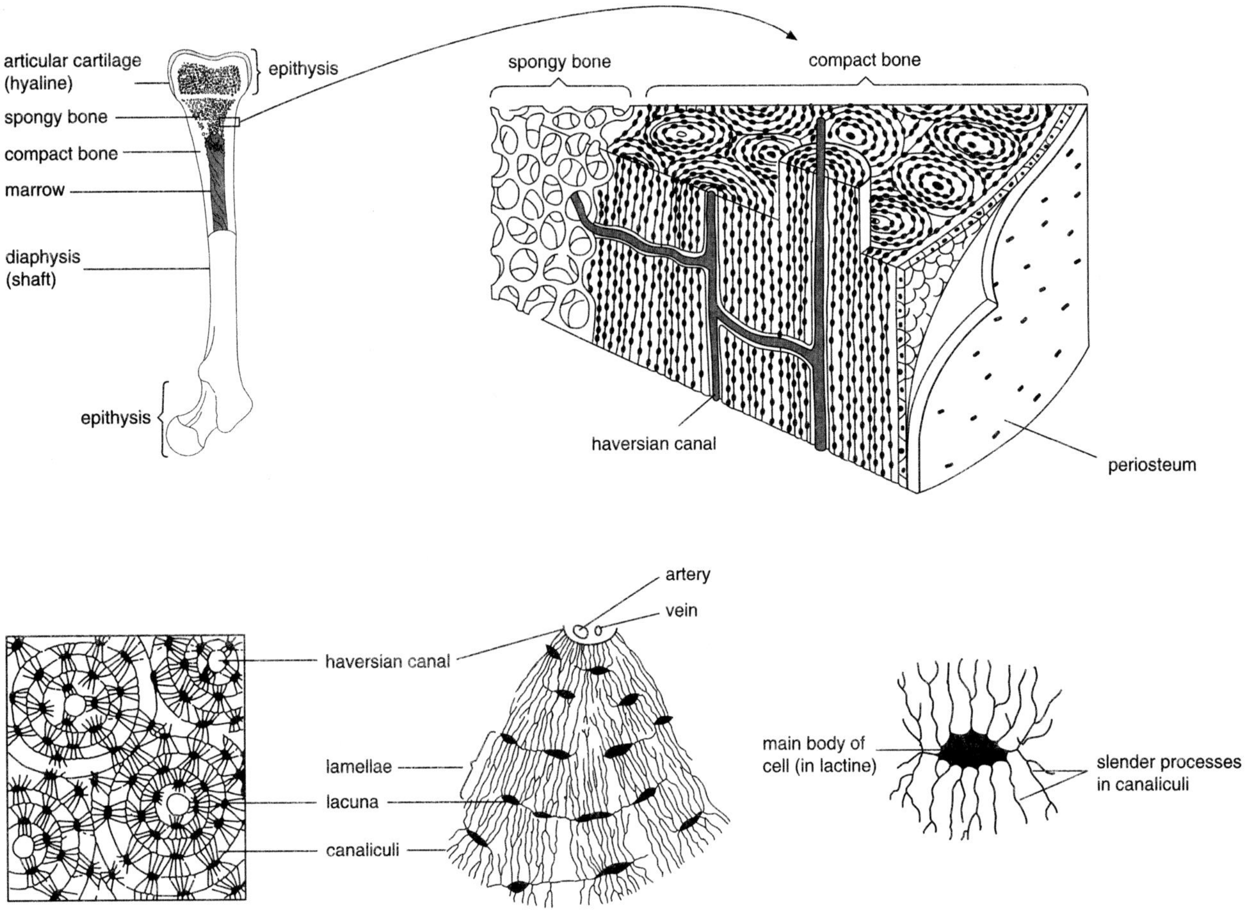

Fig. 13 (a) Structure of the Compact Bone

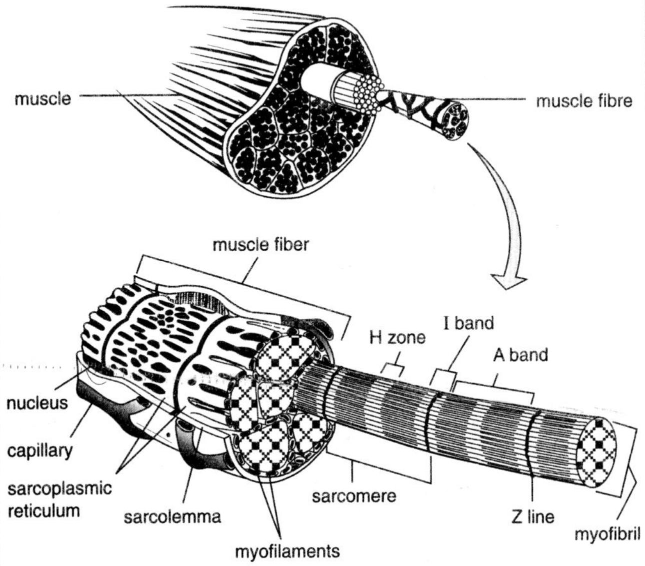

Fig. 13 (b) Structure of Muscle

Muscle Tissue

Ability to contract is an inherent property of all cells, which is necessary for the performance of basic functions involving movement. In multicellular organisms, muscle cells are specialised to enable movement of tissues or organs.

Vertebrate muscle is of three types: **skeletal, voluntary or striated muscle**, **involuntary or smooth muscle,** and **cardiac muscle.** Skeletal (striated) muscle has the largest fibres each with several peripheral nuclei and prominent horizontal stripes. Involuntary (smooth or unstriated) muscle fibres are spindle-shaped without stripes. Cardiac muscle fibres are branched with both horizontal and vertical stripes.

All type of muscle tissue are derived from the embryonic mesoderm and comprises of up to 40% of an adults body mass. All muscle types stain red (surrounding connective tissue stains blue) and consist of densely packed fibres **Fig. 13 (b)**.

Practical 57 – STRUCTURE OF MUSCLE

Skeletal voluntary, or striated muscle

Skeletal muscle in found in the trunk, head and limbs, attached to the skeleton directly or indirectly via a tendon. Powerful rapid contraction and short refractory period, cause it to fatigue quickly. It is under control of the voluntary nervous system.

Skeletal muscle consists of thousands of elongated **fibres**, lying parallel to one another. These fibres are usually cylindrical multinucleate, with nuclei positioned near the periphery of the fibres. The arrangement of the contractile proteins actin and myosin give rise to the appearance of prominent cross-striations, showing up as very long cells usually called fibres. The length of a fibre may reach as much as 35cm, with a diameter of about 10-100μm, subdivided into units called **sarcomeres.** Each fibre is bound in a plasma membrane, called the **sarcolemma,** within which is the cytoplasm known as the **sarcoplasm**. The sacroplasm contains hundreds or thousands of **myofibrils** and numerous mitrochondria. A motor nerve fibre, ending in a **motor end plate** serves voluntary muscle cell **see page 165**.

1. Using medium and high power magnification of the microscope observe prepared slides of skeletal muscle. Identify all the features mentioned above and in the **Figs. 13.1, 13.1a, 13.2**. Make detailed drawings of your observations.
2. Notice the multinucleate structure (**syncytium**) of the fibre and, in a good section, you will be able to see the striations.
3. Examine electron micrographs of skeletal muscle and note the various bands corresponding to the striations seen under the light microscope. You should be able to distinguish between the dark (**A**) band, light (**I**) band, and **H-zone** of dark band not visible in **Fig. 13.2**. Note also **sarcomere**, **sarcoplasm** and the thick filament (**myosin**) and the thin filament (**actin**).

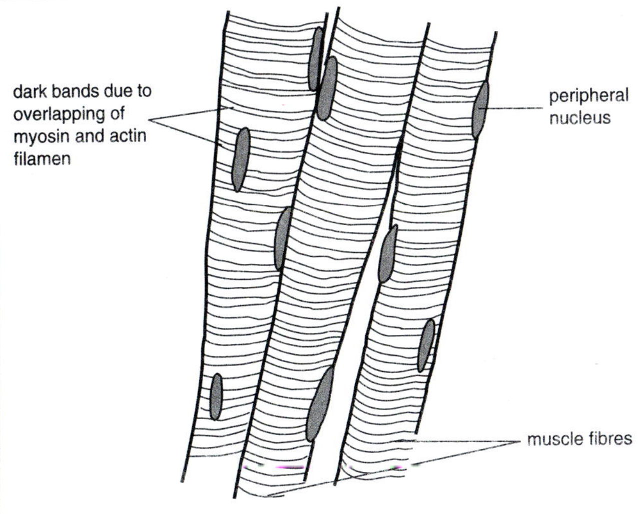

Fig. 13.1 LS Skeletal Muscle

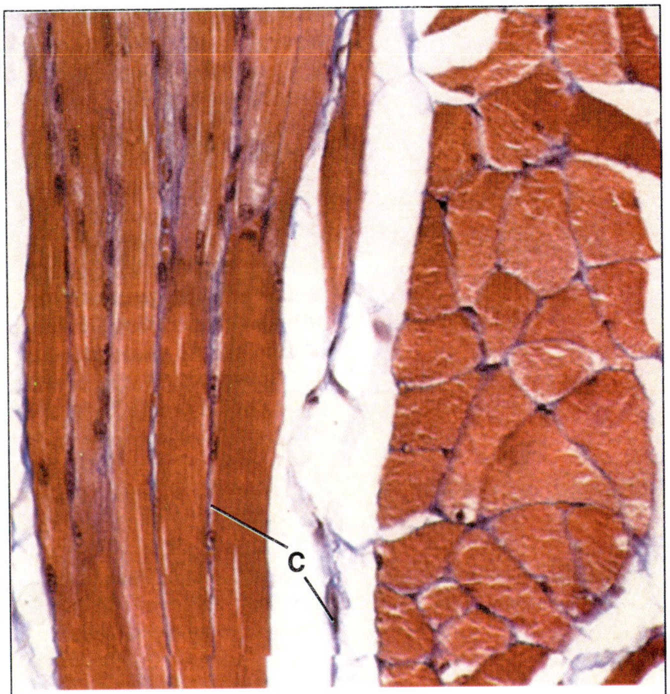

Fig. 13.1a Skeletal Muscle in Tongue.
Note the dense network of capillaries **C** between the muscle fibre shown both in transverse and longitudinal section.

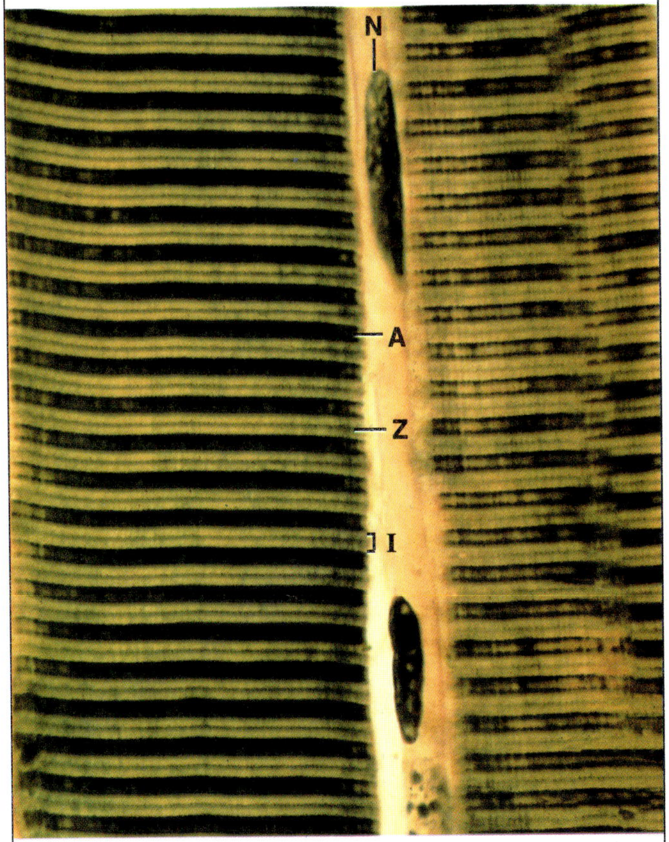

Fig. 13.2 Skeletel Muscle in Monkey Rectus (LS).
Striations are composed of alternating broad **I** and dark **A** bands. Fine lines are called **Z** bands. Note the peripheral nucleus **N**.

Smooth viceral or involuntary muscle

Smooth muscle is particularly abundant in walls of intestinal tubes and ducts of genital, urinary and respiratory tracts, walls of the blood vessels and in the iris and ciliary body of the eye. It has individual, spindle shaped (tapering at both ends) fibres which are much shorter than skeletal muscle, associated in bundles or sheets, with single elongated and centrally placed nucleus. The contractile proteins are not arranged in myofibrils as cardiac and skeletel muscle, thus the fibres are not striated. It is under direct control of autonomic nervous system. Blood vessels run longitudinally besides the fibres with a vast network of capillaries. It can sustain rhythmical contraction and relaxation, as in peristalsis, without fatigue.

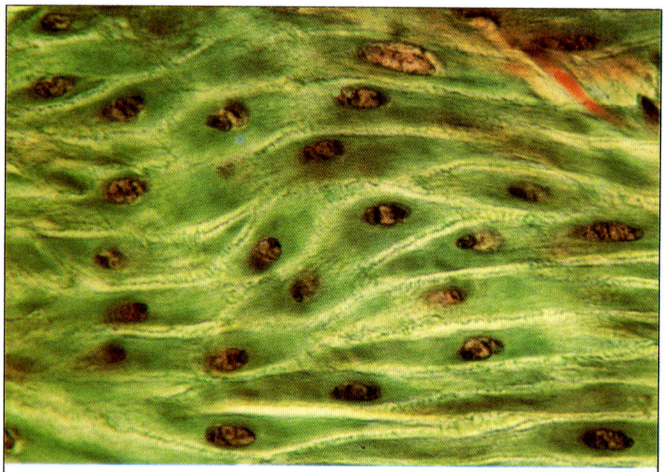

Fig. 13.3 Smooth (viceral) Muscle in Rat Stomach (LS). Elongated spindle-shaped with pointed ends, bound in irregular branching fasciculi with supporting network of connective tissue between individual fibres.

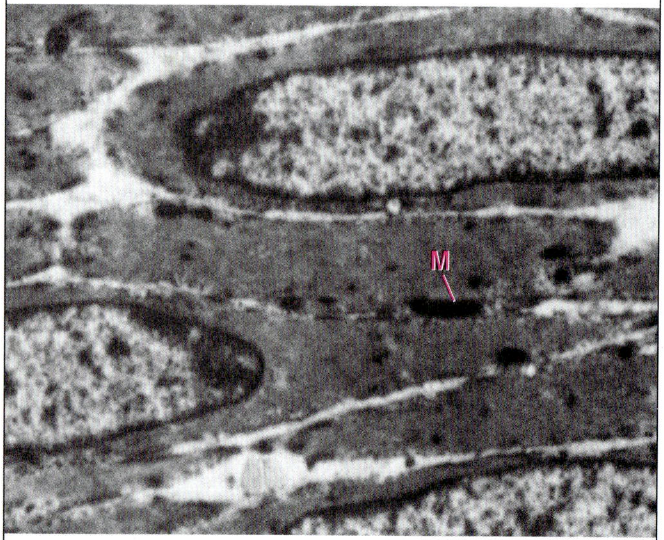

Electron Micrograph of Smooth Muscle. Organization of the short fibres with pointed ends is irregular and unstriated; mitochondria **M** are sparse.

1. Observe prepared slides of smooth muscle from different locations and note that the cells are relatively small, pointed at both ends, with only a single nucleus. The fibres are bound irregularly and the arrangement varies according to the location and functional requirement **Figs. 13.3** and **13.4**.
2. Notice in some tissues the spindle fibres are so closely arranged that it is difficult to distinguish them individually. In other they may be packed fairly loosely and the supporting network of connective tissue is clearly visible.
3. Make labelled drawings of your observations.

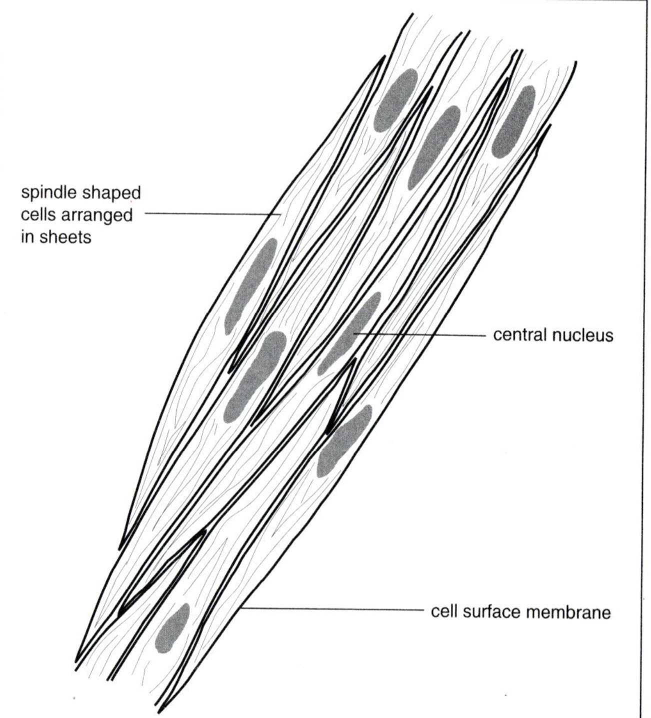

Fig. 13.4 LS Smooth Muscle

Cardiac muscle

Cardiac muscle is found only in the walls of the heart chambers. It has cylindrical branching columns of short **coenocytic** fibre (not divided into uninuclear cells); terminally branched and connected to each other by special inter-digitating surface processes the **intercalated discs.** These discs not only provide point of anchorage for the myofibril but permits extreme rapid spread of contractile stimuli from one cell to the next, causing adjacent fibres to contract almost simultaneously. Arrangement of fibres is three-dimensional to facilitate rapid rhythmical contraction and relaxation. The refractory period is long, therefore the muscle does not fatigue; contraction is not sustained. Cardiac muscle fibres have very similar contractile proteins to that of the skeletally muscle and are therefore striated in a similar manner.

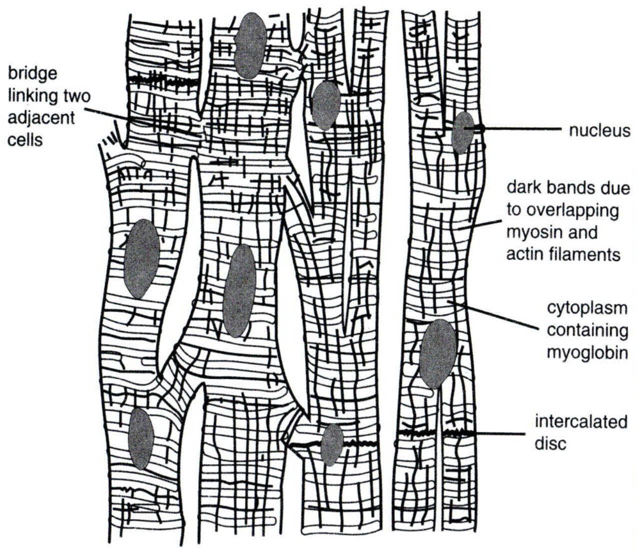

Fig. 13.5 LS Cardiac Muscle

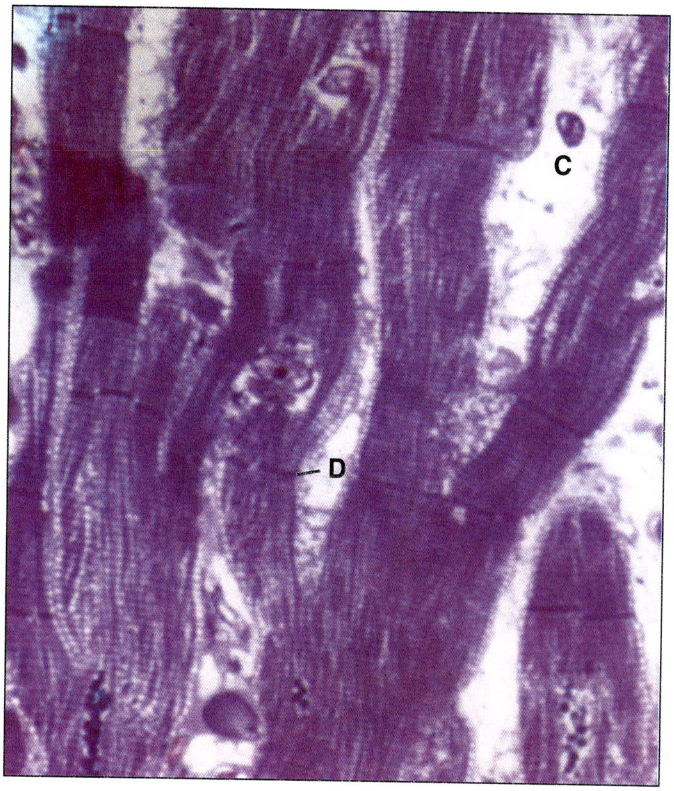

Electron Micrograph of Cardiac Muscle.
Note the branching network and the intercalated discs **D** and the ▶ rich supply of capillaries **C**.

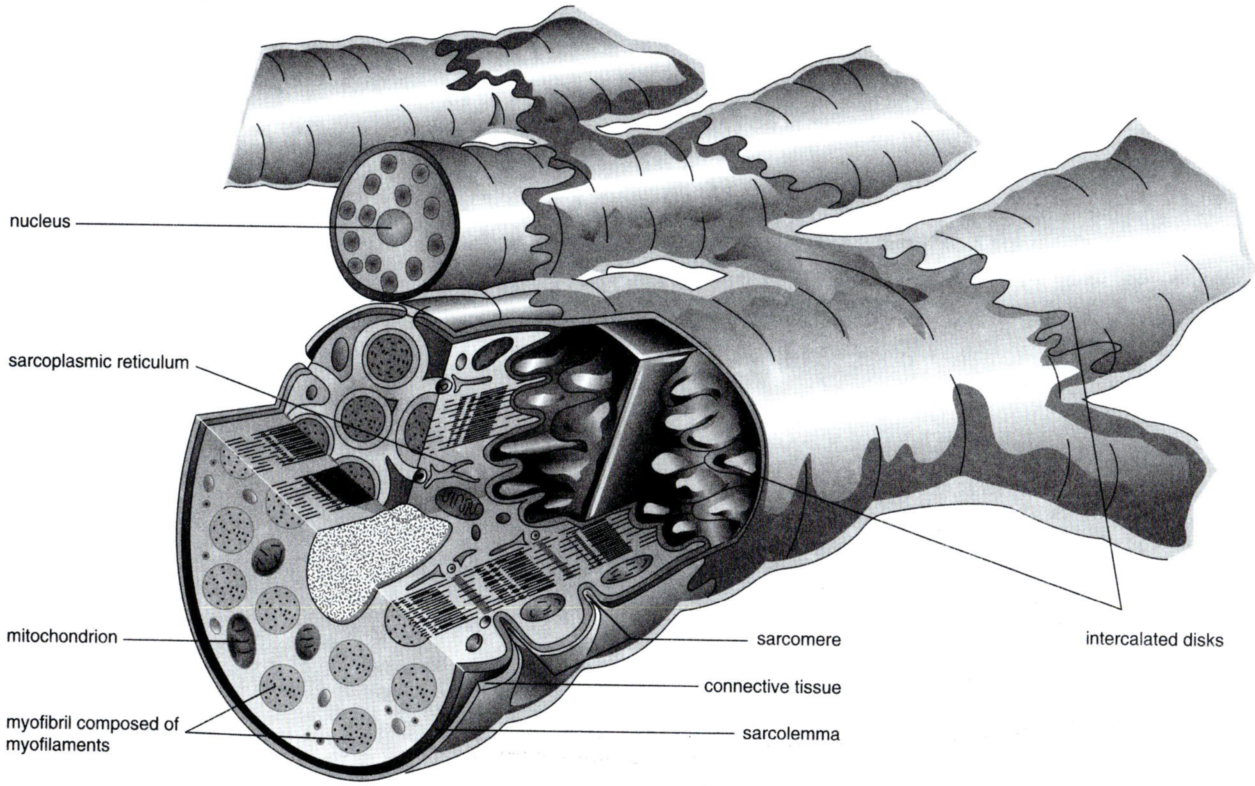

Fig. 13.5a Schematic Representation of Cardiac Muscle

1. Examine sections of cardiac muscle under medium and high power of the microscope and make annotated drawings of the tissue.
2. Examine electron micrographs and **Figs. 13.5, 13.5a** of cardiac muscle and note that each cardiac muscle fibre is surrounded by **sarcolemma**. Abundant mitrochondria are present, with a dense network of capillaries. Intercalated discs; mitrochondria and the detail of the striations can not be observed under light microscope but are clearly visible in the electron micrograph.

For consideration

(a) Explain with reference to your understanding of the structure of the striated muscle of how its structure is adapted to its function?
(b) Compare the structures of the three types of vertebrate muscles in a table. State any advantages or disadvantages of the particular muscle structure in relation to its function.
(c) Explain the presence of abundant mitrochondria and the dense network of capillaries in the cardiac muscle.

The Nervous Tissue

In general the nervous system has three overlapping functions:
(i) **sensory input** – to receive stimuli from the internal and external environment;
(ii) **integration** – these are analysed and integrated; and
(iii) **motor output** – to produce appropriate co-ordinated response to the stimuli in various effector organs.

The nervous system is divided anatomically into the **central nervous system (CNS)** comprising the **brain** and the **spinal cord**, and the **peripheral nervous system (PNS)** which constitutes all nervous tissue outside the CNS.

The nervous tissue is composed of an intercommunicating network of specialised cells called **neurones** (as many as 10^{10} in the human brain), which constitute most sensory receptors, the conducting pathways, the site of integration and analysis, and supporting cells, which protect, insulate and generally assist neurones.

The function of the nervous system depends on a fundamental property of neurones called **excitability.** As in all cells, the resting neurones maintain an ionic gradient across its plasma membrane thereby creating an electric potential. Excitability involves a change in membrane permeability in response to appropriate stimuli such that the ionic gradient is reversed and the plasma membrane becomes **depolarised**; a wave of depolarisation known as an **action potential** then spreads along the plasma membrane. The process of depolarisation follows in which the membrane rapidly re-establishes its resting potential.

Communication between neurones is controlled by a unique junction called the **synapse**. Depolarisation of the neurone causes the synapse to release chemical transmitter substances, **neurotransmitters**, the substances released as an intercellular messenger **(e.g. acetylcholine, norepinephrine or seratonin)** into the synaptic cleft which initiates an action potential in the adjacent cell, a process in which **calcium ions** play a vital role.

Within the nervous system, neurones are arranged to form pathways for the conduction of action potentials from receptors to effector organs via integrating neurones. Neurotransmitters not only mediate neurone-to-neurone transmission but also act as chemical intermediates between the nervous system and effector organs, which also exhibit the property of excitability. The effector organs of voluntary nervous pathways are generally skeletal muscle, and those of involuntary pathways are usually smooth muscle, cardiac muscle and muscle-like epithelial cells within some exocrine glands.

Practical 58 – MICROSCOPIC STRUCTURE OF THE NERVOUS TISSUE

The principle function of a nerve is to transmit messages from one location to the next, which must be done correctly and rapidly. For the most part instruction from the central nervous system (CNS) are transmitted via special cells called the neurones. These are the functional units of nervous system specialised for the reception of stimuli, conduction of excitation, and transmission of the signal to other similar cells.

The neurone

Despite great variation in shape and size in differen parts of the nervous system, all neurones have the sam basic structure as shown in the idealised **Fig. 13.6**. Th neurone consists of a large cell body (**perikaryon** containing the nucleus surrounded by cytoplasm. Mos striking features of the neurones are the fibre-lik extensions from the cell body called **dendrites**.

Dendrites function as a major site of information input into the neurone, which either end in specialised sensory receptors, as in primary sensory neurones, or form synapses with neighbouring neurones from which they receive stimuli.

Each neurone has a single **axon** extending from the **cell body (perikaryon)**, the axon can be of variable length, terminating on other neurones or effector organs e.g. muscles, by a variable number of small knobs called **terminal buttons Figs. 13.6–13.8**. The axons of neurones in the PNS may be **myelinated** (e.g. in cranial or spinal nerve). In such neurones the fibres are totally surrounded by fatty **myelin sheath** formed by **Schwann cells,** which provide both structural and metabolic support. The sheath is constricted at various intervals along the length by **nodes of Ranvier.** One Schwann cell nucleus is visible in the sheath between a pair of nodes. Surrounding the sheath is a tough inelastic membrane, **neurilemma.**

In non-myelinated fibres in the CNS there is no specific cellular support but fibres are indirectly supported by the mass of surrounding tissue.

In general, the cell bodies of all neurones are located in the CNS (hence the grey appearance) with the exception of most primary sensory neurones and the terminal effector neurones of the autonomic nervous system in which case the cell bodies lie in aggregations called **ganglia** in peripheral sites.

Nerve cells are frequently organised into a **reflex arc**. A typical reflex arc consists of receptors (afferent),

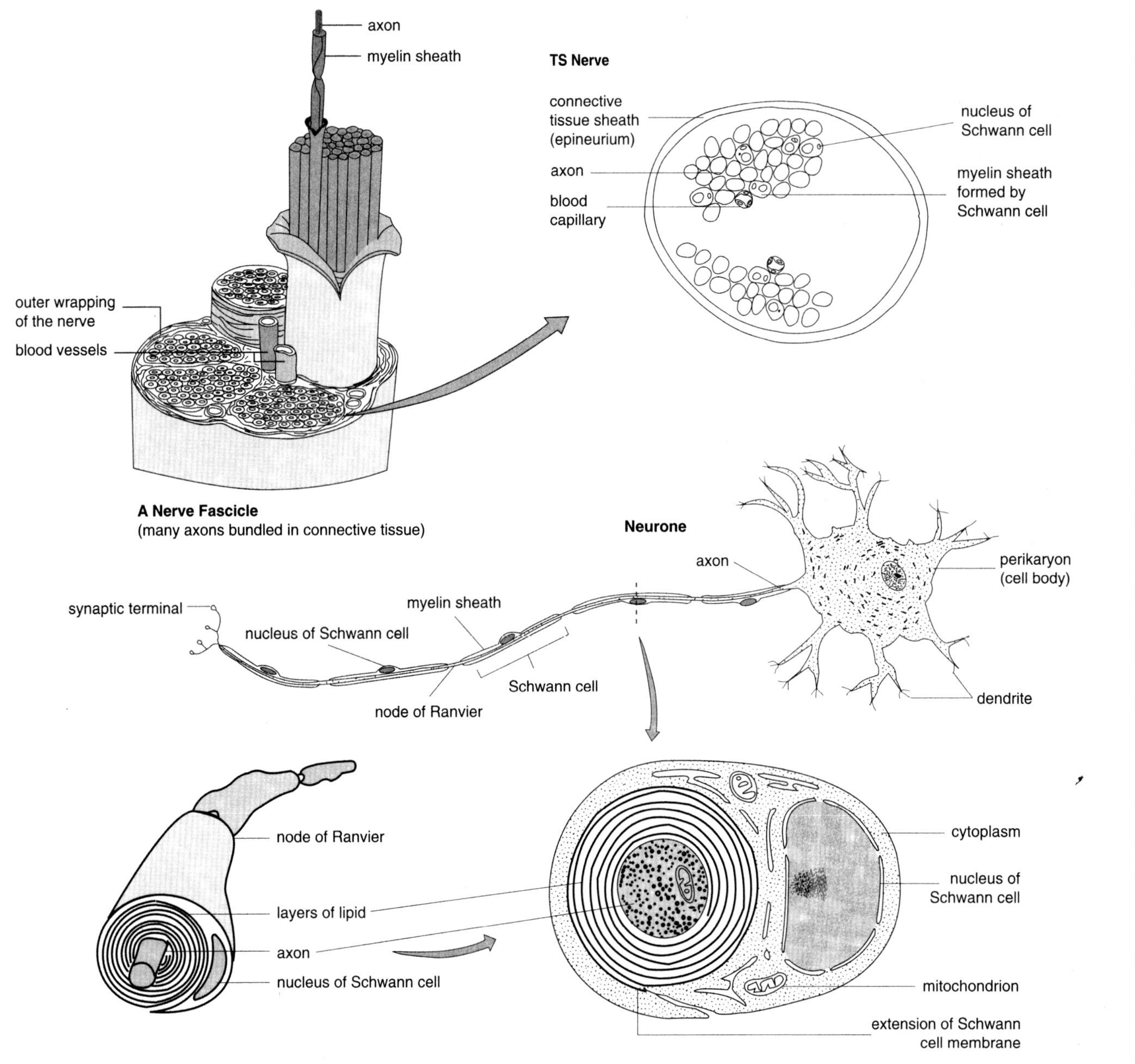

Fig. 13.6 Structure of the Nerve

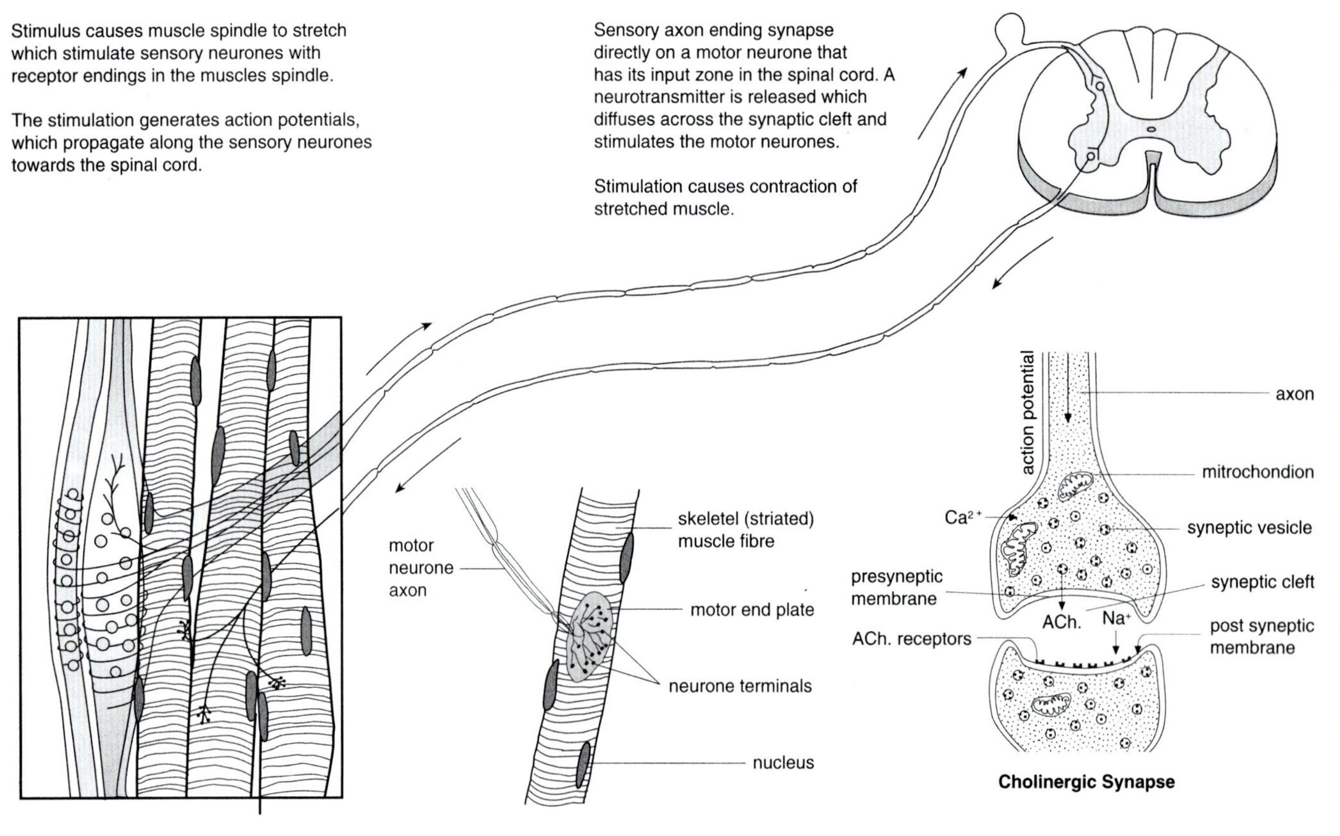

Fig. 13.7 Reflex Response to Muscle Stratching

intermediate, motor neurones, and effectors. **Fig. 13.7.** Reflex arc provides the anatomical basis of **reflex action.** Successive reflex arcs are interlinked by longitudinal neurones.

Procedure

1. Examine prepared slids of nervous tissue to identify the neurones, axons, and dendrites.
2. Examine prepared slides of the brain to locate different types of neurones. Use **Figs. 13.10–13.13** to help you make labelled drawings of your observations.
3. In the cerebral cortex notice the pyramid shaped **pyramidal cells**. You may be able to see the numerous dendrites extending from the cell body.
4. In the cerebellum you will notice the characteristic branched **Purkinji cells**. These are large pear-shaped cells with extensive connections.
5. Examine a prepared slide of the whole myalinated sheath. Draw and label the cell body, axon, and dendrites. Because of the nature of the tissue and the length of the axons, (for example in the sciatic nerve it can extend to over a meter), a whole neurone is almost impossible to see.
6. Use electron micrographs and **Figs. 13.6–13.9** to identify **Schwann cell, node of Renvier** and **myelin sheath.**
7. Examine a transverse section of the **spinal cord** under low power and using **Figs. 13.14, 13.15** draw

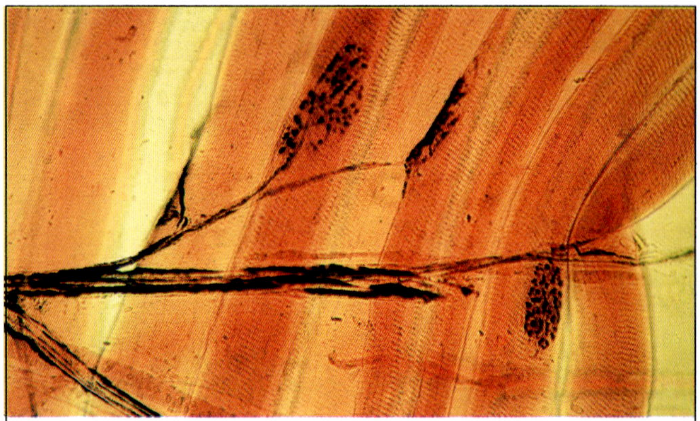

Fig. 13.8 Motor End Plates (snake muscle).

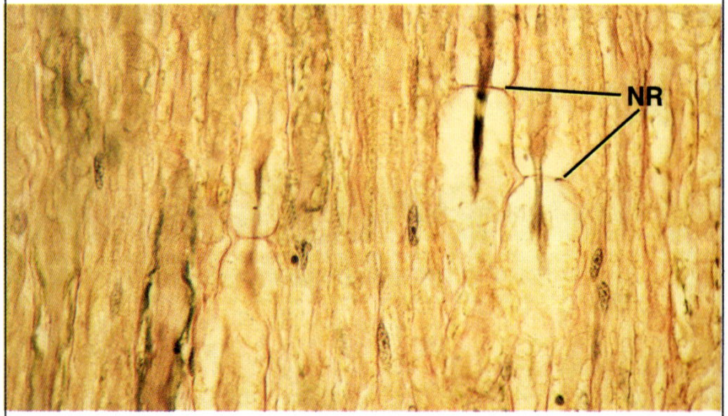

Fig. 13.9 LS Nodes of Renvier NR.

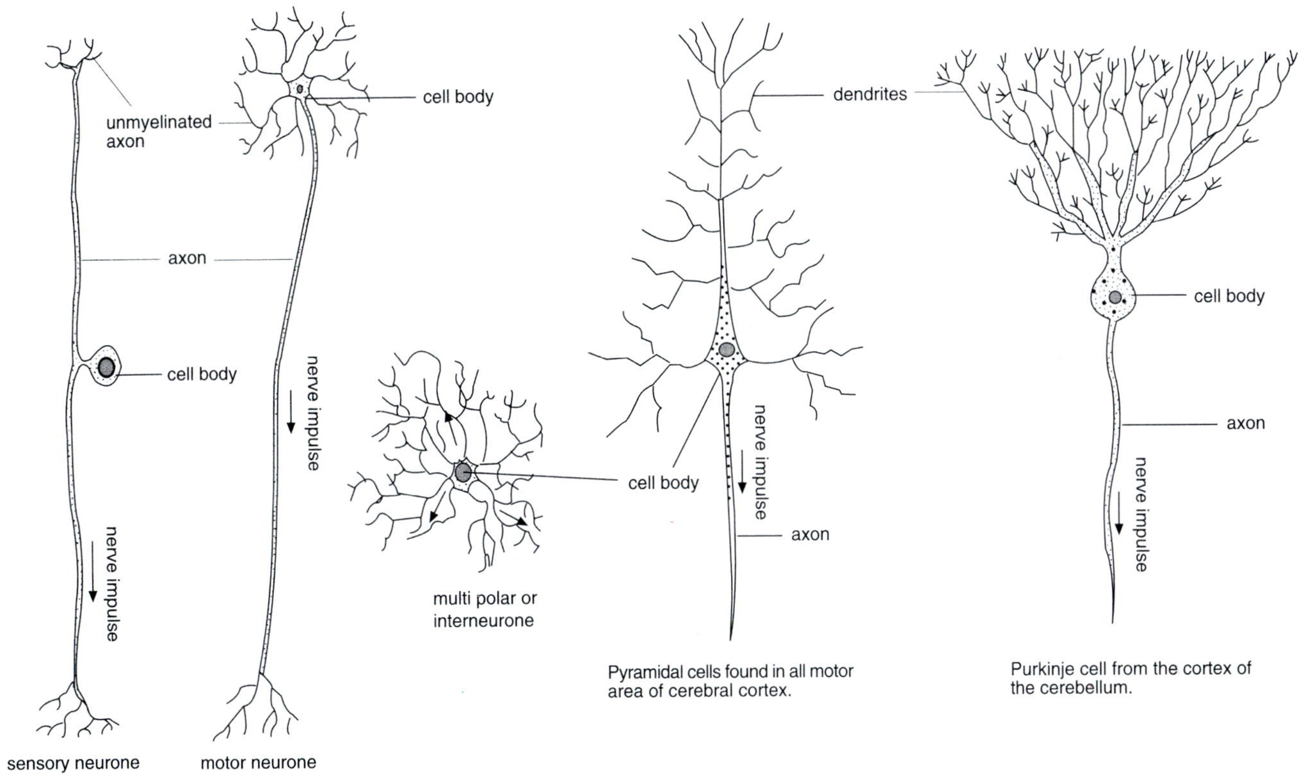

Fig. 13.10 Different types of Neurons

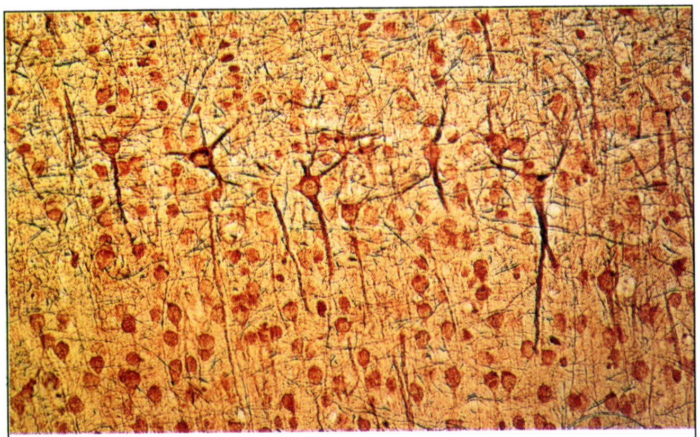

Fig. 13.11 Crebrum Pyramidal Cells (LS).

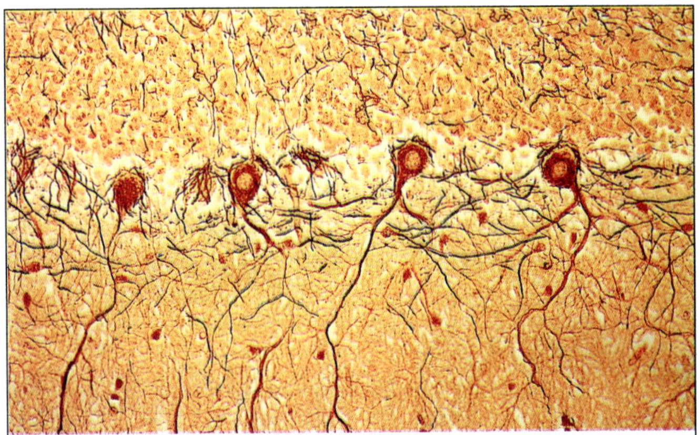

Fig. 13.12 Purkinje Cells.

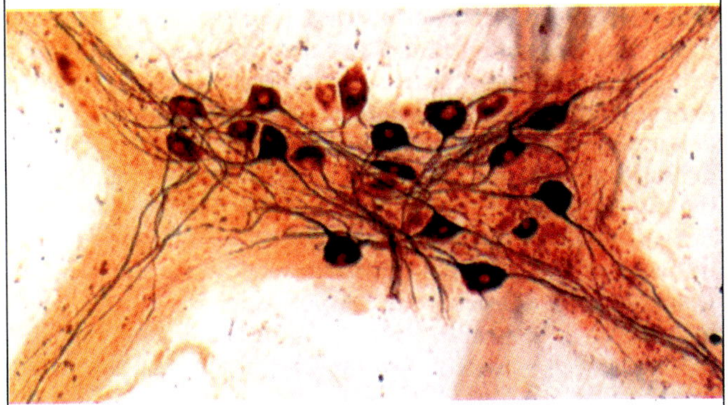

Fig. 13.12a Neurones in Peripheral Ganglion.
Note the prominent cell bodies with cytoplasmic processes and axons.

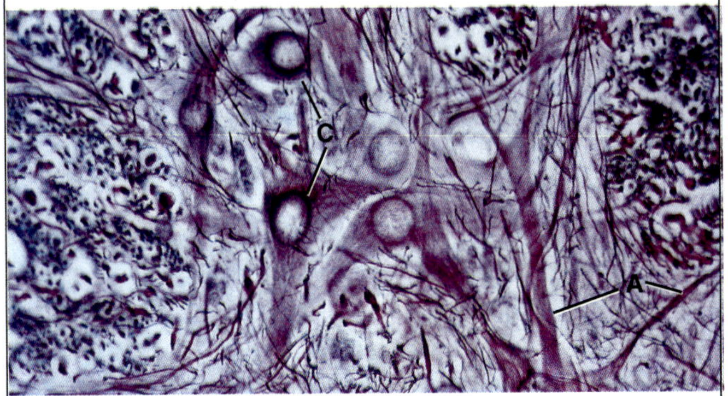

Fig. 13.13 Multipolar Neurones.
Note the dendrites, the elongated axons **A**, cell body **C** with a prominent nuclei.

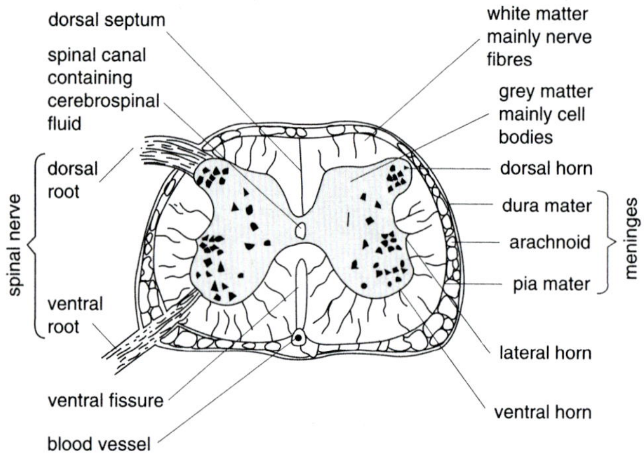

Fig. 13.14 TS of Spinal Cord

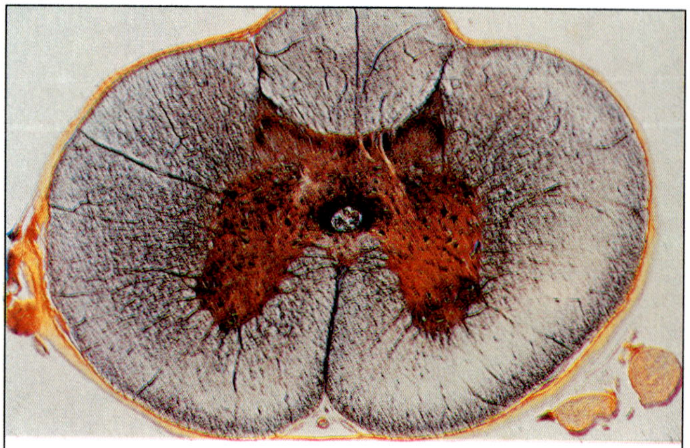

Fig. 13.15 Spinal cord lumber region (TS). Butterfly-shaped central grey matter ventral horns, dorsal horns, central canal and the white matter of the spinal cord are visible. The meninges lining the outside the section are also clearly visible.

a plan diagram to show the **butterfuly** or **H-shaped grey matter**, surrounded by **white matter**. The grey matter is made up of cell bodies of nerve cells, the white matter consists of nerve fibres that are orientated parallel to the long axis of the spinal cord. The fatty sheath (**myelin sheath**) that surrounds the fibres causes the whiteness. The arms of the 'H' that extend dorsally (towards the back of the body) are called **dorsal** or **sensory horns** while those towards the front are called **ventral** or **motor horns**. The cross of the 'H' is the **grey commissure** and the intermediate grey. The **central canal** is continuous with the ventricles of the brain **Figs. 13.14, 13.15**.

8. In a good section you may be able to distinguish the **meninges**, notice the thick **dura mater**, vascular **arachnoid**, and thin **pia mater**. Blood vessel may also be visible.

9. Observe the grey matter under high power and locate the cell body of a neurone, observe the nucleus, nucleolus and the **dendrites**. In an appropriately stained cell **Nissl's granules** may be visible.

For consideration

(a) In sections from the brain only parts of neurone, axons and dendrites are visible. How do you think the diagrams of the whole neurone have been pieced together?

(b) Does observing the structure of the nervous tissue under the microscope help in your understanding of its functions?

(c) What is the function of the pyramid and Purkinji cells?

(d) Explain how the structure of the neurone is adapted to its functions?

Reference: UCLES, Question 3, 9th Nov. 1997.

Endocrine Tissue

Endocrine glands are the sites of synthesis and secretion of substances known as **hormones**–chemical signals that communicate regulatory messages within an animal, which are dissipated throughout the body by the blood stream where they act on specific **target organs.** In conjunction with the nervous system, hormones co-ordinate and integrate the function of all physiological systems, affecting bioenergetics, metabolism, growth, development, behaviour and homeostasis.

The effect of one hormone is often countered by an antagonistic (opposing) signal, often another hormone. An example is the insulin and glucagon, interaction, which through feedback mechanism maintains blood sugar levels within a set point.

Endocrine glands are in general composed of secretory cells of epithelial origin supported by connective tissue, rich in blood and lymphatic capillaries. The secretory cells discharge hormones into the interstitial spaces from where they are rapidly absorbed into the circulatory system. Thus a characteristic feature of all endocrine glands is a very rich vascular supply. Unlike exocrine glands endocrine glands have no ducts and are therefore called **ductless glands.**

Reflecting their active synthetic function, endocrine secretory cells are generally characterised by prominent nuclei and prolific cytoplasmic organelles and hence appear darkly stained in histological sections.

Some endocrine glands exist in the form of discrete organs e.g. pituitary, parathyroid and the adrenal glands. Other endocrine tissues are found in association with exocrine glands e.g. pancreas, or within complex organs e.g. kidney, testis, ovary, placenta, brain and gastrointestinal tract.

Practical 59 – MICROSCOPIC STRUCTURE OF THE ENDOCRINE SYSTEM

Pituitary gland

The pituitary gland sometimes called the master gland is a specialised appendage of the brain. It is the most complex of the endocrine glands, secreting numerous hormones, many of which control the activities of other glands. All the secretion of the pituitary gland is directly controlled by the hypothalamus, the activity of which is under direct control of the central nervous system (CNS), and is controlled by a feedback mechanism from the levels of circulating hormones produced by the pituitary-dependant glands.

1. Examine a longitudinal section of the entire pituitary gland under low power, identify the anterior and posterior lobes.
2. Study **Fig. 13.16** and then look at a section under high power, observe and draw the nerve cell bodies in the hypothalamus, portal blood vessels in the anterior lobe and axons in the posterior lobe.

Adrenal Gland

The adrenal glands are adjacent to the kidneys. Each gland is composed of two distinct types of cells, both of different embryological origins and functions. Eighty percent of the gland is made up of the **adrenal cortex**, which is essential for life. Its main functions are control of water and electrolyte metabolism and hence maintenance of osmotic concentration of body fluids; carbohydrate and protein metabolism as well as involvement in anti-inflammatory reactions and antibody production **Figs. 13.17, 13.18.**

To the centre of the gland is the **adrenal medulla**, which is a soft tissue composed of strands of cells surrounded by blood capillaries, richly supplied by nerves. These cells secrete **noradrenalin** and **adrenaline**. The action of these hormones is widespread and prepares the animal for 'fight or flight' situations.

3. Examine prepared slids of the entire adrenal gland. Observe the cortex and the medulla under low and high power.

Adrenal Medulla

4. Observe the adrenal medulla under high power and notice the numerous capillaries, which have thin lining of pavement endothelium. The cells surrounding the capillaries are columnar and elongated at right angles to the walls of the blood vessels. They are called **chromatin** cells because the

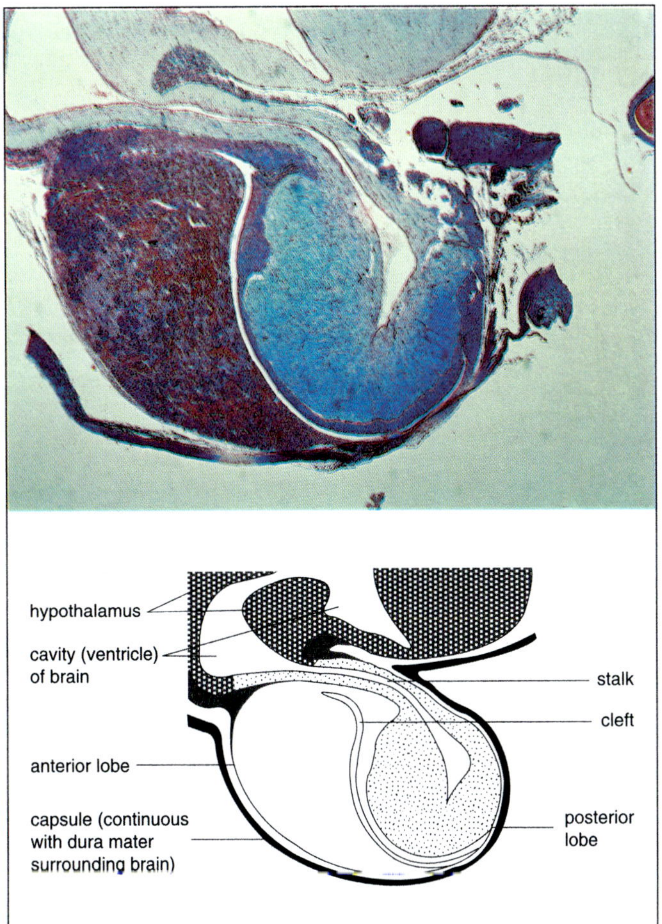

Fig. 13.16 VS of Mammalian Pituitary Gland

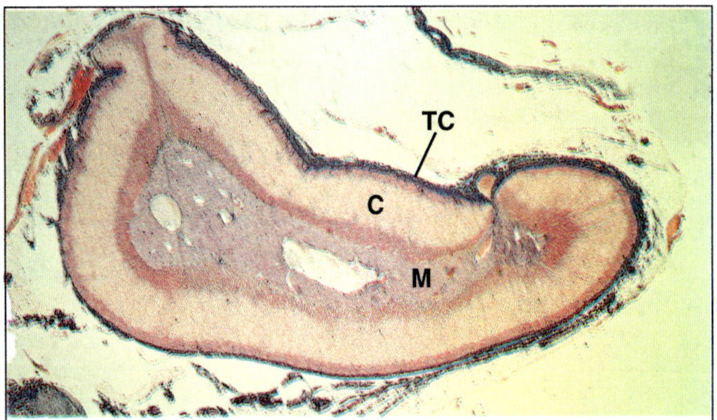

Fig. 13.17 Adrenal gland (LS).
The outer cortex **C** and the dark-stained inner medulla **M** and the dense fibrous tissue capsule **TC** stained blue are visible.

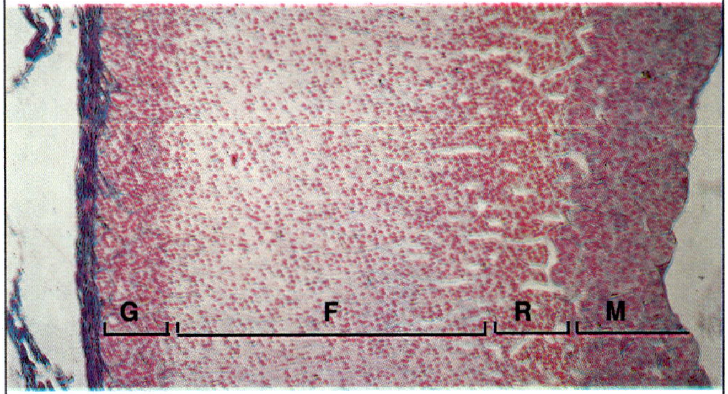

Fig. 13.18 Adrenal gland (TS) ***high power.***
Zona glomerulosa **G** just beneath the capsule, zona fasciculata **F**, zona reticularis **R** lying adjacent to the medulla **M** can also be seen under high power.

granules in their cytoplasm stain brown with chromium salts. A brown colour is also given by adrenaline when mixed with chromium salts.

5. Observe and draw the chromatin cells, which have prominent nuclei and cytoplasmic granules and are adjacent to the blood vessels.

Thyroid Gland

The thyroid gland is located in the neck in front of the upper part of the trachea. **Fig. 13.19**. It is an H-shaped structure and produces hormones of three types:
Iodine containing hormone **triiodothyonine** (T_3), **thyroxin** (T_4), and **calcitonin**. Thyroid hormones (T_3 and T_4) regulate the basal metabolic rate and have an important influence on growth and maturation particularly of the nervous tissue. The secretion of these hormones is regulated by the thyroid stimulating hormone (TSH) secreted by the pituitary. Calcitonin regulates blood calcium levels in conjunction with parathyroid hormone.

The thyroid gland is unique amongst the human endocrine glands in that it stores large amounts of thyroid gland secretions in an inactive form within extracellular compartments called **follicles Figs. 13.20, 13.21** (in contrast other endocrine glands store only small amounts of secretions in intracellular sites). These follicles are the functional units of the thyroid gland, irregular spherical structures composed of single layer of cuboidal epithelial cells, (responsible for the synthesis and secretion of the iodine containing hormoneT_3 and T_4), bound by a basement membrane. The follicles are of variable size and are usually stained pink in histological sections.

6. Examine the thyroid gland and draw the follicles, each surrounded by a single layer of cuboidal cells. The cavity (lumen) of each follicle contains **thyroglobulin**. Note the location of small blood vessels and capillaries in relation to the follicles.

For consideration

(a) Compare the adrenal medulla and thyroid gland, and present the similarities and the differences in a table.

(b) How is the hormone production in these glands controlled?

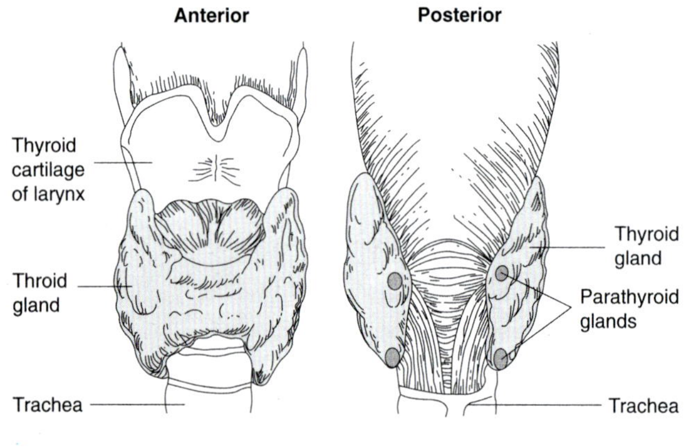

Fig. 13.19 The Thyroid Gland

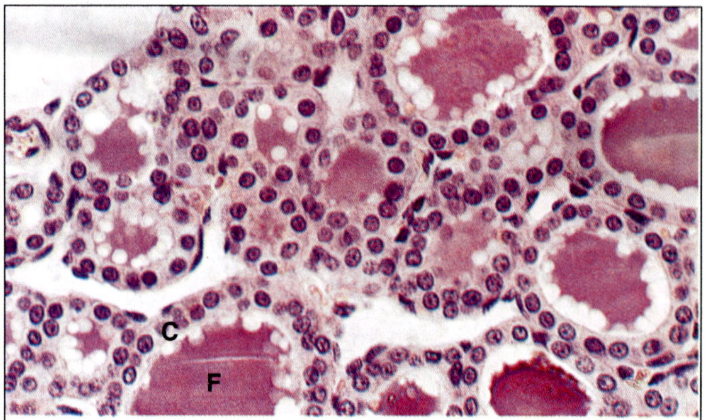

Fig. 13.20 Thyroid vesicles.
Thyroid follicles **F** are lined by simple cuboidal epithelium **C** and a filled with glycoprotein complex.

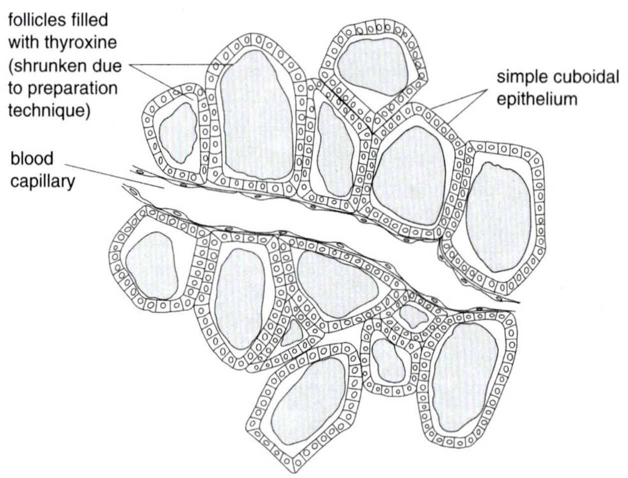

Fig. 13.21 TS Thyroid Gland

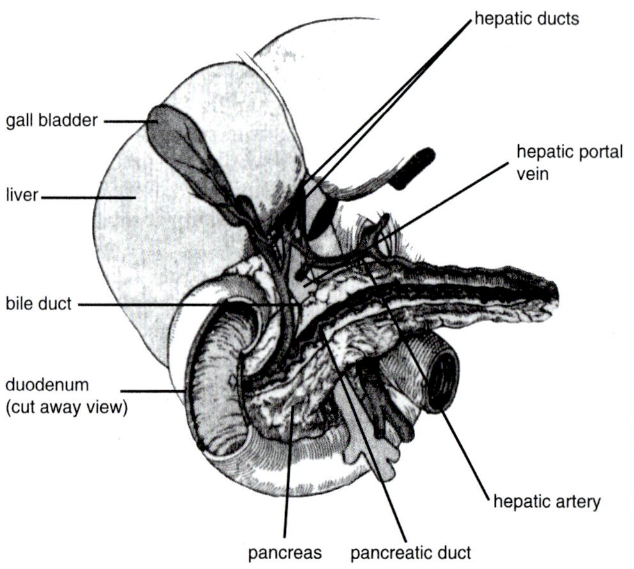

Fig. 13.22 The Liver, Pancreas and Duct System

Practical 60 – MICROSCOPIC STRUCTURE OF THE PANCREAS

The pancreas **Fig. 13.22** has both endocrine and exocrine functions. It consists mostly of exocrine **acinar** cells that produces digestive enzymes and exports them to the small intestine via the pancreatic duct. Scattered amongst this exocrine tissue are clusters of endocrine cells called the **islets of Langerhans**. Each islet has a group of **alpha (α) cells**, which secretes the hormone **glucagon**; and groups of **beta (β) cells**, which secretes the hormone **insulin**. **Fig. 13.23** Insulin and glucagon are antagonistic hormones that regulate the glucose levels in the blood within a narrow range. The antagonistic effects of glucagon and insulin are vital to glucose homeostasis, a mechanism that precisely manages both fuel shortage and fuel use by body cells.

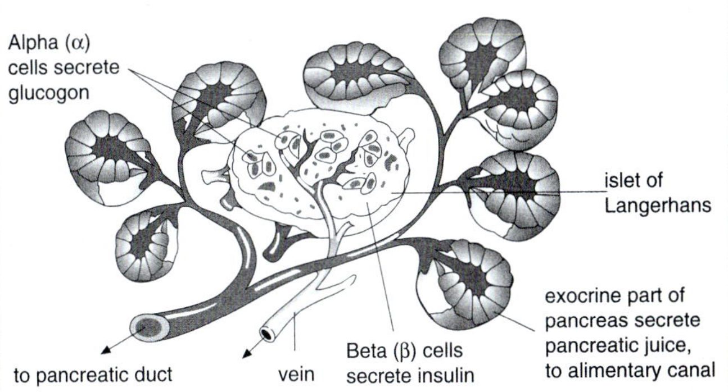

Fig. 13.23 Schematic Representation of the Pancreas

Procedure

1. Under low power observe that the bulk of the pancreas is made up of numerous secretory **acinar cells**, together with blood vessels and branches of the pancreatic duct. The secretory cells are arranged in small groups surrounding a narrow duct. This unit of structures is called an **acinus** (a group of cells associated with a branch of the duct). The cells have prominent nuclei and granular cytoplasm indicative of their secretory function **Fig. 13.25**. They secrete digestive enzymes and represent the exocrine portion of the pancreas. Amongst this exocrine tissue are distinct groups of cells, islets of Langerhans which differ, from the surrounding exocrine cells in the following way:–
   i. **Structure**–the islet cells are arranged in small groups, the diameter of an islet is approximately 200μm (0.2mm), whereas the enzyme secreting cells are irregular chains, which are 6-8 times smaller than the islet cells.
   ii. In a section stained with haematoxylin and eosin, the cytoplasm of islet cells stains light pink whereas the surrounding enzyme secreting cells stain much darker.
2. Under high power the islet cells appear as irregular chains of hormone secreting cells with highly stained cytoplasm and prominent nuclei. Between the chains of secretory cells are capillaries lined with pavement endothelium: flattened nuclei of endothelial cell can also be seen in places **Fig. 13.25**.
3. On careful observation of a good section with specific staining techniques, two different types of secretory cells can be seen in the islets of Langerhans.
   i. Numerous small **β cells**, fill the interior of the islet, these secrete **insulin**.
   ii. And the larger, fewer **α cells**, which stain darker, secrete **glucagon** are located to the periphery of the islet. Notice the intimate association between the hormone secreting cells and the capillaries, a basic requirement of an endocrine gland.
4. Record your observations with labelled drawings.

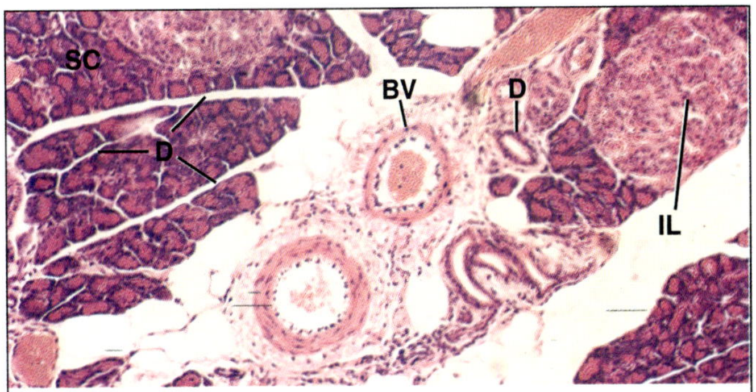

Fig. 13.24 Pancreas.
The section shows blood vessels **BV** and ducts system **D**. Clumps of secretory cells **SC**, islets of Langerhans **IL**.

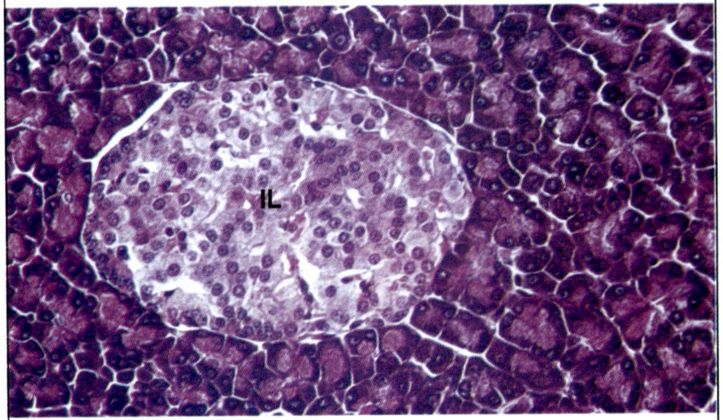

Fig. 13.25 Islet of Langerhans IL.
The endocrine cells of the IL are poorly stained with granular cytoplasm; in contrast the large cells of surrounding exocrine pancreatic acini stain strongly, reflecting high activity.

For consideration

(a) Relate the microscopic structure of the pancreas to its functions?
(b) Describe the difference in structure of the:
   i. α and the β cells,
   ii. Exocrine cells and the islet cells.
(c) If you were to examine an electron micrograph of the islet of Langerhans what special features would you expect to find?

Reference: UCLES, Question 3, 20th May, 1997.

Transport In Animals

In larger organisms diffusion alone is not sufficient to fulfill all the tissue requirements. As a result **circulatory systems**, ranging from water-filled canals to blood filled vessels have developed. The circulatory system mediates the continuous movement of all body fluids. Its principal functions are to transport oxygen and nutrients to the tissues and carbon dioxide and other metabolic waste products from the tissues. The circulatory system is also involved in temperature regulation and the distribution of molecules such as hormones and cells involved in the immune system.

The **blood vascular system** constitutes a network of vessels through which a flow of blood is maintained by continuous pumping of the **heart**. The circulation of most animals, with tubular blood vessels, is described as a **closed circulation.** The mammal has a **double circulation Fig. 13.26**, blood flowing through the heart twice for every complete circuit of the body. The mammalian circulation with its heart, **arteries**, **capillaries**, and **veins** is well adapted in structure and properties for delivering oxygen at high speed to the tissues and for transporting blood to and from the heart.

The **arterial system** distributes blood under high pressure from the heart to the network of capillaries, which are the main sites of interchange between the tissue and blood. The **venous system** returns the blood under low pressure from the capillaries to the heart. The **lymph vascular** system is merely a passive drainage system for returning excess extracellular fluid called **lymph** to the blood vascular system.

The heart, a superb pump, is divided into left and right sides, and is further divided into four chambers: two **atria** and two **ventricles**. Blood is pumped at high speed through the heart by a series of electrical and mechanical events, which makes up the **cardiac cycle**. The ventricles have thick muscular walls, and **valves** prevent blood flowing in the opposite direction. The **sino-artial node (pacemaker)** initiates the heartbeat, though it is **myogenic** (originates in the muscle) controlled by the cardiovascular centre in the hindbrain. The **sympathetic nerve** accelerates the heart, while the **vagus** slows it down. The heart automatically pumps into the arteries the same amount of blood as it receives from the veins, despite variations in the frequency with which it beats. Microscopic structure of the **cardiac muscle** is very similar to that of skeletal (striated) muscle but adjacent fibres are interconnected. It contracts repeatedly without fatigue.

The whole circulatory system has a common basic structure:

i. An inner lining **tunica intima** comprising of a single layer of extremely flattened epithelial cells called **endothelium** supported by a basement membrane and delicate connective tissue.

ii. An intermediate muscular layer, the **tunica media**.

iii. An outer connective tissue layer called the **tunica adventitia**.

Greatest variation is exhibited in the muscular layer, for example, it is totally absent in the capillaries, but comprises the whole mass of the heart. Blood flow is primarily influenced by variation in the muscular layer.

Mammalian blood, the transport medium is composed of **red blood cells (erythrocytes)**, **white blood cells (leukocytes)** and **platelets** suspended in **plasma**.

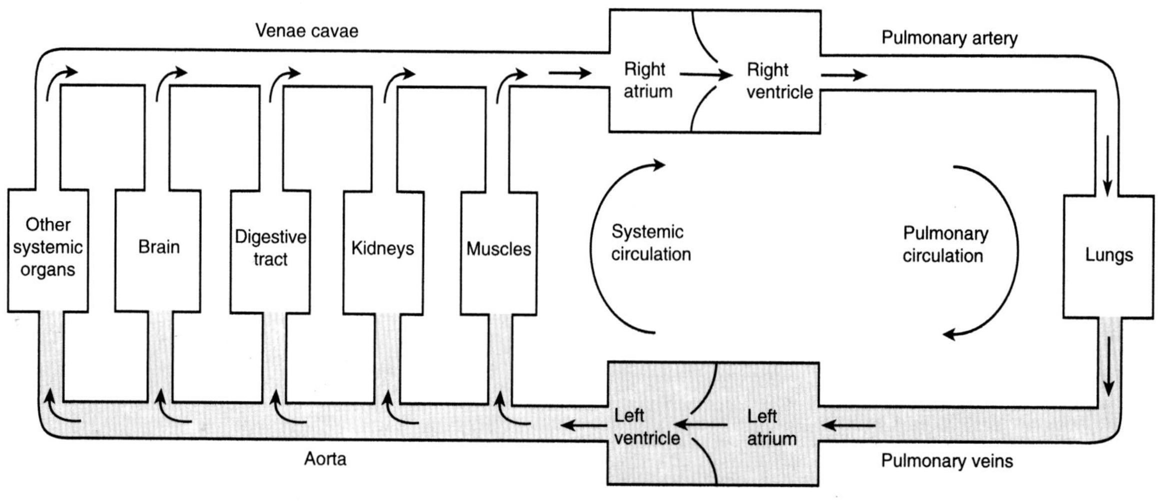

Fig. 13.26 Mammalian Circulation

Practical 61 – THE STRUCTURE OF THE MAMMALIAN HEART

Internal transport in vertebrates is accomplished by closed circulatory system called the **cardiovascular system**. The components of the cardiovascular system are the heart, blood vessels and the blood. Blood is circulated to the lungs and to the rest of the body by the pumping action of the heart via arteries, capillaries and veins. In this investigation you will observe the general structure of the most efficient pump in the world: **the heart.**

Procedure

You are provided with a sheep's heart for dissection. There is also a complete heart/lung set for general reference. Make careful observations and frequent reference to it.

1. Identify the: **ventral** (front) and **dorsal** (back) sides of the heart (the ventral side is more rounded); the four chambers; and all the blood vessels entering and leaving the heart. Note the main veins enter the heart via the dorsal side.
2. Using **Figs. 13.27, 13.28** identify the inferior and superior **vena cava**; **pulmonary artery** and **vein**; and the **aorta**. Note also the **coronary vessels** that supply the **ventricle** muscle. Note that the aorta is a thick-walled rubbery tube. The outer surface of the heart often shows an accumulation of fat, largely around the main blood vessels and over the upper part of the ventricles. Carefully remove this fat.
3. Make annotated diagrams of the external appearance of the ventral and dorsal sides of the heart.
4. Insert a rubber tube into the vena cava, connect the other end to the tap and turn on the tap. Observe the flow of water from the right side of the heart.
5. Now insert the tube into the pulmonary vein, and see the flow through the left side. Turn off the tap.
6. Insert the tube into the pulmonary artery. Carefully turn on the tap, observe how the heart swells and water pressure builds up in the heart. Also notice that hardly any water leaves the heart.
7. Now start dissecting the heart and make labelled drawings to show all the structures you are asked to identify. Hold the heart in your left hand and using a sharp scissors cut down the aorta. Locate the valves at the base of the aorta, at its junction with the ventricle wall. Note the **semilunar valves Fig. 13.28.**
8. Cut open the ventricle and observe the valves that separate the ventricle from the **atrium**. Observe the **tendineae chordae (heartstrings)**.
9. Cut open the left atrium starting at the pulmonary vein. Note the difference in the thickness of the walls of the atrium and the ventricles.

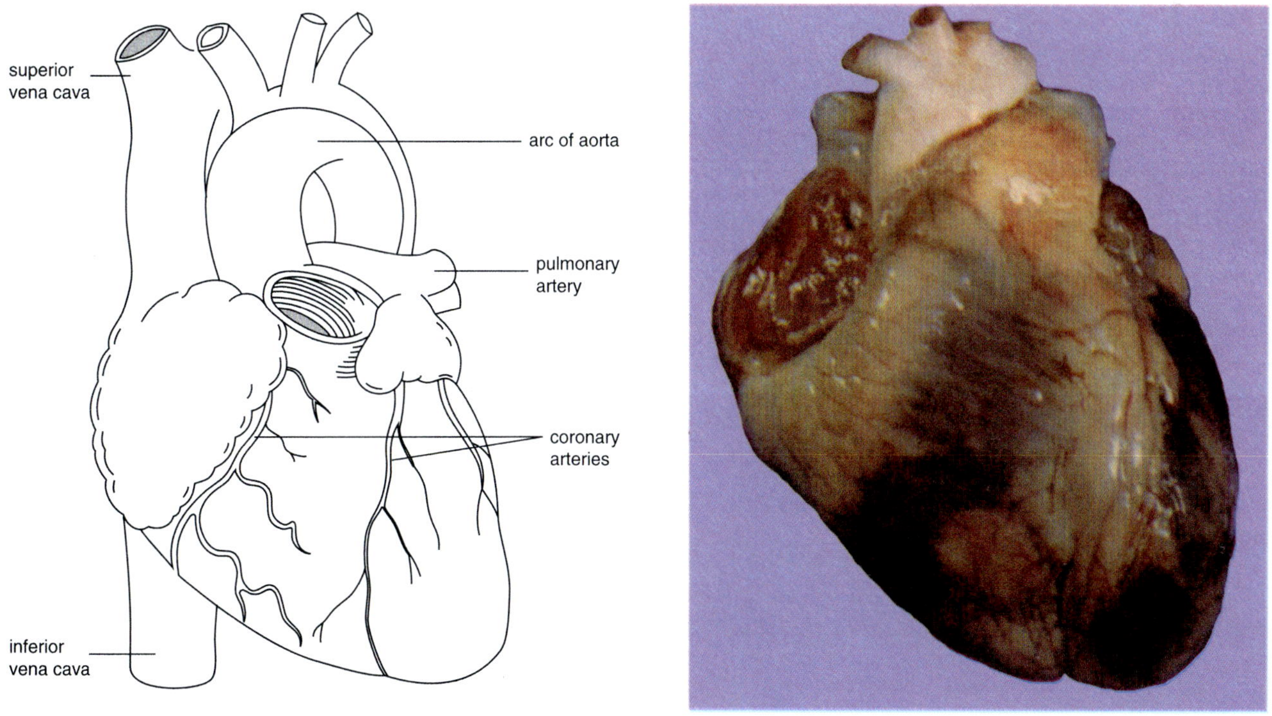

Fig. 13.27 External Appearance of the Human Heart

10. Starting at the pulmonary artery cut open the right ventricle, and locate the semilunar valves, and the **tricuspid valves**.
11. Make labelled diagrams to show all the major structures of the heart.
12. You should be able to locate the following structures and understand their functions: Aorta, pulmonary artery and vein, coronary artery and vein, left and right atrium, left and right ventricles, bicuspid valve, tricuspid valves, semilunar valves, inferior vena cava, superior vena cava, tendineae chordae.

For consideration

(a) What and where is the **pericardium**?
(b) Why is the right ventricle larger than the left ventricle?
(c) Explain the terms: diastole, systole.
(d) Which two nerves of the autonomic system regulate the heart beat?
(e) What does 'myogenic' mean?
(f) Where is the pacemaker (sino-atrial node) and what is its function?
(g) Where is the sino-ventricular node and what is its function?
(h) What is **acetylcholine** and what is its function?
(i) What is the structural and functional difference between the bicuspid and tricuspid valves?
(j) What is the function of the chordae tendineae?
(k) What type of tissue is the chordae tendineae made of?
(l) Where and what is the **bundle of His**?
(m) What other body system plays a direct role in regulating the heartbeat?

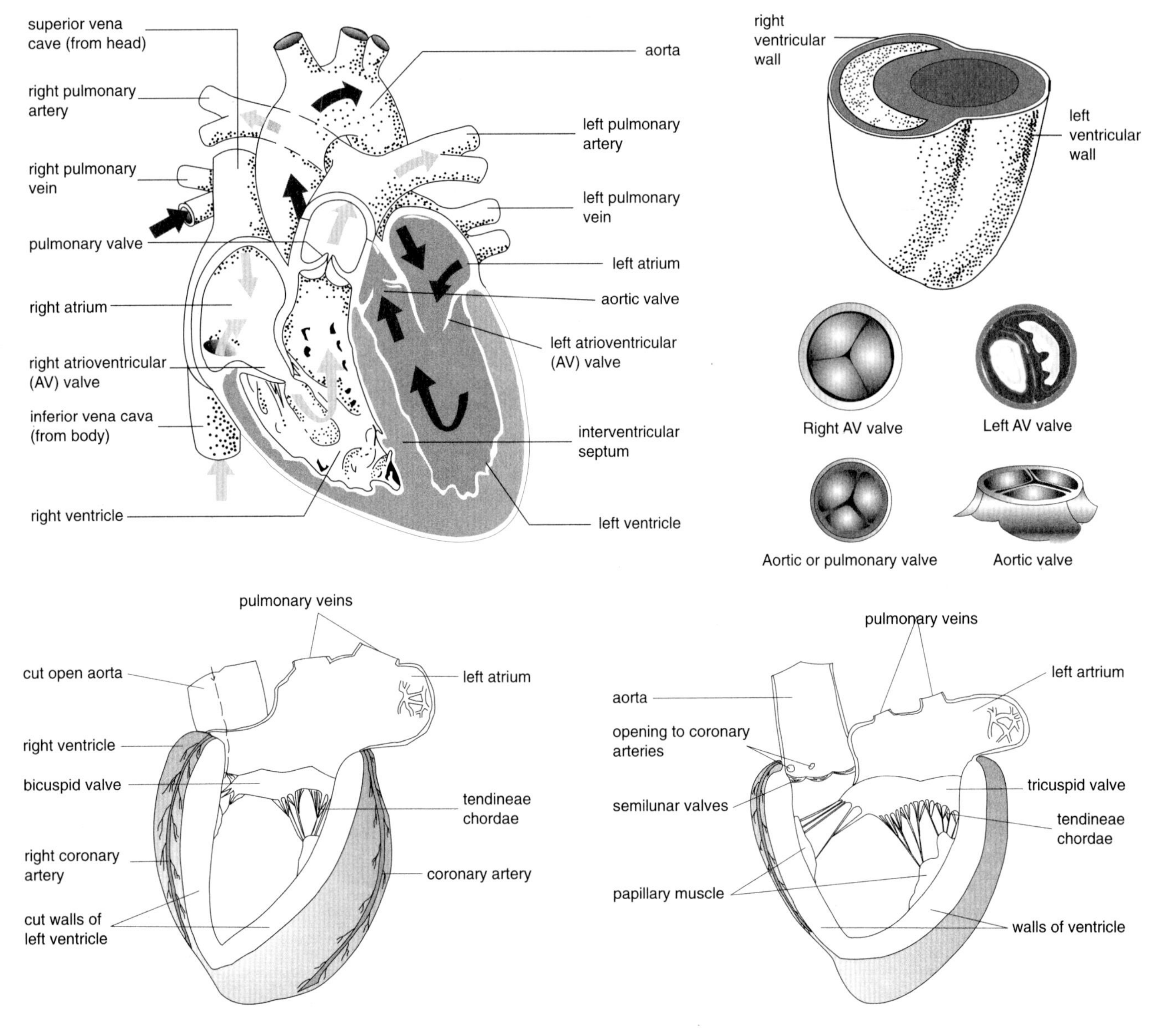

Fig. 13.28 Internal Structure of the Mammalian Heart

Practical 62 – STRUCTURE AND PROPERTIES OF THE CARDIAC MUSCLE

The general structure of the cardiac muscle is similar to the striated muscle but the primary difference is in their electrical and membrane properties. The junctions between the cardiac muscles contain specialised regions called **intercalated discs**. Thus, an action potential generated in one part of the heart rapidly spreads to the whole heart. When the heart beats, a wave of contraction spreads rapidly over the heart wall so that all the muscle fibres contract at about the same time. The wave of contraction is spread not by nerves but by the cardiac muscle itself i.e. it is **myogenic**. The plasma membrane of the cardiac muscle cells has pacemaker properties causing the single heart muscle cells to beat, even when isolated from the heart and placed in a culture medium. Also the action potential of the cardiac muscle lasts twenty times longer than that of the skeletal muscle.

Procedure

1. Place your fingers on the radial artery of your left hand and count your pulse rate per minute. Try and work out how many times the heart will beat in your life from birth till you are seventy years old.
2. Clench your fist and open it repeatedly at the same rate as your pulse for one minute. Note how your arm feels.
3. Examine a prepared slide of the cardiac muscle under low and high power of the microscope. Note that the fibres are made up of chains of cells, each containing a single nucleus. Dark and light bands similar to those of skeletal muscle are clearly visible. Notice in particular the intercalated discs, the bridged connections between adjacent fibres and numerous mitrochondria. Using **Figs. 13.29** and **13.4, 13.5** make labelled drawings of your observations.
4. Compare electron micrographs of cardiac muscle with electron micrographs of striated muscle and notice that the light and dark bands are similar. The intercalated discs are in position to the Z-membrane.

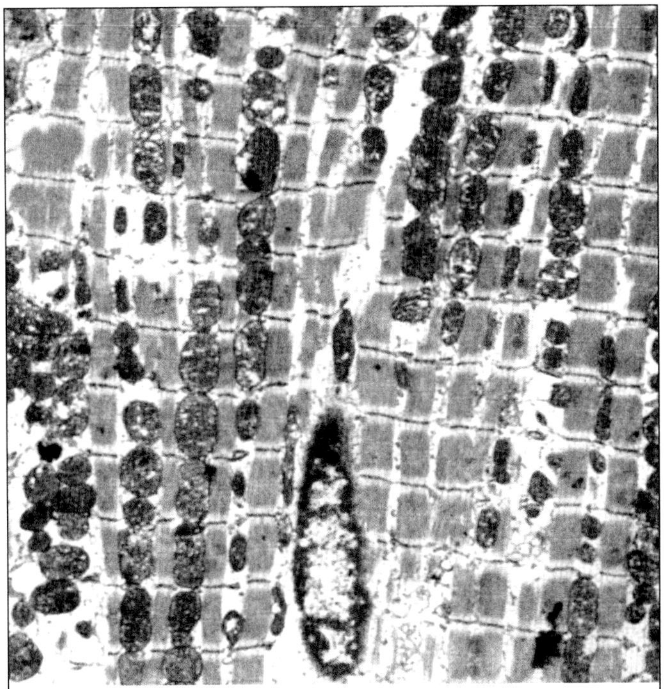

Fig. 13.29 Electron Micrograph of Cardiac Muscle.
Note the banding pattern of the muscle fibres is identical to that of skeletel muscle, the fibre are not arranged into columns but form branching network.

5. Make labelled drawings from the electron micrograph and use **Fig. 13.5** to help you identify as many features as possible on the micrograph.

For consideration

(a) From your observations in steps 1 and 2 in this investigation, what can you say about the properties of the cardiac muscle in comparison with the striated muscle?
(b) Why are there so many mitrochondria in the micrographs of the cardiac muscle?
(c) Make notes on how the structure of the cardiac muscle is adapted for its functions.

Reference: UCLES, Question 3, 19th May, 1992.

Practical 63 – MICROSCOPIC STRUCTURE OF BLOOD VESSELS

The **circulatory system** mediates the continuous movement of all body fluids. It comprises three main types of blood vessels namely the **arteries**, **veins** and the **capillaries**, which in the human body extend to a total distance of 100,000 km. **Arteries** carry blood, at high pressure to organs away from the heart. Within these organs the arteries branch into **arterioles**, which convey blood to a network of **capillaries**. The capillaries converge into **venules**, which converge into **veins**. Veins return the blood to the heart (at low pressure) **Fig. 13.26**. Before observing the structure of the blood vessels consider the functions of the vessels to see if you can predict their structure.

Procedure

1. Examine transverse sections of a large artery and vein under the microscope. Notice that there are three layers of tissue in their walls, consisting of **endothelium, smooth muscle** and **connective tissue, Figs. 13.30–13.33**. Examine the following layers in detail:
   i. **Tunica intima of endothelium:** thin, lined with

squamous endothelium and composed of delicate collagen and elastic fibres mainly longitudinally arranged.

ii. **Tunica media of smooth muscle:** thicker, consisting of tough circular elastic fibres and smooth muscle, interspersed with collagen fibres. In appropriately stained sections, the elastic fibres appear as dark wavy lines.

iii. **Tunica externa (or adventitia) of connective tissue:** varies in thickness, contains a mixture of irregularly arranged elastic and collagen fibres and blood vessels (vasa vasora).

2. Compare the artery and vein with regard to the relative amounts of elastic fibres, collagen fibres and smooth muscles of their walls. Note the tunica adventitia of arteries contain mainly elastic fibres stained black; the tunica adventitia of veins contain mainly collagen fibres. The tunica media of arteries is much thicker than that of veins and contains much more smooth muscle.
3. Compare the size of the lumen of arteries, veins and capillaries **Figs. 13.30** and **13.34**. The lumen of the

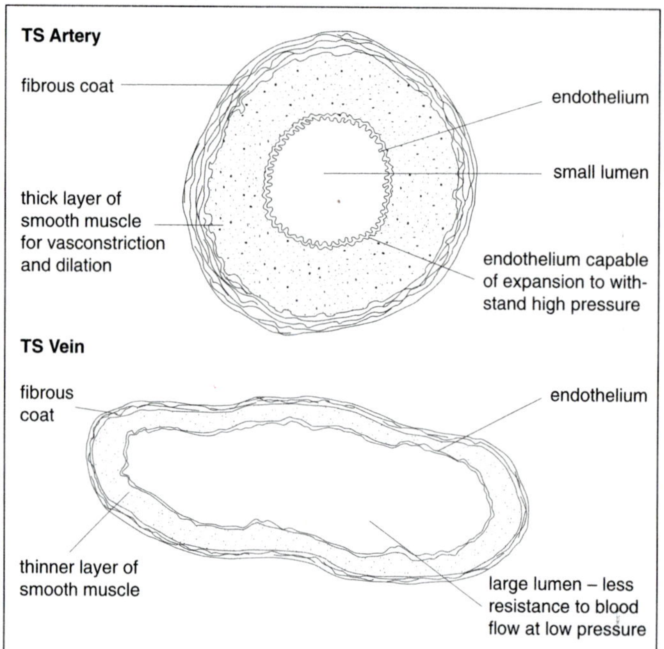

Fig. 13.30 Structure of Blood Vessels

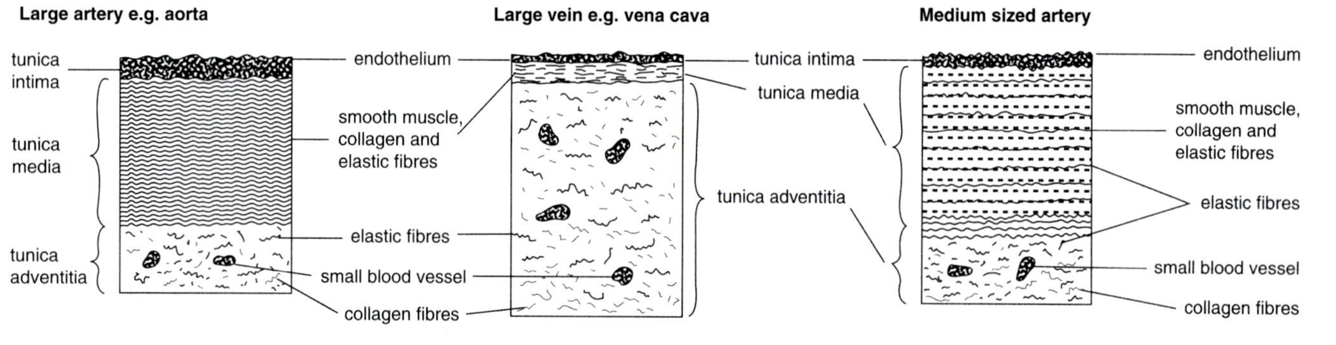

Fig. 13.31 Structure of the Blood Vessel Wall

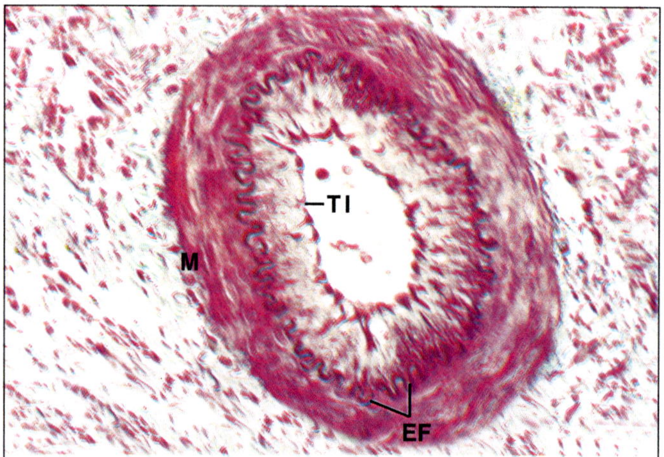

Fig. 13.32 Aorta TS.
Note the well defined tunica intima **TI**, the elastic fibres **EF** stained black and the thick layer of mascular tissue **M**.

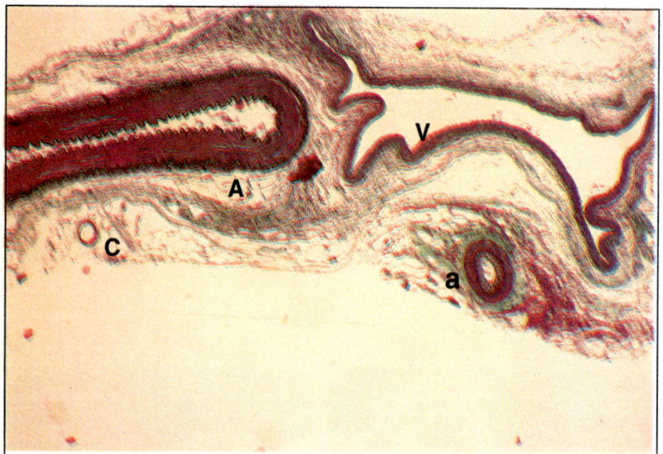

Fig. 13.33 Artery, Vein and Capillary.
Artery **A**, arterioles **a**, a large vein **V** and a capillary **C** are visible. Note the structural differences in the vessel walls and the poorly developed tunica intima in the vein.

vessel is controlled by the circulary muscle in the artery wall. Blood vessels of the brain have no connective tissue which reduces the tensile strength of the vessel and any sudden increase in pressure may result in vessels rupturing hence causing a haemorrhage.

4. Using a micrometer slide and a graticule (**see page 20**) measure the size of the walls, and of the lumen in the three types of blood vessels.
5. Examine a transverse section of an arteriole. As arteries get smaller their walls become thinner and contain progressively less elastic tissue relative to smooth muscle. The smallest arterioles have an endothelium surrounded by a layer of smooth muscle, then a thin layer of connective tissue.
6. Note the vasa vesora – small blood vessels situated in the walls of the artery and vein. Examine a capillary in a prepared section of an organ such as a lung or kidney. Notice that the wall consists of a single layer of squamous epithelial cells.
7. Now examine an electron micrograph of a section through a capillary wall. Locate one or more endothelial cells. Notice that the cell is bulbous in the vicinity of the nucleus, but flattened peripherally.
8. If available, examine the tail of a tadpole or a young fish under the microscope. Notice red blood cells flowing through capillaries in single file. Compare the velocity of blood-flow in a capillary with that of an artery.

Comparison of the Structure and Functions of Blood Vessels

Artery	**Capillaries**	**Vein**
Small overall diameter, small lumen	Small diameter	Large overall diameter, large lumen
Transports blood **from** heart	Links arteries to veins, site of exchange of materials between blood and tissue	Transports blood **to** heart
Rapid oxygenated blood flows at high pressure (10-16kPa) and pulsatile	Slowing, mixed oxygenated and deoxygenated blood flow, pressure falling (4-1kPa) and non-pulsatile	Slow deoxygenated blood (except in pulmonary vein), low pressure (1kPa), non-pulsatile
Valves absent	Valves absent	Semilunar valves present
Thicker wall with greater overall content of elastic fibres	Thin single cell walls, muscular and connective tissue layer absent	Thinner wall with smaller overall content of elastic fibres
Tunica intima thicker	Only sqamous epithelium present	Tunica intima thinner
Tunica media thicker and more muscular	Absent	Tunica media thinner and less muscular
Tunical adventitia (or externa) thinner with high elastic fibre content relative to collagen	Absent	Tunica adventitia (or externa) thicker with low elastic fibre content relative to collagen
Vasa vasora are small blood vessels situated in the wall of the artery and vein which are located further away from the inner surface of wall	Absent	Vasa vasora penetrate closer to inner surface of wall

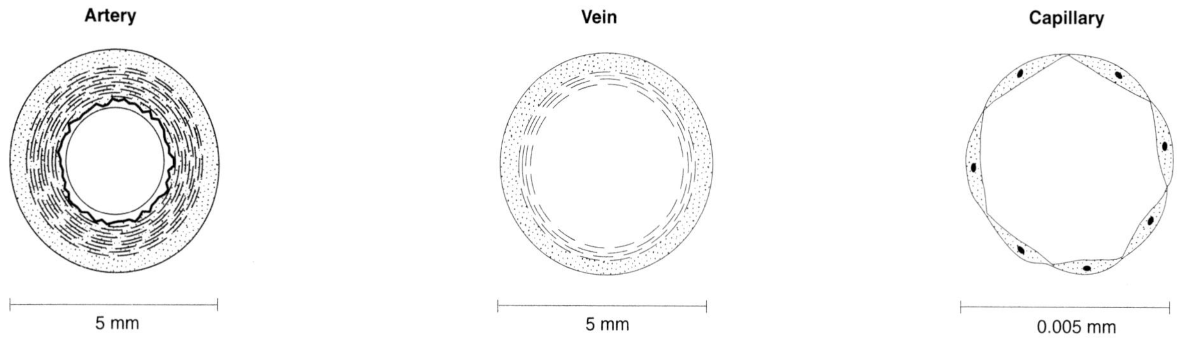

Fig. 13.34 TS of Blood Vessels

For consideration

(a) In the table on **page 177** the structure of a typical mammalian artery is compared with that of a vein. On the assumption that your own observations agree with the information given in the table, comment on the functional significance of each of the difference.

(b) How will the structural differences of the blood vessels affect their functional properties?

(c) Arterioles have an endothelium surrounded by a layer of smooth muscle, then a layer of connective tissue. Venules, on the other hand, have an endothelium surrounded by connective tissue, but there is no muscle present. Why the difference?

(d) How do capillaries manage without any muscle or connective tissue in their walls?

(e) Which of your observations made during this investigation help you to answer this question?

(f) What causes fluid to leave the capillary at the arteriole end?

(g) What causes the change in hydrostatic pressure as blood flows through the capillary?

(h) What structure is absent from the diagrams, which is attached to the interior walls of arteries and veins and why is it needed for the successful operation of the circulation?

Reference: UCLES, Question 3, 6th Nov. 1996.

Blood

Blood is a complex fluid tissue consisting of several different cell types: **erythrocytes**, red blood cells (RBC), **leucocytes**, white blood cells (WBC) and **platelets** suspended in a clear fluid matrix called **plasma**. Dissolved food substances and oxygen are transported to the plasma by the red blood cells.

Formed Elements of Human Blood

Cell Type			Description	Function
Erythrocyte (Red Blood Cells)			Biconcave disk; no nucleus; 7-8μm in diameter; 4.2 to 5.8 million/mm³.	Transports oxygen as oxyhaemoglobin and carbon dioxide as carbonic anhydrase.
Leucocytes (White Blood Cells)			Spherical cells with a nucleus 5000 to 10,000/mm³.	Five types of leucocytes; each with specific functions.
	Granulocytes	Neutrophil	Spherical cell; with two to five lobed nucleus connected by thin filaments; cytoplasmic granules stain a light pink or reddish purple; 12-15μm in diameter; 60% to 70% of leucocytes.	Phagocytosis of micro-organisms and other substances.
		Basophil	Spherical cell; nucleus with two indistinct lobes; cytoplasmic granules stain blue-purple; 10-12μm in diameter; 0.5% to 1% of leucocytes.	Releases histamine which promotes inflammation, and heparin which prevents clot formation.
		Eosinophil	Spherical cell; nucleus often bi-lobed; cytoplasmic granules stain orange-red or bright red; 10-12μm in diameter; 1% to 4% of leucocytes.	Releases chemicals that reduce inflammation; attacks certain worm parasites.
	Agranulocytes	Lymphocyte	Spherical cell with large round nucleus; cytoplasm forms a thin ring around the nucleus; 6-8μm in diameter; 20% to 30% of leucocytes.	Produces antibodies and other chemicals responsible for destroying micro-organisms; contributes to allergic reactions, graft rejection, tumour control, and regulation of the immune system.
		Monocyte	Spherical or irregular cell; nucleus round, kidney or horse-shoe shaped; contains more cytoplasm than the lymphocyte; 10-15μm in diameter; 2% to 8% of leucocytes.	Phagocytic cell in the blood; leaves the circulatory system and becomes a macrophage, which phagocytises bacteria, dead cells, cell fragments and other debris within tissues.
Platelet			Cell fragment surrounded by a cell membrane and containing granules; 2-5μm in diameter; 150,000 to 400,000/mm³.	Forms platelet plugs; releases chemicals necessary for blood clotting.

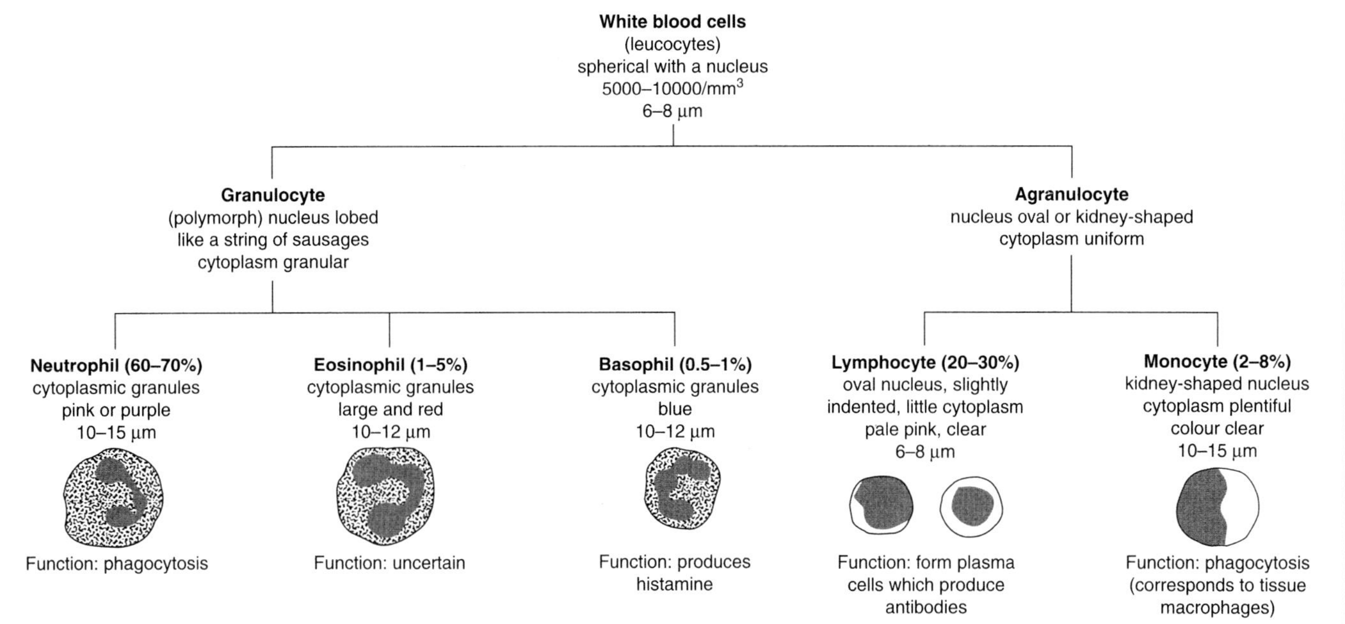

Fig. 13.35 Different Types of White Blood Cells found in Human Blood

Practical 64 – OBSERVING RED BLOOD CELLS IN HUMAN BLOOD

Red blood cells (RBC) or erythrocytes are by far the most numerous blood cells and are amongst the simplest of cells. There are about 5.5 x 10^6 (5.5 million) erythrocytes per mm^3 of human blood and up to 25 trillion in 5 litres of human blood. The structure is highly befitting their function. They are biconcave disks, thinner in the centre than its edges. The human RBC lack a nucleus at maturity and their cytoplasm is less elaborate than that of most cells. They lack mitrochondria and generate their ATP exclusively anaerobically and yet at the chemical level they perform the specialised job of taking up oxygen in the lungs and transporting it to the tissues. As small as a RBC is, it carries about 25 million molecules of haemoglobin. Bear this in mind as you examine them.

This investigation involves making a slide of your own blood. If you find it impossible to prick yourself use a prepared slide of human blood.

Caution: ***use a sterilised lancet and dispose of it in a beaker of disinfectant.***

Procedure

1. Sterilise the skin of your finger or thumb by rubbing it with cotton wool soaked in ethanol. Put an elastic band round it.
2. Using a sterile lancet, obtain a drop of blood and prepare a smear as shown in **Fig. 13.36**.
3. Allow the smear to dry, then examine it under the microscope first under low power, then high power. Record your observations by drawing what you see. You will see large numbers of red blood cells. Note the shape and colour of the cells.
4. Examine a single red blood cell in as much detail as you can.
5. Using an eyepiece graticule and a micrometer slide (**see page 20**), measure the diameter of a red blood cell and compare it with an animal cell.

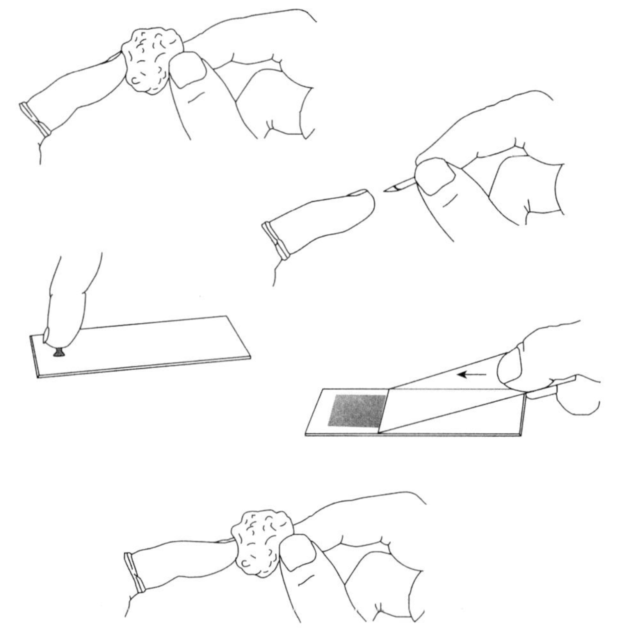

Fig. 13.36 Preparation of Blood Smear

6. Examine a prepared slide of a frog's blood under the microscope and compare it to human blood cells.
7. Examine transmission and scanning electron micrographs of red blood cells **Fig. 13.37**.

For consideration

(a) Each haemoglobin molecule carries four oxygen molecules. Calculate the number of oxygen molecules in a single RBC when its haemoglobin is saturated with oxygen.

(b) There are about 5.5×10^6 (5.5 million) erythrocytes per mm^3 of blood. Each heartbeat pumps about 60 cm^3 of oxygenated blood from the left ventricle into the aorta and then to the capillaries of the body. Calculate the number of oxygen molecules carried by the blood, which leaves the left ventricle with each contraction, assuming that all the haemoglobin molecules are saturated with oxygen.

(c) Assuming that the heartbeat is 72 per minute. Calculate the number of oxygen molecules supplied to the tissues and the oxygen demand of the tissues per day.

(d) Assume that all oxygen is required to oxidise glucose. The equation for aerobic respiration indicates that six moles of oxygen are required to release 2880 kJ of energy:

$$C_6H_{12}O_6 + 6O_2 \rightarrow 6CO_2 + 6H_2O \; -2880\text{kJ mol}^{-1}$$

(e) If the daily energy intake of normal healthy man is 12000 kJ how many moles of oxygen does he need daily to fulfil his energy requirements?

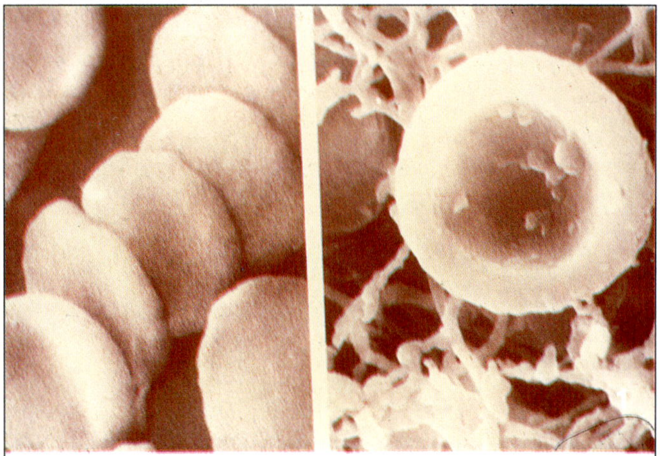

Fig. 13.37 Red Blood Cells (*Erytherocytes*)
SEM showing the biconcave disc-shape of RBCs.

(f) How many molecules of oxygen does this represent? (**Avogadro number = 6×10^{23}**).

(g) Is your estimate of the oxygen supplied consistent with your estimate of the oxygen required? If not, explain any discrepancy.

(h) Of what relevance is the calculation you carried out on oxygen supply and demand?

(i) Why do you think it is better to have haemoglobin inside the cells rather than free in the plasma?

(j) In the electron microscope red blood cells show little internal organisation i.e. the usual cell organelles are absent. Comment on this in relation to its functions.

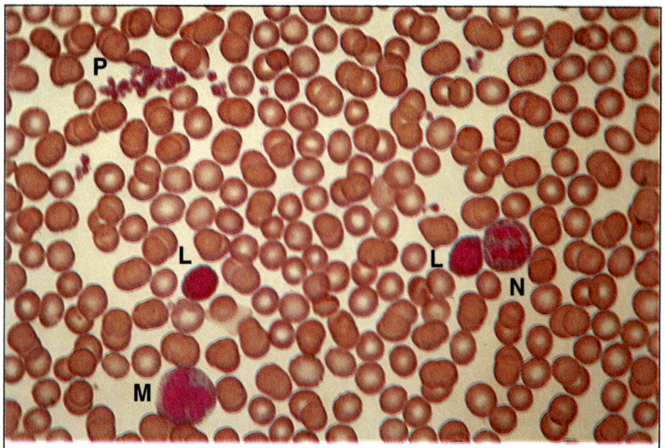

Fig. 13.38 Blood film (human) showing red blood cells, lymphocytes **L**, monocyte **M**, neutrophil **N** and platelets **P**.

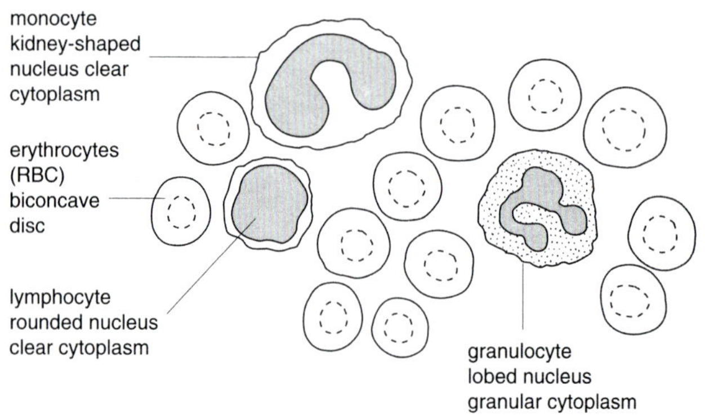

Fig. 13.39 Human Blood Cells

Practical 65 – OBSERVING WHITE BLOOD CELLS IN HUMAN BLOOD

Blood is a complex circulating tissue consisting of red and white blood cells and platelets suspended in a fluid medium, called the plasma. There are five major types of white blood cells or **leucocytes**: **monocytes, neutrophils, eosinophils, basophils** and **lymphocytes.** Collectively they combat all infections. Normally there are between 5,000-10,000 leucocytes present in a mm^3 of blood, mostly in transit. Leucocytes can easily be distinguished from RBC as they are quite large and possess a nucleus. Platelets are comparatively very small and clump together.

No staining is required to see the red blood cells, but to distinguish the leucocytes and the platelets staining is necessary.

Procedure

Stain a blood smear with Leishman's stain or Wright's stain which consists of a mixture of eosin and methylene blue as follows:

1. Wipe two clean glass slides with a swab of ethanol.
2. Sterilise a finger using an ethanol swab. Using a clean lancet prick and draw a drop of blood **Fig. 13.36.**
3. Place the blood on the glass slide and make a blood smear.
4. Allow the smear to air dry; add eight drops of stain to the smear. Leave for about 45 seconds.

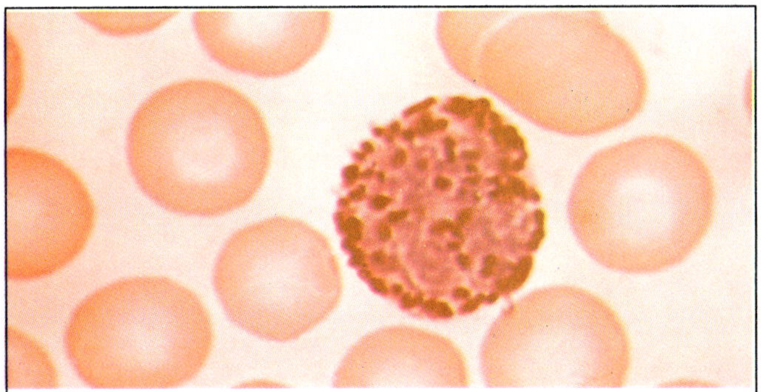

Fig. 13.40 Basophil
Bi-lobed nucleus. Dark pink granular cytoplasm of uniform size.

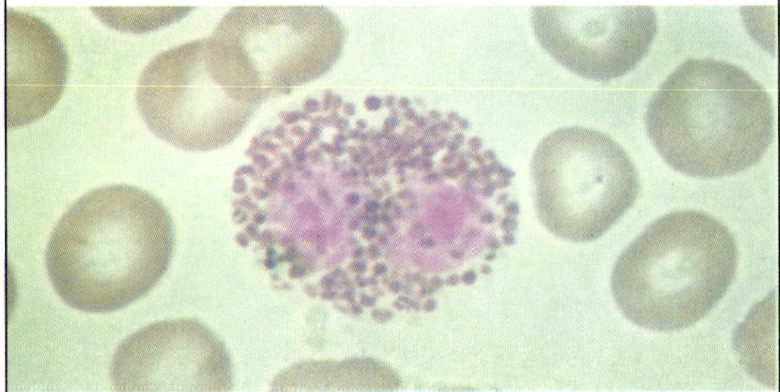

Fig. 13.41 Eosinophil
Least common leucocyte. Bi-lobed nucleus. Deep blue granular cytoplasm.

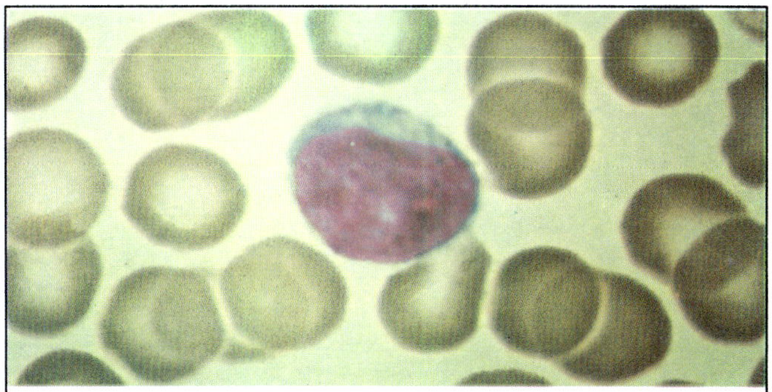

Fig. 13.42 Lymphocyte
Smallest leucocyte, round densely stained nucleus and a small amount of basophilic, pale, clear nucleus.

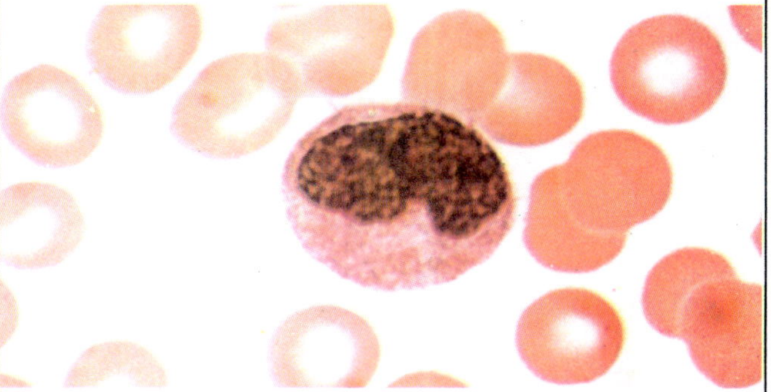

Fig. 13.43 Monocyte
Large, often indented nucleus stains less intensely than other leucocytes. The large cytoplasm is granular due to many lysosomes.

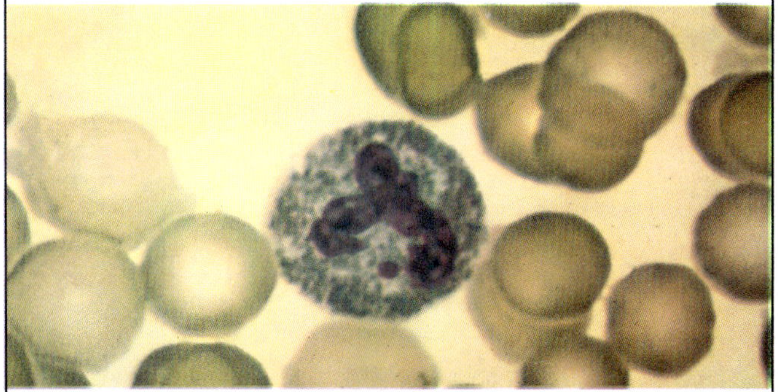

Fig. 13.44 Neutrophils
Most common leucocyte. Highly lobulated nucleus, as many as five lobules in mature nutrophil connected by a thin thread.

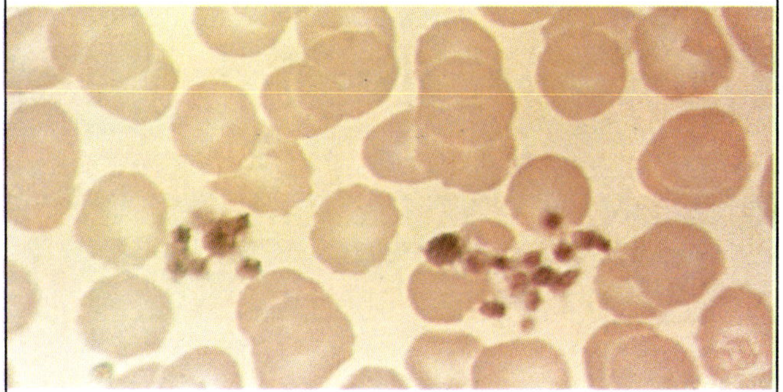

Fig. 13.45 Platelets or thrombocytes.
Small, non-nucleated cells. Appear as single or clumps of purple dots.

5. Add eight drops of distilled water to the stain; mix by rocking the slide. Leave for about 10 minutes.
6. Wash off the excess stain under a gentle stream of water.
7. Blot dry with filter paper and observe under low and high power of the microscope without a coverslip.
8. If you want to preserve the smear a coverslip can be added using Canada balsam.
9. White blood cells stain blue-purple and have a prominent nucleus. Platelets will appear as small groups of purple dots, try to identify five types of white blood cells, by referring to **Figs. 13.40–13.45**.
10. Distinguish between the **granulocyte** (**polymorph**) with its granular cytoplasm and **lobed nucleus** (which looks like a string of sausages) and the **agranulocytes** with its non-granular cytoplasm and large spherical or bean-shaped nucleus. Generally the most common type of granulocyte is the neutrophil, and the most common type of agranulocyte is the lymphocyte.

For consideration

(a) Which are the most numerous of the five types of white cells in your own blood smear?
(b) Leucocytes spend a lot of their time outside the circulatory system in the plasma. How do they get there and why?
(c) Is any type absent altogether as far as you can see? If so, explain why?
(d) Leishman's stain consists of a mixture of acidic eosin (pink) and alkaline methylene blue (blue). Can you explain why the three types of granulocytes stain differently with these stains, and why they are given their respective names?

Reference: UCLES, Question 3, 9th Nov. 1994.

Practical 66 – ESTIMATING THE NUMBER OF WHITE BLOOD CELLS IN HUMAN BLOOD

Red blood cells and white blood cells can be counted using a **haemocytometer**. Such counts are clinically important, because abnormally high or low blood cell count could be indicative of certain diseases.

Haemocytometer

For details on how to use the haemocytometer **see page 30**. Examine the haemocytometer slide under low power and identify the **type-B squares**. These are the squares you should use for your white cell count. Each type-B square has an **area of 1/25 mm^2**, and **the volume represented by a type-B square is 0.0004 mm^3.**
The pipette used for white blood cells is larger of the two, the one with the mark II above the bulb. Make sure the slide and pipette are clean.

Caution: ***Organise yourself before you begin, if you delay in adding the stain, the blood will clot inside the pipette, and you will have to start all over again.***

Procedure

Work in pairs.

1. Sterilise a finger using an ethanol swab. Using a sterilised lancet prick and draw a large drop of blood **Fig. 13.36**. Do not squeeze out the blood too vigorously, this will force out a lot of tissue fluid which will dilute the cell concentration.
2. With the rubber tubing attached to the pipette, suck the blood up to the 'I' mark. Quickly dry the tip of the pipette. If the 'I' mark has been passed, touch the tip of the pipette with filter paper until the blood drops back to the 'I' mark.
3. Carefully suck up Turk's solution until the **contents of the pipette reach the 'II' mark**. If the 'II" mark is passed, you have to empty the pipette and start again.
4. Close the two ends of the pipette with thumb and finger and rock the pipette for at least one minute to mix the blood and Turk's solution thoroughly. Blow out about six drops to expel excess Turk's solution. **Your blood sample is now diluted 1/10.**
5. Put one drop of diluted blood from the pipette onto the centre of the slide, on top of the grid and place the coverslip on top.
6. Place the slide on the bench and press firmly. You should be able to see the Newton's rings. Wait for a few minutes to allow the cells to settle.
7. Meanwhile rule out the grid of type-B square on paper or use a graph paper.
8. Observe the slide under the microscope and count the white blood cells in at least ten type-B squares.
9. Write the number of cells in each square on your grid. **Note: In each square, count all the cells which lie entirely within it, plus those that are touching or overlapping the top and left hand sides. Do not include those touching or overlapping the bottom and right hand sides even if they are within the square.**
10. Calculate the average number of cells in a type-B square. Take into consideration the dilution factor and the volume represented by a type-B square, calculate the number of white cells per mm^3 **see page 30.**
11. Calculate the number of white blood cells in your blood.

For consideration

(a) In what circumstances would you expect there to be, temporarily or permanently, an abnormally large number of white blood cells in the bloodstream?
(b) Turk's solution stains the white cells but red blood cells are rendered invisible, how does this occur?

Practical 67 – STRUCTURE OF THE MAMMALIAN RESPIRATORY APPARATUS

For respiration to take place, **gaseous exchange** with the environment is essential, the mechanism of which varies from organism to organism. In small flattened organisms the **surface volume ratio** is large enough for gas exchange to take place by **diffusion** across the surface. Larger more compact organisms, with a smaller surface volume ratio, have developed special **respiratory surfaces** for efficient gas exchange.

In plants the respiratory structures are the stomata and lenticles with a network of intercellular spaces, whereas in animals the respiratory surfaces range from the **tracheal system** of insects to **gills** in fishes to highly complex **lungs** in the mammals.

In humans air is drawn by expansion of the thorax into the **lungs Fig. 13.46** where gas exchange takes place by diffusion across greatly folded and highly vascularised **alveolar** surface.

The rate of respiration reflects the demand for oxygen by the organism and can be measured with a simple **respirometer Fig. 10.3** or a **spirometer Fig. 10.4** for humans.

Structurally and functionally the respiratory apparatus of the mammal can be divided into two components. The **respiratory surface,** where the gaseous exchange takes place and the **respiratory tract**, the tubes through which the gases move to and from the respiratory tract are intimately connected to the blood stream. For gas exchange to take place efficiently the respiratory tract should remain open and free from obstruction for ease of gas movement.

Structure of Respiratory Tract

1. If a whole mammalian lung is available with the trachea intact, attach a piece of rubber tube to the end of the trachea and blow to see how the lung tissue expands when fully inflated.
2. Examine the **trachea**. Note the **C-shaped cartilage rings** and that the cut in the C-shaped cartilage rings are on the dorsal side, adjacent to the oesophagus.
3. Dissect the trachea and try and follow the tube as far as possible into the lung tissue. Observe the difference in diameter and the structure of the wall of the tube along its path.
4. Using a prepared slide of the transverse section of the trachea and **Figs. 13.49, 13.50** identify and make labelled drawings of the structures of the tracheal wall under low and high power. Note the following:
   i. **pseudostratified ciliated columnar epithelium** interspersed with **goblet cells** on the inner lining of the tracheal wall;
   ii. location of the **mucus glands** in the **submucosa**, below the epithelium;
   iii. location of the blood vessels.
5. Examine the transverse section of **bronchioles**. Note the absence of the cartilage rings. At this point the bronchial wall consists of smooth muscle, connective tissue, possessing **elastic fibres**, and an inner lining of ciliated epithelium interspread by mucus secreting goblet cell.

Structure of the Respiratory Surface

1. Examining the fresh lung tissue, note that the tissue is spongy, slimy, moist and very soft to touch.
2. Using **Figs. 13.50–13.55** examine a prepared slide of a mammalian lung, under low power and high power. Notice how numerous the alveoli in the section are. There are over 700 million alveoli in the lung of a mammal, with a total surface area of 80-90 m^2.
3. Note the **squamous epithelium** lining the alveolus outside which is a dense network of capillaries (all of which originate from the pulmonary artery and will rejoin the pulmonary vein). Collagen and elastic fibres are also present.
4. **Blood vessels** can be distinguished from other cavities by the fact that they contain red blood cells.
5. **Arteries** can be distinguished from **veins** by the thickness of the muscular walls and the capillaries are lined by a single layer of **pavement epithelium.**
6. **Bronchi** and the **bronchioles** can be distinguished by the fact that the bronchi are larger, and contain **glands** and cartilage in their walls. Bronchioles are smaller and have no glands or cartilage in their walls, and are lined with ciliated epithelium.
7. Examine electron micrographs of the alveoli **Figs. 13.53, 13.55** and note that the boundary between alveolus and the capillaries is only two cells thick, note also the giant **alveolar cells** in the alveolus cell walls, which secrete **surfactant** inside the alveolus **Fig. 13.47.**

For consideration

(a) Why is the lung tissue moist and slimy and why is this important?

(b) Comment on the location and function of:
   i. ciliated cells;
   ii. C-shaped cartilage rings;
   iii. pseudostratified epithelium;
   iv. pavement epithelium in the capillaries,
   v. squamous epithelium in the alveoli;
   vi. elastic fibres in the bronchiole;
   vii. the mucus secreting cells;
   viii. the muscle fibres in the walls of the trachea and bronchi.

(c) What is surfactant and what is its function?

(d) The diameter of the capillaries is smaller than the diameter of the red blood corpuscles passing through them. How does this help oxygen uptake, and how are they able to pass through?

(e) How is the structure of the lung adapted to perform the function of rapid gaseous exchange?

Reference: UCLES, Question 3, 2nd Nov. 1992.
Reference: UCLES, Question 3, 23rd May, 1995.
Reference: UCLES, Question 3, 4th Nov. 1998.

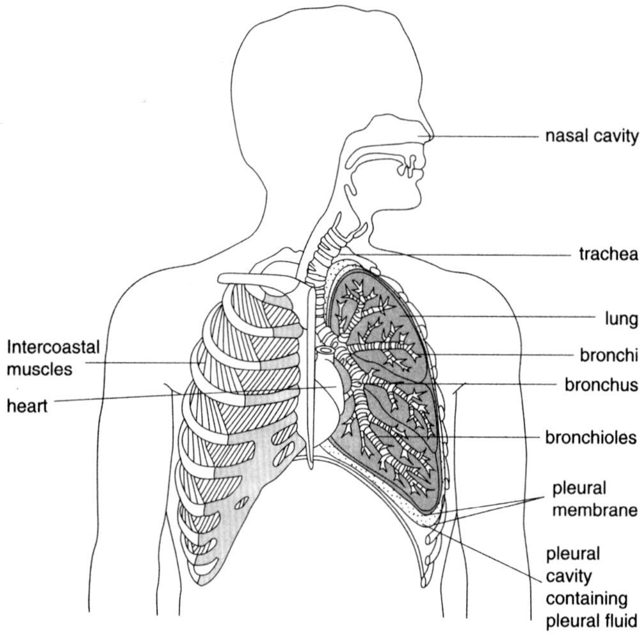

Fig. 13.46 Human Respiratory System

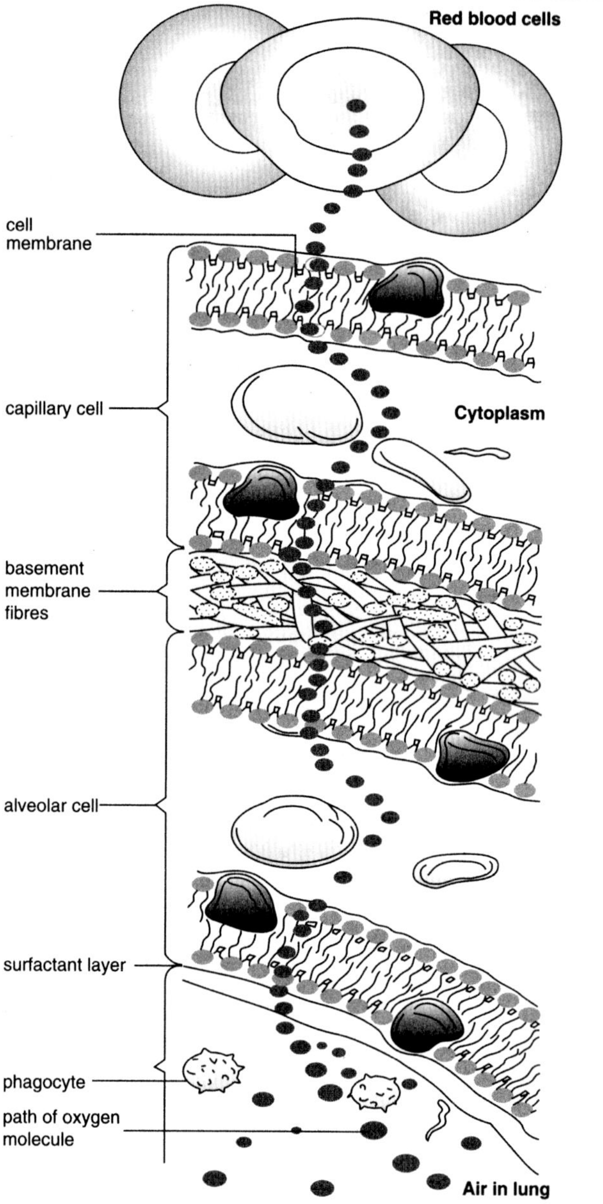

Fig. 13.48 Oxygen Diffusing into Blood

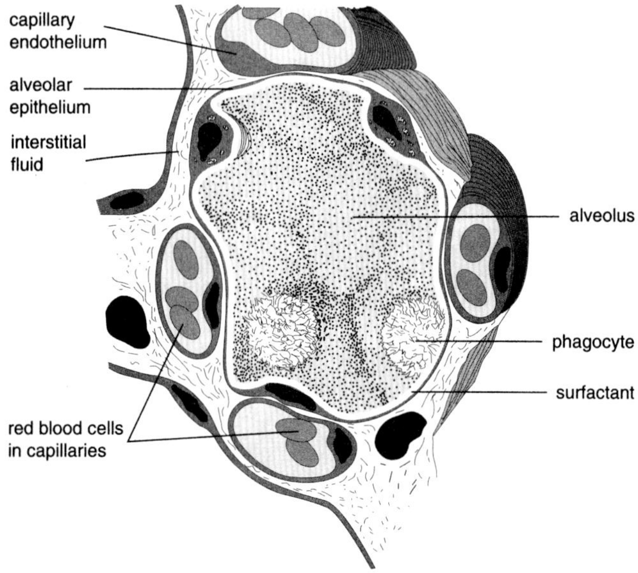

Fig. 13.47 Alveolus and Associated Pulmonary Capillaries

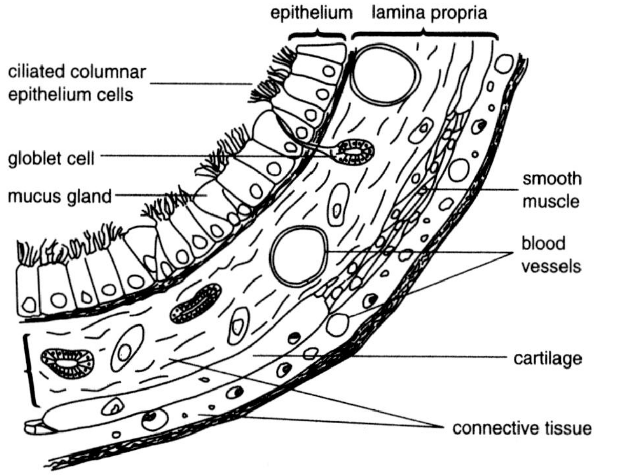

Fig. 13.49 TS of Tracheal Wall

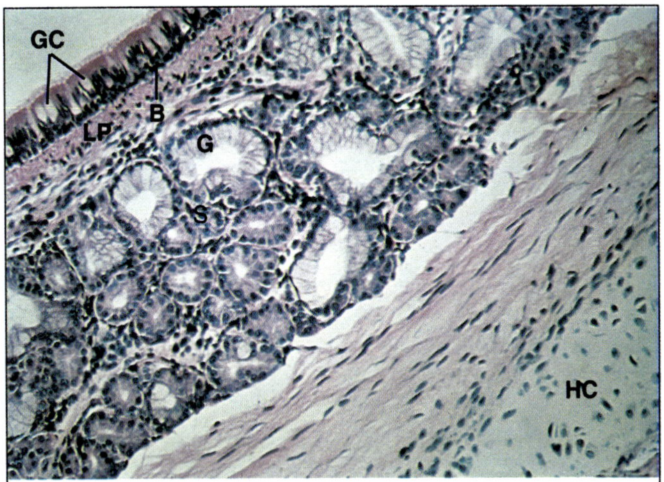

Fig. 13.50 Tracheal Epithelium and Glands.
Tracheal epithelium is psedostratified and ciliated containing goblet cells **GC**. Beneath the basement membrane **B** is the lamina propria **LP** consisting of highly vascularised connective tissue. Underlying the **LP**, loose submucosa **S** containing sero-mucus glands **G**, beneath which is hyaline cartilage **HC**.

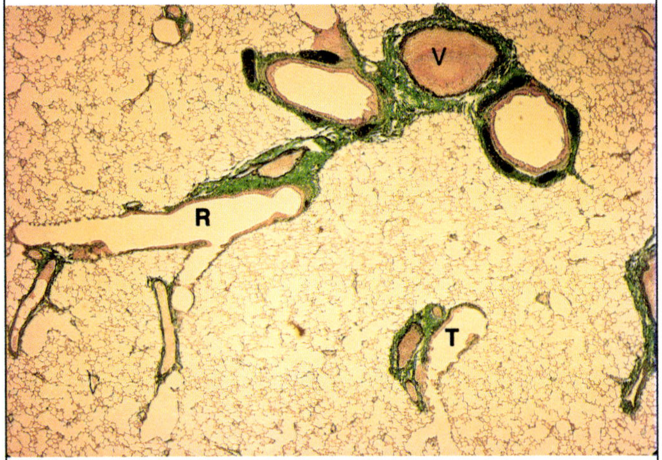

Fig. 13.51 Mammal lung (TS).
Terminal bronchiole **T** divides to form respiratory bronchioles **R.** Surrounding each alveolus is a rich network of capillaries supplied by pulmonary vessels **V**.

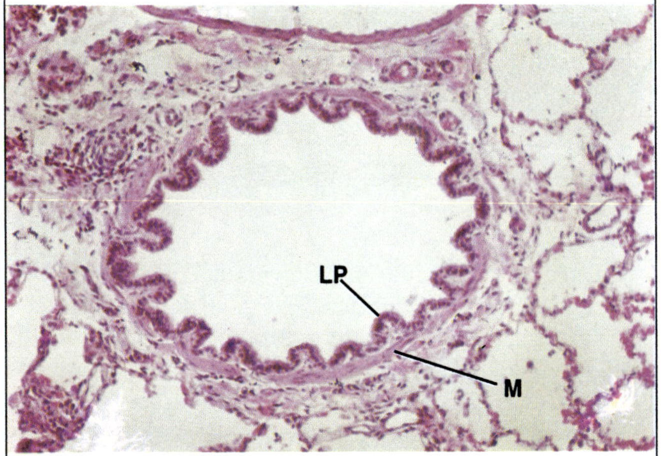

Fig. 13.52 Bronchiole.
Bronchiole has no cartiliginous support, lamina propria **LP** is thin, elastic and completely surrounded by smooth muscle layer **M.**

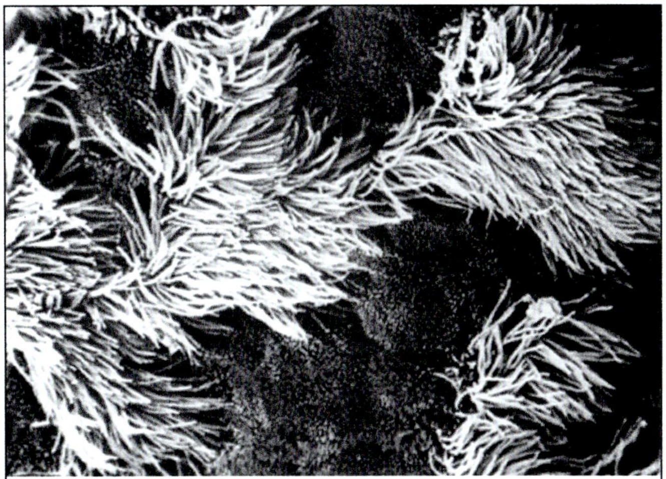

Fig. 13.53 EM of Lung of Alveolous showing Tracheal Epithelium.
The ciliated epithelia are clumped together amongst goblet cells **G.**

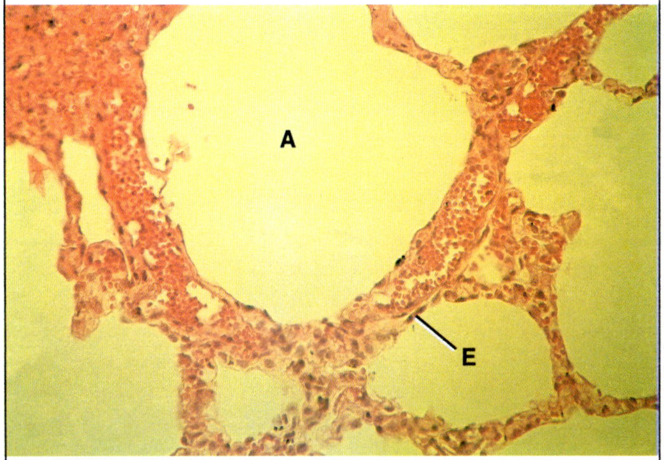

Fig. 13.54 Lung Alveoli A in man (TS).
Note the thin inner lining of epithelium **E** covering the entire alveolus **A**. Capillaries from plexus surround each alveolus.

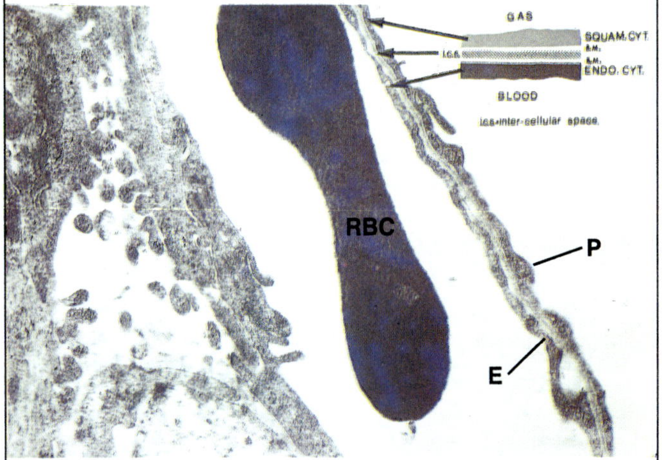

Fig. 13.55 Electron micrograph of alveolar wall between two alveoli.
Note the capillary endothelium **E**, red blood cells **RBC** and the pneumocytes **P** of the alveolar surface.

Practical 68 – MICROSCOPIC STRUCTURE OF THE GASTROINTESTINAL TRACT

The gastrointestinal tract is primarily involved in reducing food for absorption. The process occurs in five distinct phases within defined regions of the tract: **ingestion**, **fragmentation**, **digestion**, **absorption** and **elimination** of waste products.

The gastrointestinal system is essentially a muscular tract lined by mucus membrane, which exhibits regional variations in structure reflecting the changing functions of the system from the mouth to the anus.

After ingestion, fragmentation takes place in the **mouth** (facilitated by saliva) and is completed in by the muscular action of the **stomach** (aided by secretions from the stomach wall) where digestion begins.

Digestion is the process by which food is broken down by enzymes to molecules, small enough to be absorbed into the circulation. Proteins are broken down to amino acids, carbohydrates to glucose and the fats to lipid and glycerols. The amino acids and glucose are absorbed directly into the intricate network of associated capillaries of the **villi** and the lipids and glycerols, too large to enter the circulation directly enter via the **lacteals** at the centre of the villi.

Major part of the digestion takes place in the **duodenum** where enzymes from a large exocrine gland the **pancreas** enters the duodenum together with **bile** from the liver **Fig. 13.22**. When the digestion is almost completed in the duodenum, the duodenal content pass into the **jejunum** where process of digestion is completed and process of absorption takes place.

The unabsorbed semi-liquid is passed on into the **large intestine** where water is absorbed from the liquid residue, which becomes progressively more solid and is eventually excreted via the **anus**.

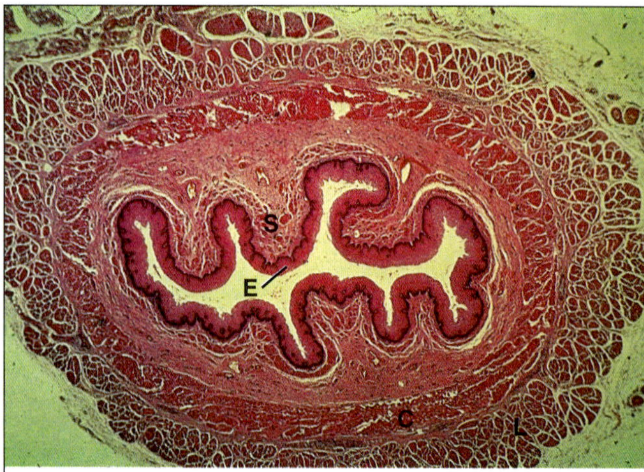

Fig. 13.56 Oesophagus.
The luman is lined by stratified squamous epithelium **E**. Submucosa **S** is highly vascular containing mucous glands. Muscularis is composed of circular **C** and longitudinal **L** smooth muscle.

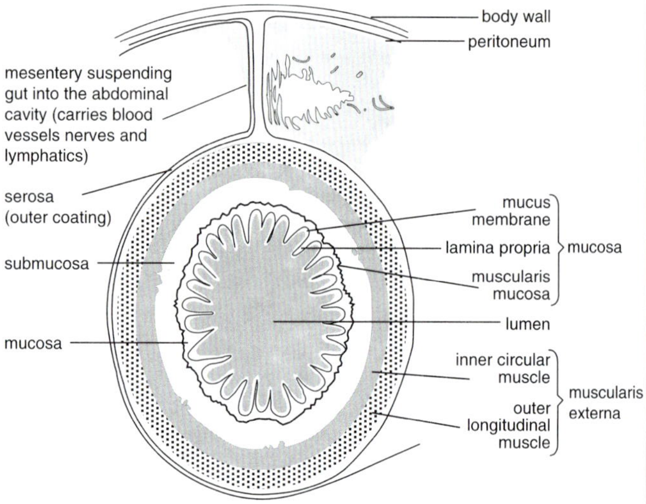

Fig. 13.57 Layers of Digestive Tract Wall

The structure of the gastrointestinal tract conforms to a general plan, which is consistent from the oesophagus to the anus.

A mucus membrane essentially lines the tract. The arrangement of the major muscular components remains relatively constant throughout the tract whereas the mucosa shows marked variations in the different regions of the tract.

Although the mammalian gastrointestinal tract shows regional differentiation, **Figs. 13.56, 13.57**, its wall can always be distinguished into four distinct layers:

i. The **mucosa:** consists of three distinct layers, an epithelial lining, (which shows various degrees of folding, is **protective**, **secretary**, and/or **absorptive**); a supporting connective tissue layer and a thin smooth muscle layer, the *muscularis mucosa,* which produces local movements of and folding of the mucosa.
ii. The **submucosa:** a layer of loose connective tissue supports the mucosa and contains the large blood vessels, lymphatics and nerves.
iii. The **muscularis propria:** the muscular wall proper consists of smooth muscle, which is subdivided into inner and outer longitudinal layers. The opposing action of these muscle layers is the basis of peristaltic contraction.
iv. The **adventia:** this outer layer of connective tissue conducts the major blood vessels and nerves. It is continuous with the connective tissue of the mesenteries and in other sites it is continuos with the surrounding connective tissue. Where the adventia is exposed to the abdominal cavity it is referred to as **serosa**, and is lined with simple squamous epithelium.

Glands are found throughout the tract at various depths in the tract wall. In some parts the mucus lining is arranged into glands, which have a variety of secretary functions. In other regions, glands penetrate the muscularis mucosa to lie in the submucosa. The pancreas and liver are large glands draining into the gastrointestinal lumen but lying entirely outside the tract wall.

Small intestine

Small intestine in humans is about 4-6 m in length, comprising the **duodenum**, **jejunum** and the **ileum**. It is the principal site for absorption of digestion in the gastrointestinal tract. The duodenum into which opens the **pancreatic** and **bile ducts Fig. 13.22**, leads into jejunum and then to ileum which is about 5m long. The submucosa of the duodenum is highly folded. The mucosa possess finger-like projections called **villi** whose walls are richly supplied with blood capillaries and lymph vessels and contain smooth muscle. Throughout the small intestine certain mucosal cells secrete mucus. Submucosal **Brunner's glands** also secrete mucus and alkaline fluid in the first part of the duodenum, which protects the intestinal mucosa from the acid pH of the stomach and provides the optimum pH at which the intestinal enzymes are active.

1. Examine a transverse and a longitudinal section of the ileum under low power. Observe and draw various layers of the wall mentioned above.
2. Examine your section under high power and answer the following questions:
   i. What sort of cells occur in the epithelium lining of the villi and the **crypt of Lieberkuhn** and what are their functions?
   ii. In what way is the epithelium adapted for absorption of the products of digestion?
   iii. What functions are performed by the various muscles, which are visible in your section?
3. Examine a section of the wall of the duodenum.
   i. How does it differ from that of the ileum?
4. Look at an electron micrograph of a section of small intestine. Notice in particular numerous microvilli projecting from the free surface of the cell.
   i. In what plane have they been cut? Identify other structures in the micrograph. If the structures are lettered state what each letter stands for.

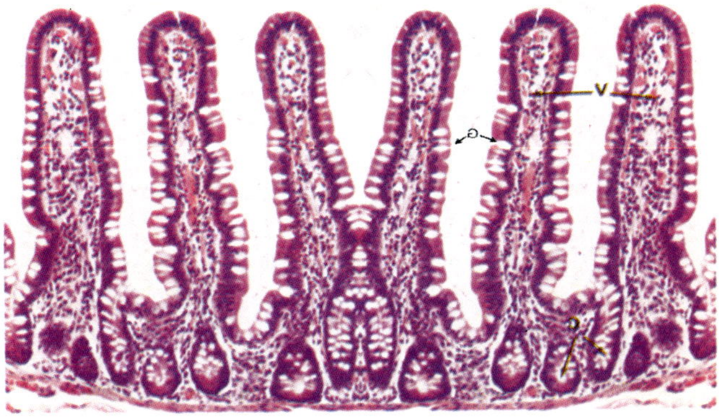

Fig. 13.58 Intestine Villi.
Intestine villi **V** are lined by simple columnar epithelium which are continuous with that of the crypts **C**. Note the mucus secreting gastric glands **G**.

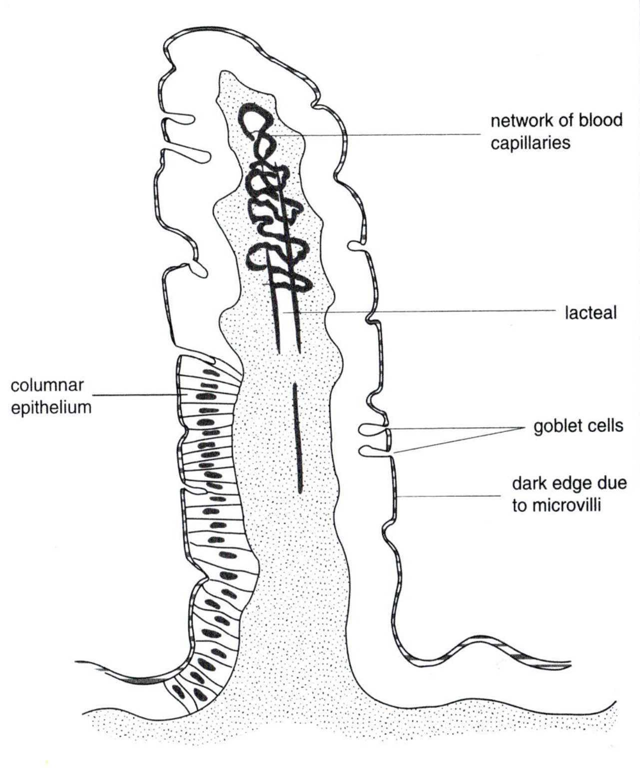

Fig. 13.59 Villus

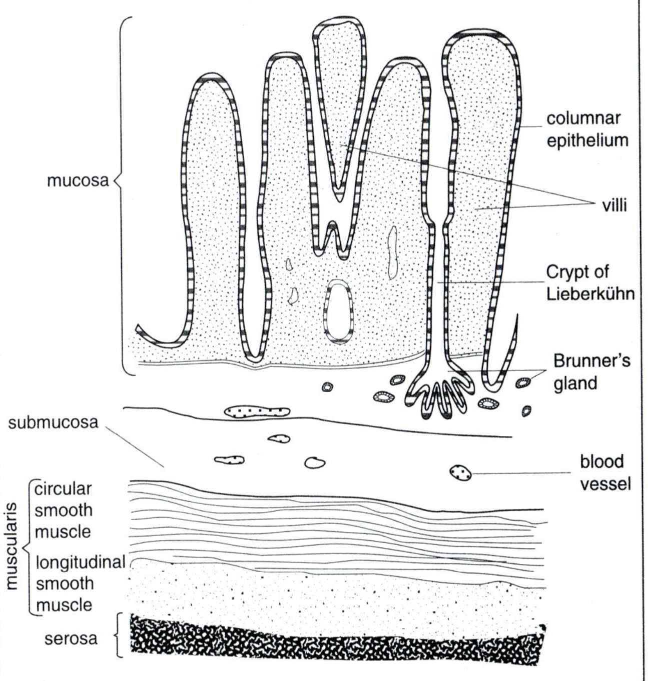

Fig. 13.60 TS Ileum Wall

Stomach

5. Examine a vertical section of the stomach. Identify various layers of the wall and compare them with the ileum. The mucosa possess millions of tubular glands, which open into gastric pits on the mucosal surface.

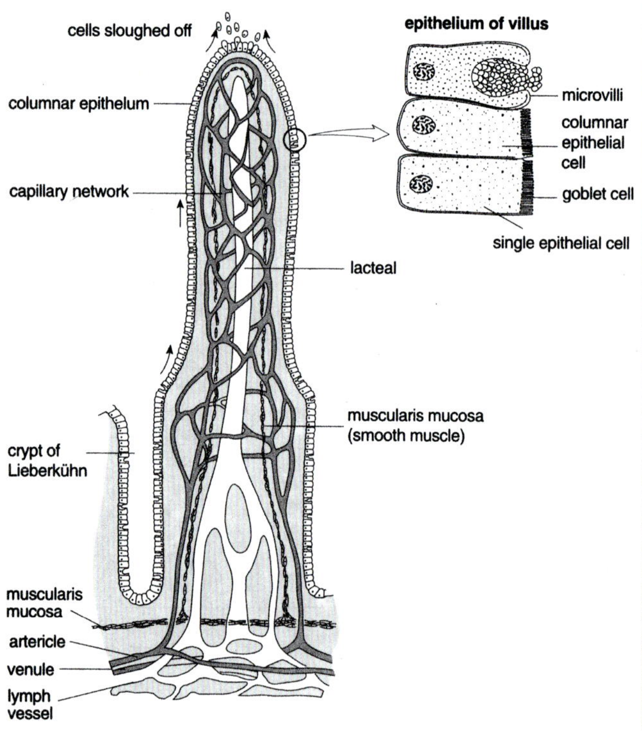

Fig. 13.61 Structure of the Villus

In the main body of the stomach these are lined with **parietal (oxyntic cells), zymogen** or **chief (peptic) cells** and **mucus cells.** Parietal (oxyntic) secrete a 0.04-0.05% HCl solution, making the pH of stomach 1-2.5, zymogen or chief (peptic) cells secrete enzymes pepsinogen and prorennin. In the distal stomach, near the pylorus, peptic and oxyntic cells are absent.

6. Examine and draw gastric glands in detail. Identify the epithelial cells lining the **gastric glands**, noting mucus secreting cells lining the neck and **gastric pits**, pear shaped parietal (oxyntic) cells at intervals along the length of the gland and closely packed chief (peptic) cells lining the deeper part of the gland.
   i. In what way is the wall of the stomach adapted for its function?
   ii. What is the function of the hydrochloric acid in the stomach?
   iii. What is the function of the pepsinogen?
   iv. What would happen to the activity of the intestinal enzymes if the pH in the duodenum remained at 2?

Other regions of the gut

In humans the bulk of water and inorganic salts are absorbed in the large intestine. Mucosal epithelial cells secrete mucus, which lubricates the solidifying food residue of **faeces**.

6. Examine and draw sections of the oesophagus, colon and rectum. Note the following:
   Oesophagus–inner lining of the stratified epithelium, outer layer of stratified circular muscles.

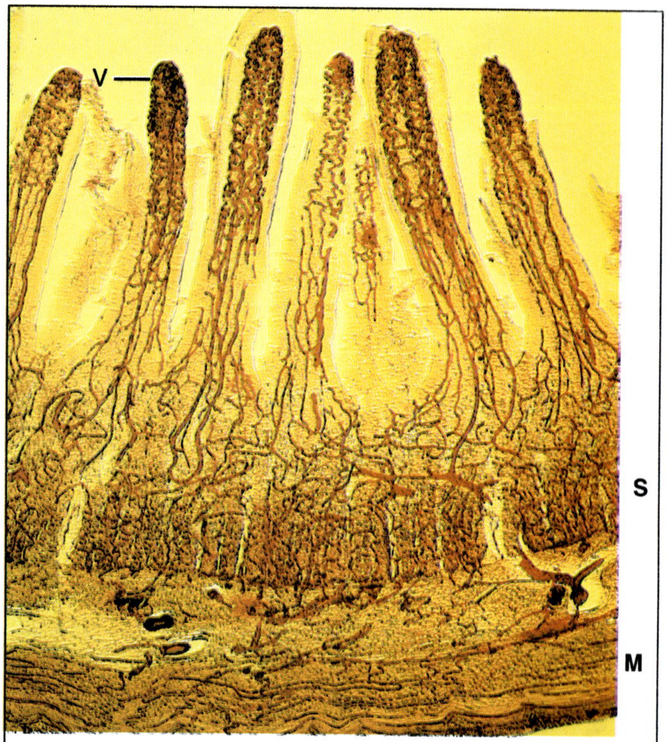

Fig. 13.62 Ileum (cat) Injected with Dye to Show Blood Vessels (TS).
Note the dense capillary network in submucosa **S**. Long branching capillaries extend upto the tip of the villi **V** with its brush borders. Note also the blood supply to the muscular wall **M**.

   Colon, rectum–walls contain simple tubular glands lined by numerous goblet cells.
   Compare their structure in relation to their functions.
7. Observe micrographs of various sections and identify as many structures as possible.

Reference: UCLES, Question 3, 24th May, 1994.
Reference: UCLES, Question 3, 4th Nov. 1998.

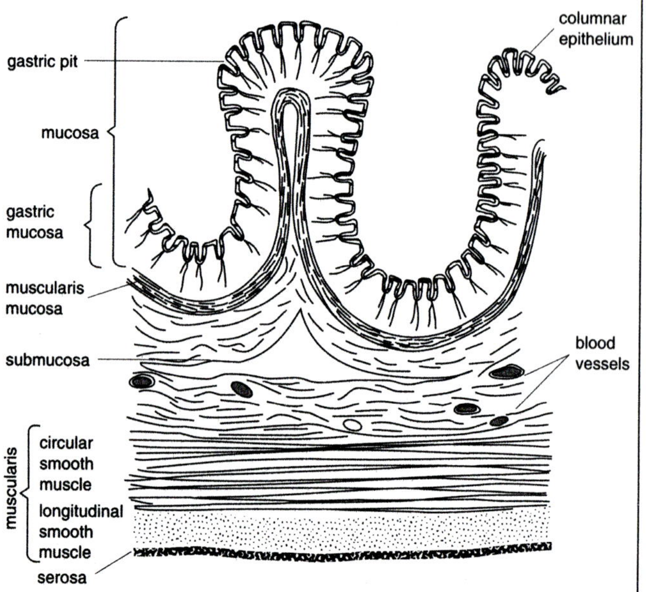

Fig. 13.63 LS Stomach Wall

Practical 69 – MICROSCOPIC STRUCTURE OF THE LIVER

Liver is a large organ, which lies immediately beneath the diaphragm. It makes up about 3-5% of the body's weight. Despite the numerous metabolic activities carried out by the liver its histological structure is fairly uniform and simple. The cells of the liver show no structural or functional differentiation and are called **hepatocytes**. The only other cells found in the liver are nerve cells and associated lymph and blood vessels.

The liver has a unique dual blood supply. Blood vessels from the **hepatic portal vein**, carrying absorbed materials from the alimentary canal, and the **hepatic artery**, carrying oxygenated blood, join together to form **'venules'** which supply blood to the hepatocytes. Smaller blood vessels called **sinusoid** originate from the venules to form a massive network of capillaries before joining together and eventually meeting the hepatic vein. The venules and the hepatocytes form functional units called **acinus**. The blood vessels criss-cross with channels called **bile canaliculi.** These form branching networks that join to form the **bile duct,** which eventually leave the liver as the **common hepatic duct**.

The liver has numerous functions; together with the kidneys; it regulates the metabolites and the composition of all body fluids.

Two of the liver's most important functions are:

i. Secretion of bile into the bile duct, which carries it to the gall bladder to the duodenum where bile salts speed up fat digestion.
ii. Maintains blood glucose at a constant level of 90mg cm^3 blood in humans.

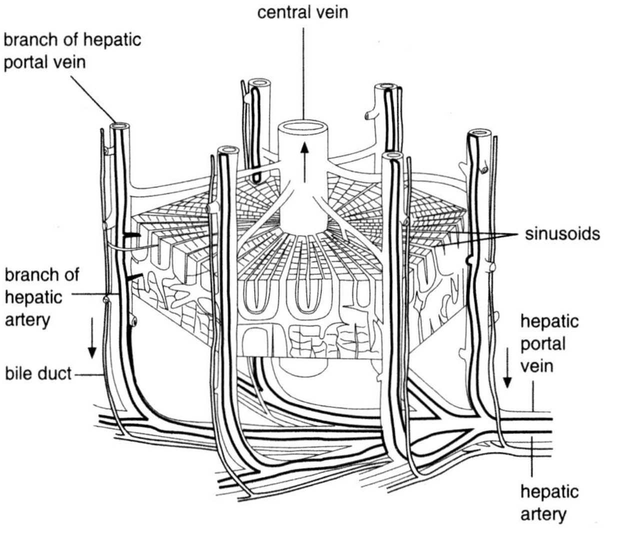

Structure of the Liver

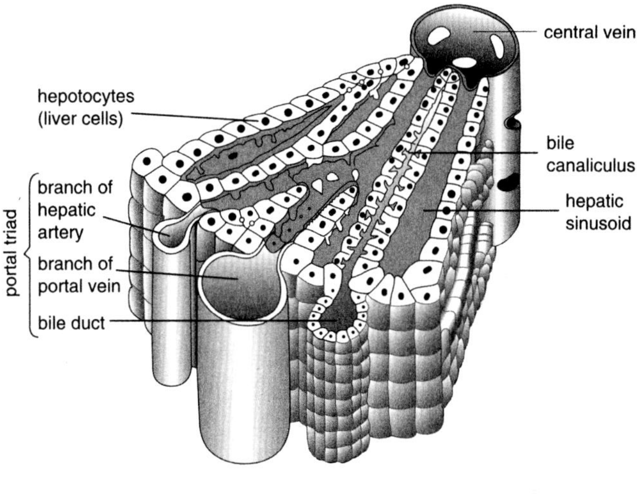

Section of a Liver Lobule

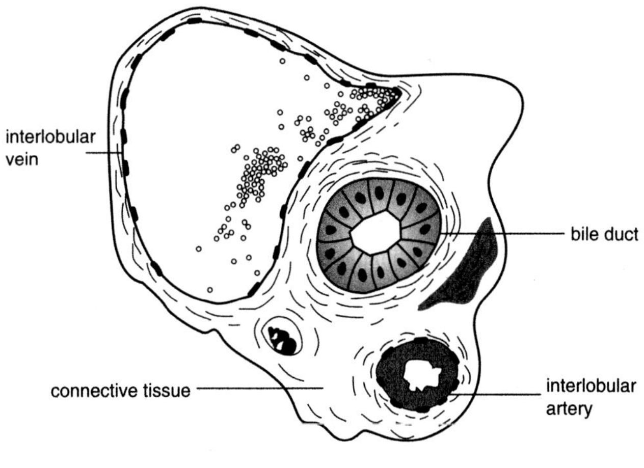

Fig. 13.64 Portal Tract between Lobules

Procedure

1. Examine a transverse section of a pig's liver under low power **Figs. 13.65, 13.66** (Human and other mammals' livers do not have distinct lobules.) Observe the closely packed **lobules** enclosed in connective tissue. Each lobule is hexagonal in shape, roughly 1.0 mm in diameter. A **central vein** is at the centre of the lobule and receives blood, which flows along the sinusoids from the portal vein and artery. Around the interlobular vein radiating rows of hepatocytes are arranged **Fig. 13.64.**
2. Between the lobules are the **interlobular blood vessels**, consisting of:
   i. an **arteriole** (branch of hepatic artery), small lumen, thick walls,
   ii. a **vein** (branch of hepatic portal vein), large lumen, thin walls,
   iii. and a **bile ductule** (branch of bile duct), intermediate in size, with distinct lining of cuboidal epithelium.

   Make labelled drawings of a liver lobule and interlobular blood vessels.

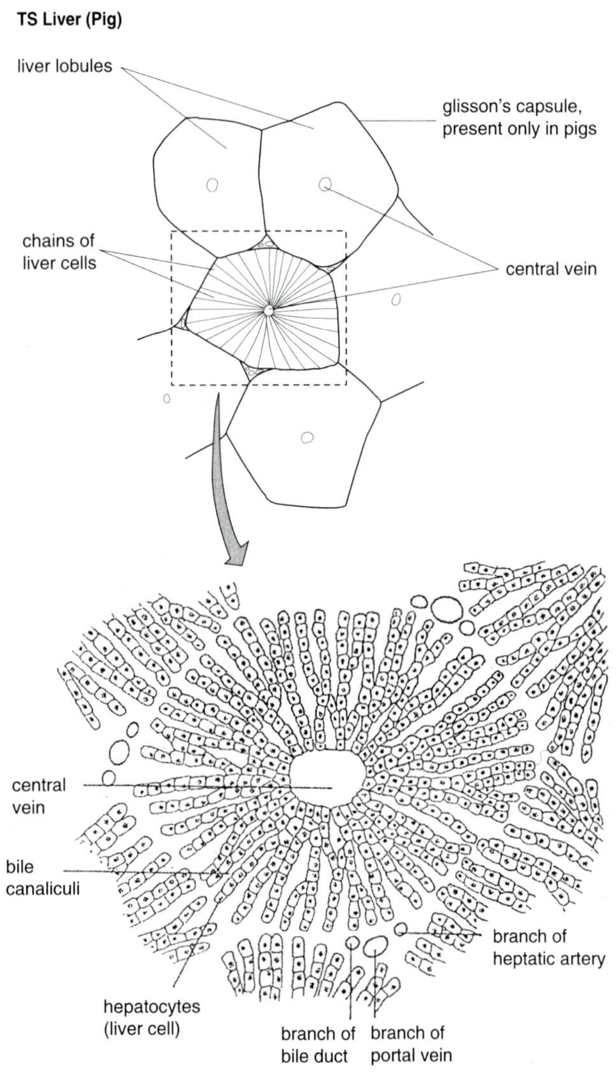

Fig. 13.65 Section of a Liver Lobule

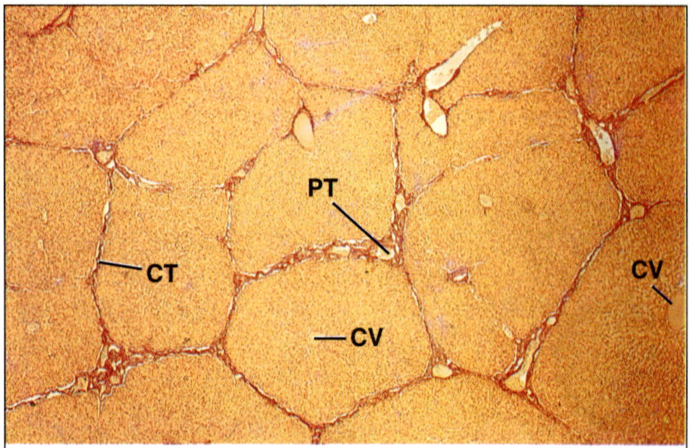

Fig. 13.66 Hepatic Lobule Pig's Liver (TS).
The hexagonal boundary of the lobule is defined by connective tissue **CT** (not visible in humans). Sinusoids **S** originate at the lobule margin and converge upon the central vein **CV**. Vessels of portal tract **PT** are visible.

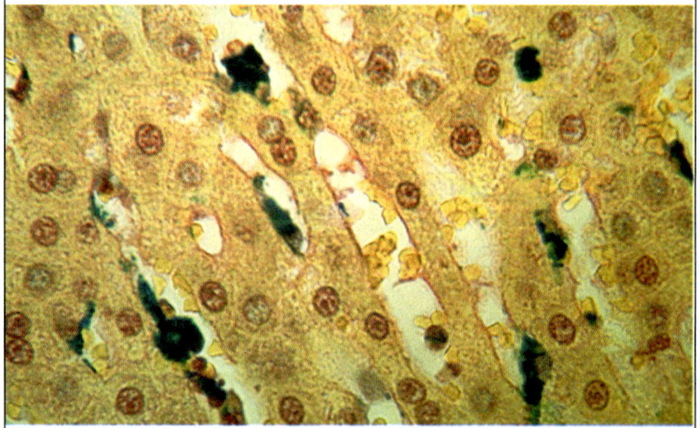

Fig. 13.67 Liver Parenchyma showing Kupffer Cells.
The phagocytic cells of the liver are called Kupffer cells (dark deposits), which participate with spleen in removal of spent RBC and other debris from circulation. Large hepatocytes with distinct neuclei with prominent nucleoli and chromatin granules are visible.

3. Examine the hepatocytes under high power, forming chain of cells. Each hepatocyte is regular in shape with prominent nuclei and granular cytoplasm, indicative of high activity **Figs. 13.65, 13.67**.
4. Observe the sinusoids lined with pavement epithelium. Between the chains of hepatocytes are phagocytic **Kupffer cells**. These cells are involved in the breakdown of old (spent) erythrocytes and ingestion of other pathogens.
5. Examination of an electron micrograph will reveal Golgi apparatus, many mitrochondria, lysosomes, lots of star-shaped **glycogen** granules and fat droplets. Make drawings of your observations.

For consideration

(a) How is the structure of the liver adapted to perform its functions?

(b) Why is the liver regarded as an exocrine gland?

(c) In most exocrine glands the basic functional unit is **acinus**, a branch of the duct and its associated secretary cells e.g. in the pancreas. What comprises an acinus in the liver?

Practical 70 – EXAMINATION OF THE MAMMALIAN RENAL SYSTEM

The kidney, the blood vessels that serve them, and the structures that carry urine formed in the kidneys is the **renal system** in vertebrates. In humans a pair of bean shaped organs called kidneys about 10cm long are located at the back of the abdominal cavity. Blood enters the kidney via the **renal artery** and leaves via the **renal vein**. Urine exits the kidney through a duct called the **ureter**. The ureters of both kidneys together drain into the **bladder**. Leading from the bladder a tube called **urethra** opens outside the body near the vagina in females and through the penis in the males. In this investigation you will examine the general structure of the mammalian renal system.

1. If possible observe the renal system in a freshly dissected mammal. Observe the rich blood supply via the renal artery bringing blood to the kidney from the dorsal aorta running close to the larger, thinned-walled, renal vein, which takes blood from the kidney to the posterior vena cava. (The kidneys make up >1% of body weight, yet receive 20% of the blood pumped with each heartbeat).
2. Locate the thin thread-like **ureter**, coming out from the indented inner side of the kidney running all the way down to the **bladder**.
3. Remove the kidney from the body (or use one bought from the butcher). Carefully remove the fat and slice through the kidney horizontally **Fig. 13.68** and notice the light coloured outer **renal cortex**, and a darker inner **renal medulla**. Notice the **pyramids** (onto which collecting ducts open), **pelvis** is the expanded cavity, which is the origin of the ureter.
4. Using a fresh kidney gently massage it in warm saline (1% NaCl solution) to empty the contents.
5. Using separate $5cm^3$ syringes, inject:
   i. the ureter with warm yellow latex, then tie a thread round it,
   ii. the renal artery with warm red latex, then tie a thread round it,
   iii. the renal vein with blue latex, then tie it with a thread.

   Allow the latex to cool. It will harden like rubber.
6. Carefully slice the kidney horizontally with a sharp razor blade. Observe the distribution of the latex. The yellow latex should have filled the pelvis and collecting ducts, the red latex the arteries and the blue latex the veins. Make labelled drawings of your observations.
7. Examine thin slices under the microscope and compare them with prepared sections of the kidney. Make labelled drawings of your observations.

For consideration

(a) How could you use this technique to estimate the total length of blood vessels in the kidney?
(b) Describe the pattern of collecting ducts in the kidney?
(c) Are your sections as you expected them to be, if not explain why?

Kidneys and their associated blood supply

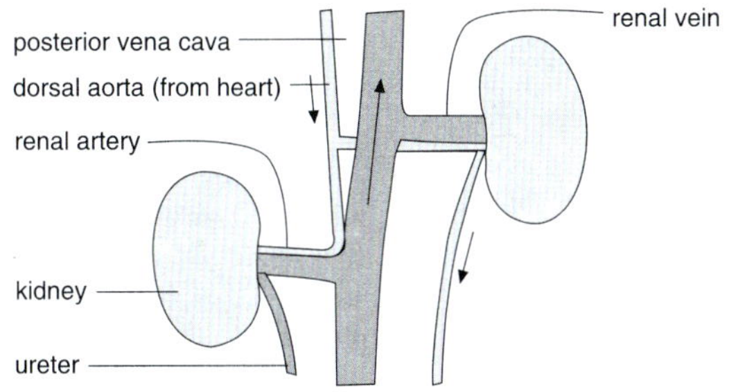

Kidney showing various planes in which it can be sectioned

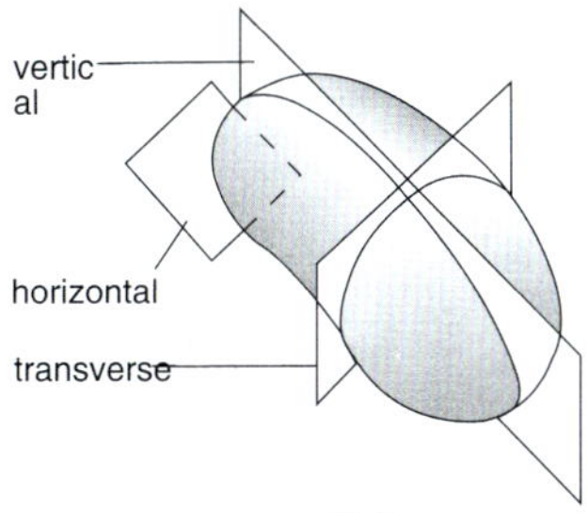

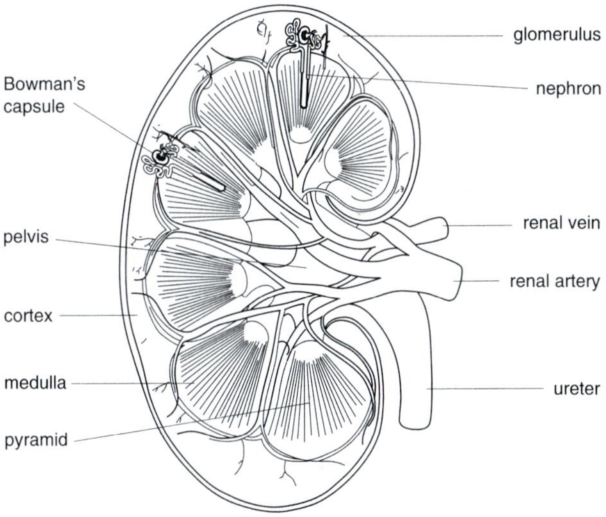

LS Section of a freshy bisected kidney

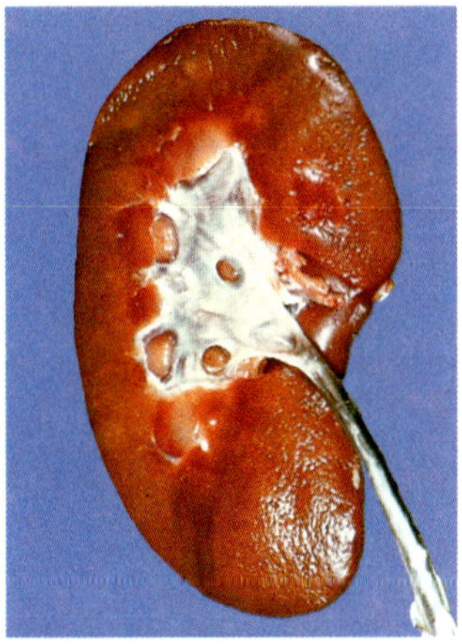

Fig. 13.68 Structure of the Kidney

Practical 71 – MICROSCOPIC STRUCTURE OF THE MAMMALIAN KIDNEY

Before examining the microscopic structure of the kidney consider its functions so that they can be related to the relevant structures.

The kidney is a major excretory, osmoregulatory, homeostatic organ of the body. It removes metabolic waste products and maintains the composition of the blood within a narrow range, by removal of substances in excess, and regulation of water balance and hence pH and body fluids. The functional unit of the kidney is the **nephron Fig. 13.71** where formation and processing of renal fluid are carried out. The kidney in humans contain about 1.5 million nephrons. Each nephron consists of two major components, the **Bowman's capsule** and the **renal tubules**.

The Bowman's capsule contains a ball of capillaries called the **glomerulus**, and a long differentiated tubule, which leads to a **collecting duct**. (Bowman's capsule and the glomerulus together comprise a **Malpighian corpuscle**) **Fig. 13.69, 13.72.**

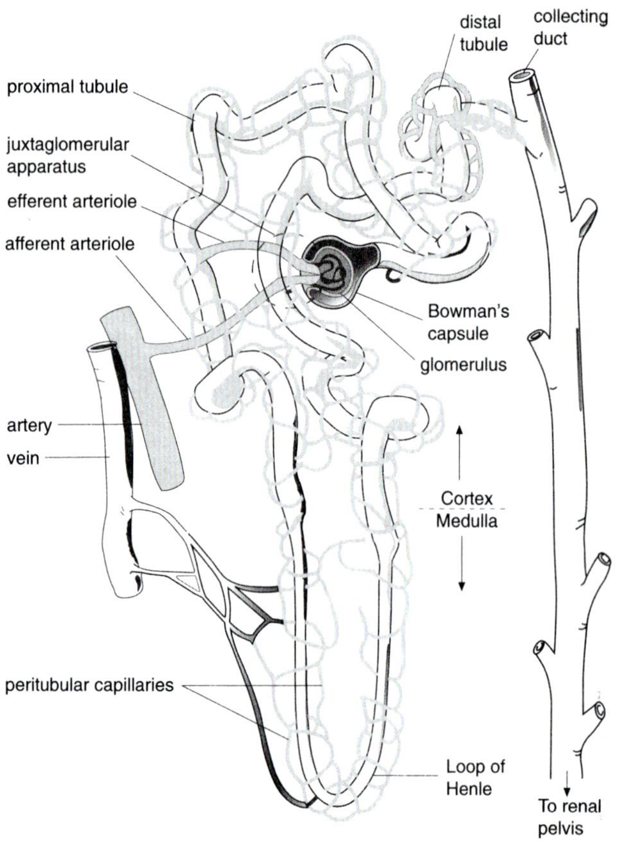

Fig. 13.71 Structure of the Nephron

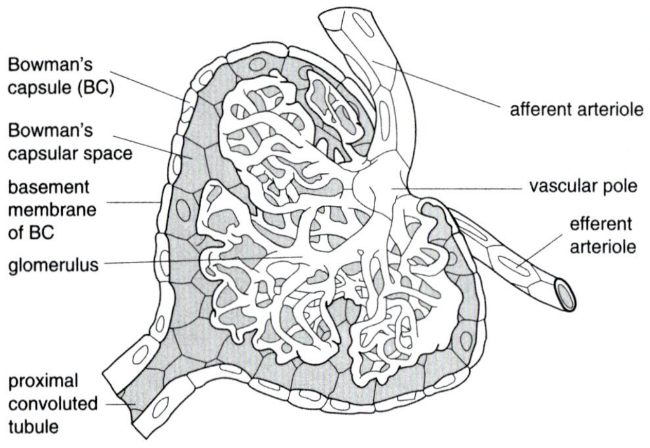

Fig. 13.69 Malpighian (renal) Corpuscle

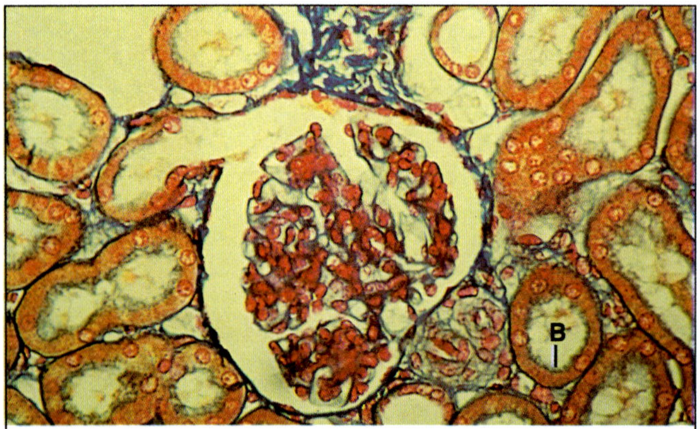

Fig. 13.70 Renal Corpuscle and Proximal Convulated Tubules. Simple cuboidal epithelium with prominent brushed borders **B** are visible. The cytoplasm of the proximal collecting tubule stains intensely indicative of high content of cell organelles, especially mitrochondria. Structure of Malpighian capsule is clearly visible.

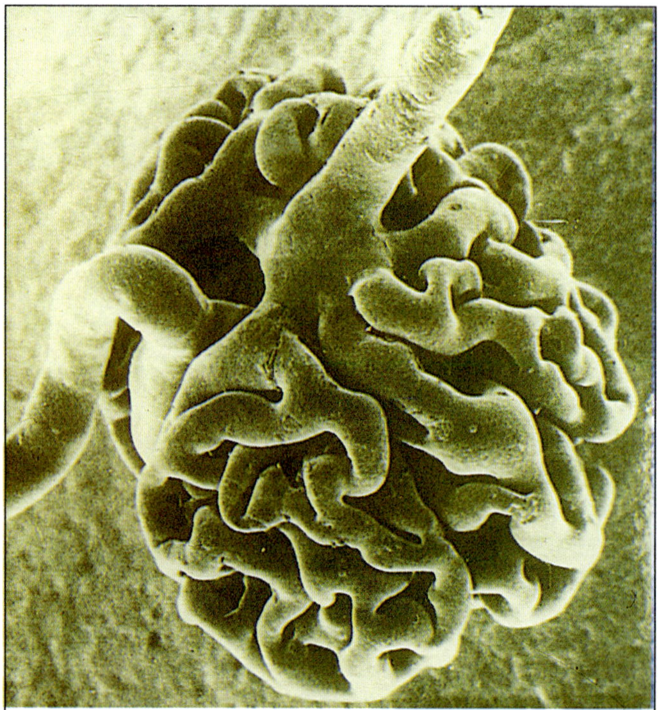

Fig. 13.72 SEM of Glomerulus shows the three dimensional tighly packed capillary loops C.

Blood is filtered across the wall of the glomerular capillaries into the cavity of Bowman's capsule (**capsular space**). The **glomerular filtrate**, (**renal fluid**) consists of plasma minus proteins.

From the Bowman's capsule, the filtrate passes through three regions of the nephron: the **proximal tubule**; the **loop of Henle**, a hairpin bend with a descending an ascending limb; and the **distal tubule**. The distal tubule empties into a **collecting duct**, which receives filtrate from lots of nephrons. Many collecting ducts empty into the **renal pelvis**, where useful substances are selectively reabsorbed back into the bloodstream, whilst harmful substances that escaped filtration are secreted from the blood into the tubule. To achieve this there is close association between the nephron and its blood supply. The nephrons are of two types, the **cortical nephrons** (80%) and the **juxtamedullary nephrons** (20%). In the human kidneys 80% of the **cortical nephrons** have reduced loop of Henle, and are almost entirely confined to the cortex. The **juxtamedullary nephrons** have long loops of Henle which extend deep into the renal medulla.

Procedure

Examine a prepared slide of mammalian kidney under low power and draw a plan diagram to show the cortex, medulla and the pelvis.

Cortex

i. Observe the cortex under low power. Notice the numerous Bowman's capsules, tubules and capillaries in the section. Find one that resembles **Fig. 13.70** and record your observations with detailed drawings, showing glomerulus, capsular space, **afferent** and **efferent arterioles**.

ii. The tubular structures visible in a section of the cortex are a mixture of proximal and distal convoluted tubules and collecting ducts. Using the information in the table on **page 193** locate and draw these tubules.

iii. Note in particular the proximal tubule, particularly its brush borders and its proximity to the capillaries.

Medulla

Examine the medulla under high power. This part of the kidney contains the **loops of Henley**, which connects the **proximal** with the **distal convoluted tubules**. Notice the descending and the ascending limbs of the loop of Henle and the long straight capillaries, **vasa recta**, running parallel with them. The wall of the thin limb is extremely similar to that of the capillaries (vasa recta). The capillaries can be distinguished by the fact that they contain red blood cells. Using the information in the table on **page 193** locate and draw the descending, ascending limb and the collecting ducts.

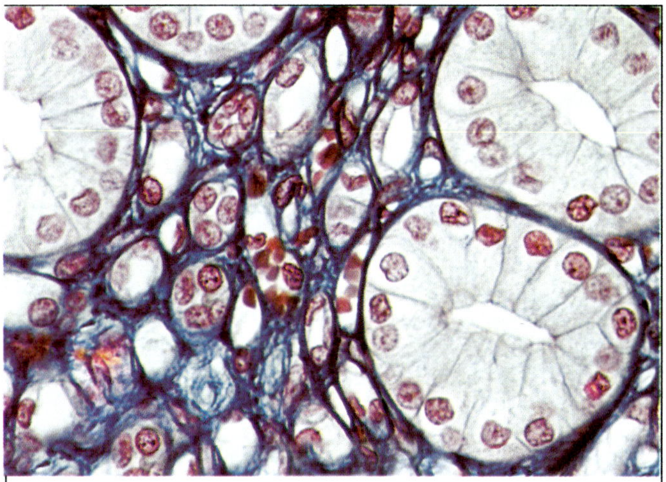

Fig. 13.73 Collecting Ducts CD, Thin Limb of Loop of Henle. Note tall columnar epithelium with distinct nuclei and absence of brushed border, thin limb of loop of Henle and vasa recta.

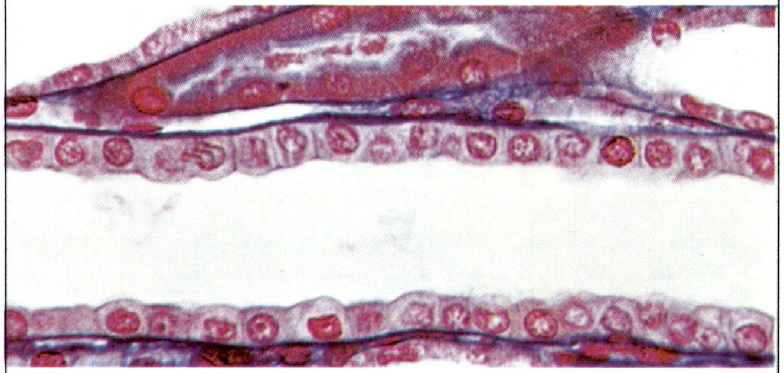

Collecting Tubules CT.
The section shows proximal section of **CT**. Note the absence of brushed borders and clear cytoplasm of the cuboidal cells with prominent nuclei indicative of reabsorption.

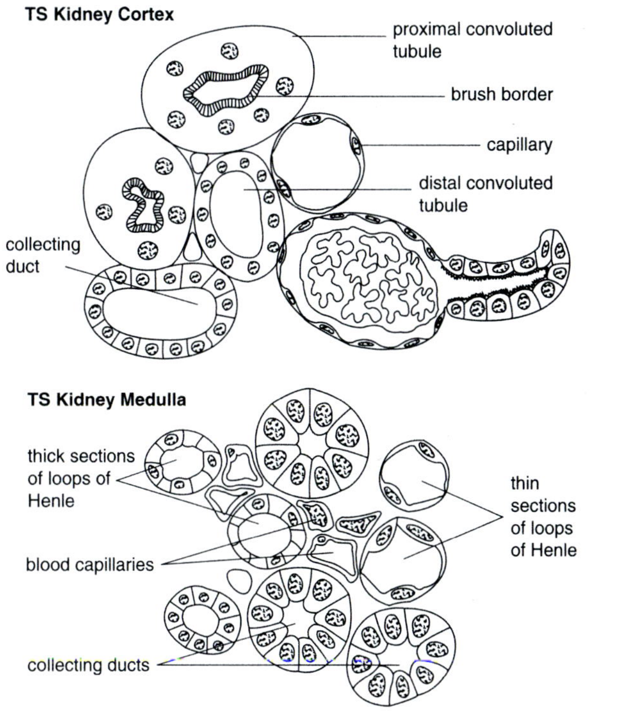

Fig. 13.74 Kidney Tubules

For consideration

(a) In what respect is the structure of the kidney adapted to perform its function of excretion and osmoregulation?

(b) How could you try and estimate the number of Malpighian corpuscles in the entire kidney from a single transverse and horizontal section?

(c) Discuss the structural difference between the afferent and the efferent arterioles in relation to their function.

Table showing comparison of various tubes of the kidney

Proximal tubule (PT)	**Distal tubule (DT)**	**Collecting duct (CD)**
Outer diameter about 60μm, Brush borders, which almost fills lumen.	Outer diameter 20-50μm. No brush border.	Outer diameter 25-60μm. Walls similar to distal convoluted tubule.
Large lining cells.	Smaller lining cells.	
Cell membranes between adjacent cells not visible. Relatively few nuclei, visible in cross-section of tubule.	Cell membranes between adjacent cells not visible. More nuclei visible in cross section of tubule since cells are smaller than those of proximal tubules. Large clearly defined lumen.	Cell membranes between adjacent cells are clearly visible. Cuboidal epithelium, clear cytoplasm as no active reabsorption takes place. Rounded nuclei.
Cytoplasm stains intensely, as lots of cell organelles present, especially mitrochondria.	Larger regular tubule, less affinity for stain.	Cuboidal to columnar cells, largest tubules.
Small, irregular lumen. Three times as long as distal tubules, so more plentiful in section.	Shorter than proximal tubule so less plentiful in section.	
Function: 75% of glomerular filtrate reabsorbs by proximal tubules.	**Function:** mainly reabsorption of sodium ions.	**Function:** water drawn out by osmosis into extracellular fluid and thence into adjacent vasa recta.

Descending limb	**Ascending limb: (plus lowest 3rd of descending limb)**	**Collecting ducts**
Outer diameter 14-20μm.	Outer diameter 30-35μm.	Outer diameter 50-200μm.
Lining of thin pavement epithelium.	Lining of cuboidal epithelium. Cell membranes between adjacent cells not visible.	Lining cells cuboidal to columnar. Cell membranes between adjacent cells clearly visible.
Nuclei flattened and bulging into lumen. (Known as thin limb).	Rounded nuclei, (known as thick limb).	Rounded nuclei.

Reference: UCLES, Question 3, 21st May, 1991.

Reference: UCLES, Question 3, 9th Nov. 1993.

Reference: UCLES, Question 3, 21st May, 1996.

Practical 72 – MICROSCOPIC STRUCTURE OF THE OVARY AND THE TESTIS

The ovaries are the sites of **oogenesis**. In a sexually mature mammal the **ova** are released in a cyclic manner at regular intervals throughout the year. In humans one ovum is released from alternating **ovary** each month controlled by the posterior pituitary.

In the non-pregnant state the female reproductive system undergoes a continuos cyclic change from puberty to menopause. When implantation is not followed by ovulation of a fertilised ovum the proliferated lining of the uterus is shed in a period of bleeding lasting from 3-10 days, known as the **menstrual cycle**. In humans the menstrual cycle is usually 28 days and ovulation occurs at the midpoint of the cycle (14th day). The ovulatory and the menstrual cycle are regulated by the hormones secreted by the ovaries **Fig. 13.75**.

The mammalian ovaries have a similar basic structure. The body of the ovary consists of a ground substance, constituting the **ovarian stroma**. In the peripheral zone of the stroma, known as the **cortex** are numerous **follicles**, which contain female gametes at various stages of development. In addition there may be **post-ovulatory follicles** of various kinds such as **corpus luteum**, **degenerative follicles** and **atretic follicles Fig. 13.76**.

During each ovarian cycle as many as 20 primordial follicles may be activated to undergo maturation, but only one follicle reaches maturity and is ovulated. The rest degenerate before the point of maturation. The reason for this wastage is not fully understood, however the follicles have an endocrine function, and it may be that the endocrine functions of the follicles is beyond a single follicle.

Both the testis and the ovary contain developing sperms and eggs respectively. In both cases diploid **primordial germ cells**, associated with the germinal epithelium, divide mitotically to form **spermatogonia** and **oogonia**, which grow and then undergo meiosis to form ultimately, **spermatozoa** and **ova** respectively.

General structure of the ovary

1. Observe the general structure of the ovary under low power and draw a plan diagram. Under high power you should be able to see developing **Graaffian follicles** at various stages. Try and interpret as many stages as possible **Figs. 13.76–13.78**.
2. After ovulation the hollow Graaffian follicle develops into a solid corpus luteum, see if you can find a corpus luteum. Make detailed labelled diagram under high power. As many as 400 000 primary follicles may be present at birth, but normally about 400 reach maturity. The rest degenerates into **atretic follicles**.

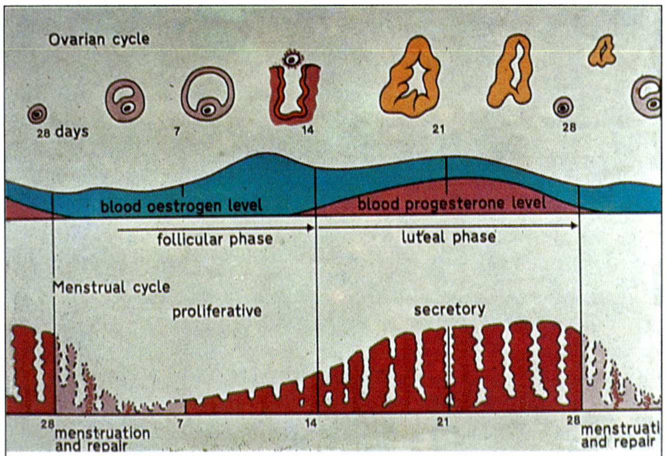

Fig. 13.75 The Hormanal Integration of the Ovarian Menstrual Cycle.

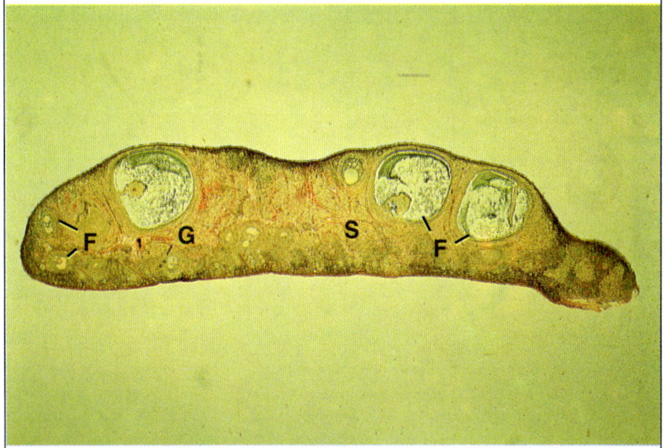

Fig. 13.76 Ovary of Rabbit (LS).
In the peripheral zone of stroma **S** numerous follicles **F** at various stages of development can be seen. Graffian follicle **G** is also visible.

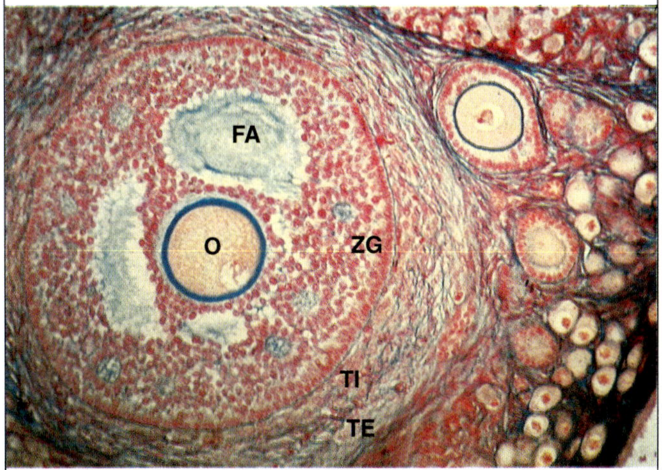

Fig. 13.77 Graffian Follicle in Rabbit (LS).
Follicular antrium **FA**, zona granulosa **ZG** an oocyte **O** are visible. Theca interna **TI** and the theca externa **TE** are well defined.

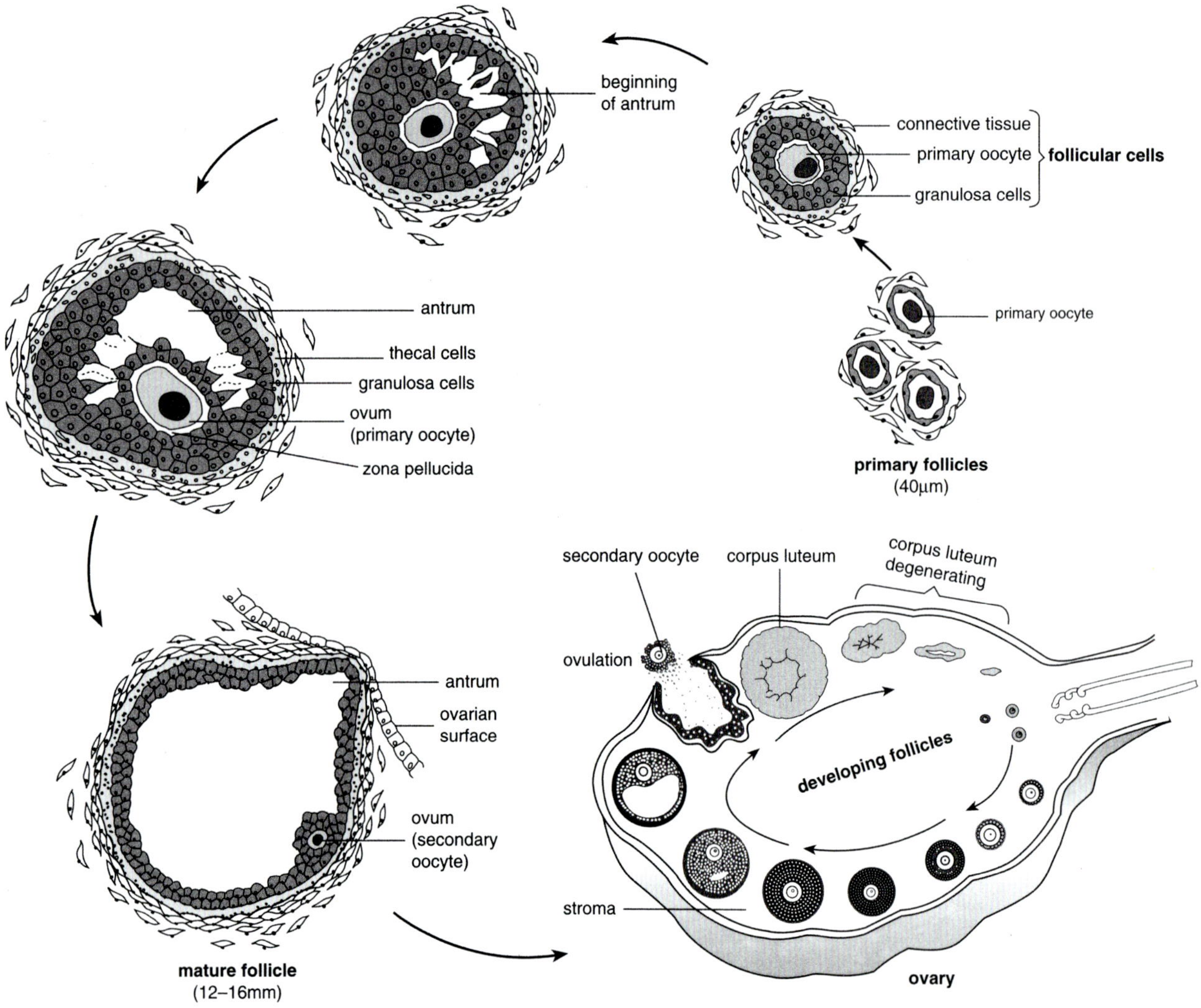

Fig. 13.78 Follicular Development in Mammalian Ovary

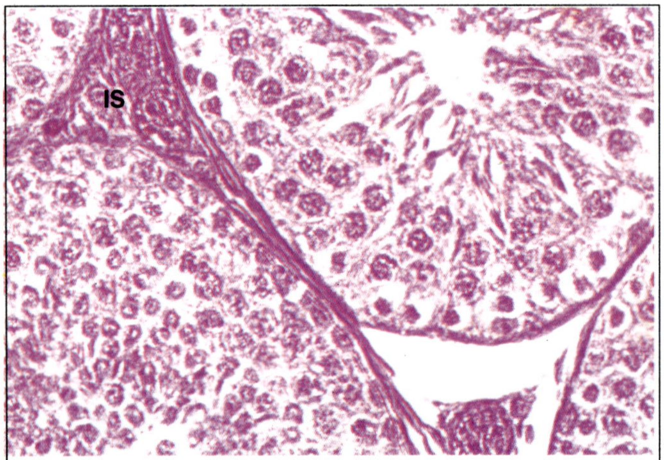

Fig. 13.79 Seminiferous Tubules (TS) ***low power.***
Highly convulated lined by stratified epithelium with cells at various stages of spermotogensis. In the interstitial spaces **IS** between tubules Leydig cells (endocrine function) are found amongst connective tissue.

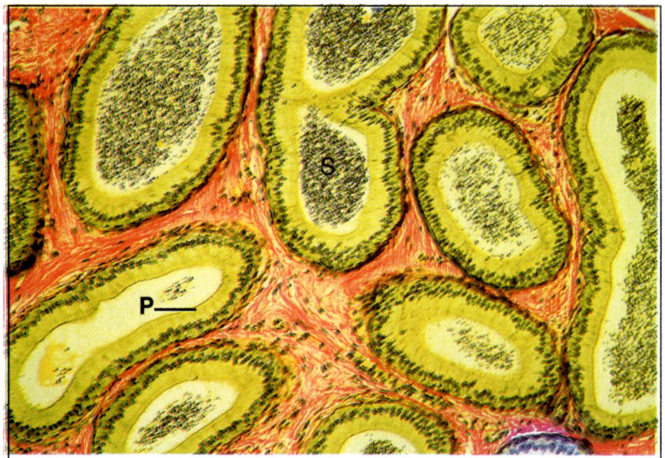

Fig. 13.80 Epididymis in Mammal (TS).
Epididymis (stores spermatozoa **S**), tube of smooth muscle lined by pseudostratified epithelium **P**.

General structure of the testis

1. Under low power numerous **semniferous tubules** (approximately 50 cm long and 200μm in diameter), highly convoluted tubules, lined by stratified epithelium located in **testicular lobules,** are seen cut in various planes.
2. On examining the walls of these tubules under high power **Fig. 13.79** two distinct population of cells are seen:
   i. Sperm development at various stages can be seen: **spermatogonia → spermatocytes → spermatids → spermatozoa**.
   In a particularly good slide you may be able to see stages of meiosis.
   ii. Non-spermatogenic cells called **Sertoli cells** or **nurse cells**, support and nourish the developing spermatozoa **Fig. 13.81**. The tails of the spermatozoa hang into the lumen of the semniferous tubules. Their heads are buried in the Sertoli cells or nurse cells.
3. Under high power you may be able to observe **Leydig cells**, (responsible for secretion of male sex hormones) either singly or in clumps in the interstitial spaces between the tubules. You may also see the tubules and capillaries embedded in supporting connective tissue. The large Leydig cells have an eosinopilic cytoplasm. Only in man do these cells contain elongated cytoplasmic crystals called **crystals of Reinke**, the function of which is not known.
4. Draw labelled drawings both at low and high power showing germinal epithelium, seminiferous tubules **Fig. 13.79**, epididymis **Fig. 13.80** and as many structures as you can identify.
5. Also draw under high power detail of spermatozoa showing nucleus, acrosome, middle piece and the tail.

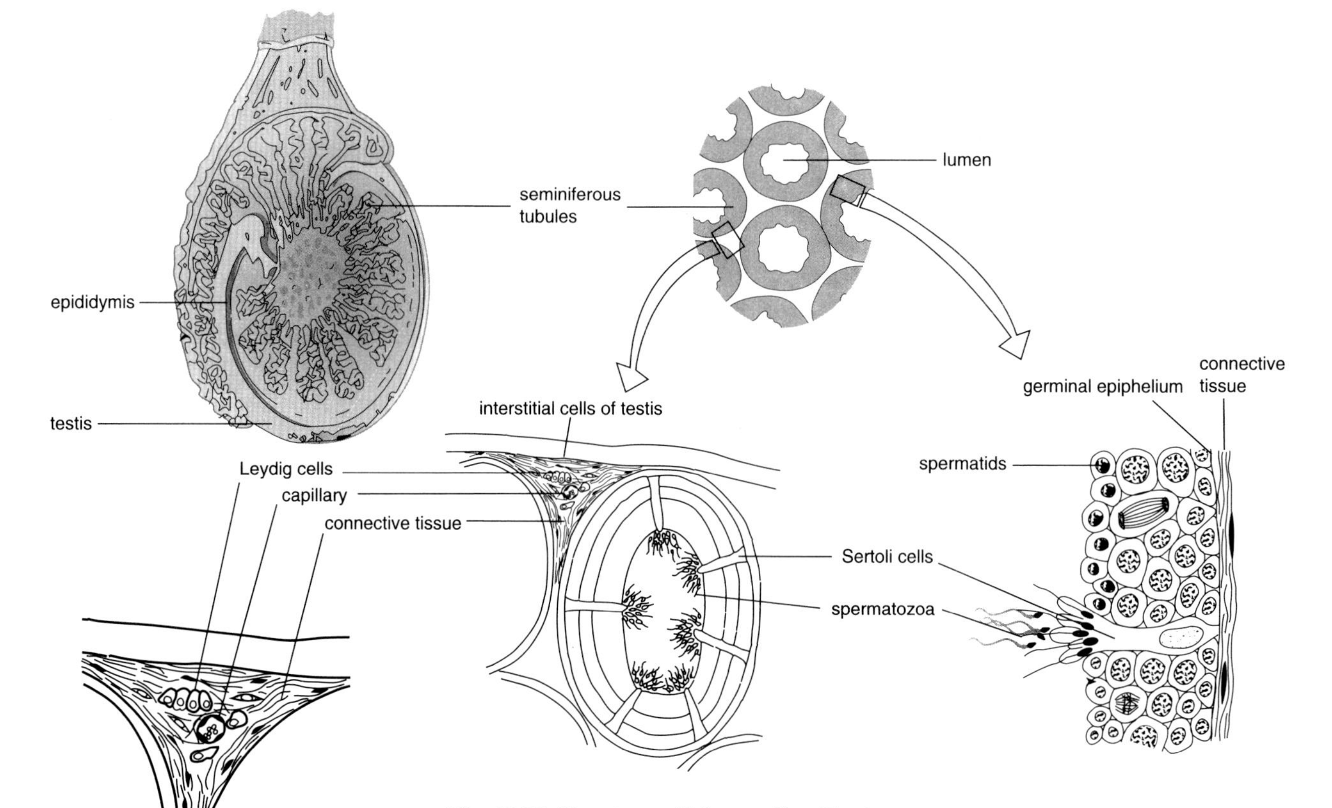

Fig. 13.81 Structure of Mammalian Testis

For consideration

(a) Why are Leydig cells close to the capillaries?
(b) How often are Graaffian follicles formed?
(c) What is the function of the corpus luteum?
(d) What are the essential similarities and differences between the development of the egg and the sperm?
(e) How are the developmental events that you have observed controlled?

GLOSSARY

abiotic factors the non-biological components of the environment, such as temperature, topography, wind speed.
absorption the taking in of fluids, in higher animals the movement of nutrients, fluids, and ions across the gut lining and into the internal environment.
absorption spectrum range of a pigment's ability to absorb various wavelengths of light.
acetylcholine a neurotransmitter substance liberated in the synapses in the CNS.
acid a substance that releases hydrogen ions (H^+) in water, pH < 7.
acinus describes a group of rounded exocrine secretory unit.
actin a globular protein that links into chains forming microfilaments in muscle and other contractile elements in cells.
actinomorphic a regular, radially symmetrical flower.
action spectrum range of wavelengths of light within which a process like photosynthesis takes place.
activation energy the minimum amount of collision energy required to bring reactant molecules to an activated condition (the transition state) at which a reaction will proceed spontaneously.
active site the region of enzyme molecule where the substrate molecule binds.
active transport movement of substances across a membrane involving a carrier protein and energy from respiration.
adrenal cortex outer region of the adrenal gland which responds to signals in reacting to stress and affects salt and water balance.
adrenal gland an endocrine gland located above the kidneys in mammals, composed of two glandular portions; an outer cortex and the inner medulla.
adrenal medulla the central part of the adrenal gland which responds to nervous inputs resulting from stress.
adrenaline a hormone secreted by the adrenal medulla and a neurotransmitter substance secreted by nerve endings of the sympathetic nervous system.
adventia outer layer of connective tissue, conducts major vessels and nerves.
aerobic respiration the main energy releasing metabolic pathway of ATP formation, in which oxygen is the final electron acceptor of electrons stripped from glucose or other organic compounds.
afferent 'bringing towards' usually applied to nerves or blood vessels.
agranulocytes two of the five types of white blood cells; lymphocytes and monocytes, with clear cytoplasm
agglutination sticking together.
alkali a hydroxide which dissolves in water to release hydroxyl ions (OH^-) pH > 7.
alpha (α) cells glucagon secreting cells of the islet of Langerhans in the pancreas.
alveolus (plural alveoli) the dead end multilobed air sacs involved in gas exchange in the lungs.
amino acids an organic molecule possessing both carboxyl and amino groups. Amino acids serve as monomers of proteins.
amphoteric having both acid and basic properties e.g. amino acids.
amylopectin a branched component of starch.
amylase a group of enzymes which decompose starch or glycogen e.g. salivary ptyalin.
anaerobic lacking oxygen, referring to an organisms' environment, or cellular process that lacks oxygen and may be poisoned by it.
anabolism the building up of complex molecules from smaller ones.
androecium collective name for the male part of the flower (stamens).
angiosperm a member of the most dominant group of land plants.
annual plant a flowering plant that completes its life cycle in one growing season.
anther the pollen-bearing male part in flowers.
antipodal cells a group of three cells found in the embryo sac.
antibiotic organic compound produced by plants which selectively kills or inhibits the growth of other micro-organisms.
aorta main artery in systemic circulation carrying oxygenated blood away from the heart.
apical meristem a mass of self perpetuating cells responsible for primary growth (elongation) at root and shoot tips.
apocarpous gynaecia in which there are separate free standing carpels.
apoplast collective name for the cell wall of a plant.
arachnoid matter one of the three layers of connective tissues in the brain—meninges; between the dura mater and the pia mater.
arteriole any of the blood vessels between arteries and capillaries.
artery a vessel that carries blood away from the heart to organs throughout the body.
ATP adenosine triphosphate, a nucleotide composed of adenine, ribose, and three phosphate groups. When it is hydrolysed, releases a large amount of free energy.
atretic follicles of the ovary, primordial follicles that degenerate.
atrio-ventricular node mass of tissue in the wall of the right atrium.
atrio-ventricular valve tricuspid or bicuspid valves found in the heart.
atrium one of two chambers in the mammalian heart.

autonomic nervous system those nerves leading from the central nervous system to the smooth muscle, cardiac muscle and glands of the internal organs and structures.

axil angle between the leaf and stem (containing a bud).

axillary bud a bud that develops between a stem and a leaf.

axon a long cylindrical extension from a neurone along which an action potential travels.

bacillus (*pl.* bacilli) a rod-shaped bacterium.

base a substance that releases hydroxyl ions (OH^-) in water and reacts with acids to form salts.

basophils fast acting white blood cells that secrete histamine and other substances during inflammation.

beta (β) cells insulin secreting cells of the islet of Langerhans in the pancreas.

biennial a flowering plant that completes its life cycle in two growing seasons.

bile an alkaline secretion of the liver cells discharged in the duodenum.

bile canaliculi a tiny channel in the liver lobule which carries bile.

bile duct a duct between bile canaliculi of the liver leading into the duodenum.

bilateral symmetry structure in which the two halves are mirror-images of each other.

biosphere all regions of the Earth and its atmosphere in which organisms live.

biotic factors the living components of the environment.

biuret test a test to check the presence of proteins based on the bases of peptide linkage.

bladder of the urinary system where urine is stored prior to excretion.

blood a fluid connective tissue, composed of water, solutes, blood cells and platelets.

Bowman's capsule the cup shaped portion of the nephron that receives the renal filtrate.

bract a modified leaf, usually having a protective role.

bronchus (*pl. bronchi*) windpipe—tube-like branch of the trachea.

bronchiole a component of the finely branched bronchial tree inside each lung.

Brunner's glands glands in the wall of the duodenum.

buffer a substance that can combine with hydrogen ions, release them or both. Buffers help to stabilise pH of fluids.

calcitonin a hormone secreted by the thyroid gland in direct response to raised calcium levels.

calyx collective name for all the sepals of the flower.

cambium one of two types of meristem that are responsible for secondary growth (increase in stem and root diameter).

canaliculus (*pl.* canaliculi) a tiny channel in the liver lobule which carries bile.

capillary a thin walled blood vessel that functions in the exchange between blood and the interstitial fluid.

capitulum disc-shaped head of a flowering stem carrying many florets in Compositae flowers such as dandelion.

carbohydrate a simple sugar or large molecule composed of sugar.

carbon cycle a biochemical cycle in which carbon moves from its largest reservoirs in the atmosphere through oceans and organisms, then back to the atmosphere.

carbon dioxide fixation first step of the light-independent reactions of photosynthesis. Carbon becomes affixed to a carbon compound that can enter the Calvin-Benson cycle.

cardiac cycle the sequence of muscle contraction and relaxation constituting a heartbeat.

carina in a pea flower the lowest two petals tacked together forming a keel or carina.

carotenoids light-sensitive, accessory pigments that transfer absorbed energy to chlorophylls. They absorb violet and blue wave-lengths but transmit red, orange, and yellow.

carpel the female reproductive part of a flower, sometimes called a pistle.

cartilage a type of connective tissue with solid, pliable intercellular material that resists compression.

caruncle of seeds, a fleshy outgrowth of the testa which overlaps the micropyle.

Casparian strip of the root, a waxy band that acts as an impermeable barrier between the walls of abutting cells.

cell fractionation a centrifugation technique to separate cell organelles.

cell sap fluid in the vacuoles of plant cells.

cell wall a rigid sometimes semi-rigid wall outside the plasma membrane, found in plants, fungi, protistas and most bacteria.

cellulose an unbranched polymer of several thousand glucose residues usually found in plants.

central nervous system the brain and the spinal cord of vertebrates.

centriole a cylinder of triplet microtubules that give rise to flagella and cilia.

centromeres a small constricted region of chromosomes having attachment sites for microtubules which help in movement of chromosomes during nuclear division.

cerebellum hindbrain region of the brain involved in maintaining posture and limb movements.

cerebral cortex thin surface layer of the cerebral hemispheres.

cerebrospinal fluid clear extra cellular fluid that surrounds and cushions the brain and spinal cord.

cerebrum forebrain in the vertebrates.

chalaza of the ovule, tissue lying at the opposite end of the micropyle next to the nucellus.

chief (peptic) cells cells found in the stomach which secrete pepsin and renin.

chitin a polymer, chemically related to cellulose usually found in insect exoskeleton.

chlorophyll light sensitive molecules that absorb light, involved in photosynthesis (green pigment).

chloroplast a plant cell organelle that specialises in photosynthesis.

cholesterol an animal lipid formed in the liver.
chondroblasts precursor to cartilage cells.
chondrocytes mature cartilage cells.
chondroitin sulphate mucopolysaccharide similar to hyaluronic acid, major component of cartilage.
chromatid one of a duplicated eukaryotic mitotic chromosome, joined together at the centromere.
chromatin dark stained material in nucleus, active in RNA synthesis.
chromatography method of separating complex mixtures.
chromatophores pigment (melanin) containing cells, found in the skin and the eyes.
climate prevailing weather conditions for an ecosystem, including temperature, humidity, wind speed, cloud cover, and rainfall.
closed circulation type of transport system found in higher animals where the blood flows within vessels.
Coccus (pl. cocci) spherical bacterial cells.
coenocytic tissue not divided into cells.
cohesion condition in which molecular bonds resist rupturing when under tension.
coleoptile the sheath surrounding the epicotyl in the embryo of grasses.
collagen connective tissue protein.
collagen fibre flexible but very strong, non-stretchable fibres found in connective tissue.
collecting duct of the kidney, terminal portion of distal convoluted tubule.
collenchyma one of the simple tissues of flowering plants; lends flexible support to primary tissues, such as those of lengthening stems.
colorimeter instrument to measure colour intensity of coloured solutions.
commensalism two-species interaction in which one species benefits significantly while the other is neither helped nor harmed to any notable extent.
community the populations of all species occupying a habitat; also applied to groups of organisms with similar life-styles in a habitat (such as the bird community).
companion cells a specialised parenchyma cell found adjacent to the sieve tube in the conducting phloem of the plant.
compensation point the point where respiration and photosynthesis are balanced.
Compositae flowers such as dandelion, with a flowering stem carrying many florets grouped together on flat disc-shaped capitulum.
conjugate protein protein combined with a non-protein part.
connective tissue a category of animal tissues, all having mostly the same components but in different proportions. These tissues contain fibroblasts and other cells, the secretion of which form fibres of collagen and elastin and ground substances.
cork cambium a type of lateral meristem that produces a tough, corky replacement for epidermis in woody plants.
corpus luteum a glandular structure which develops when ovarian follicle ruptures. Secretes progesterone and some oestrogen.
corrola collective name for the petals of a flower.
cortex in general, outer layer; the kidney cortex is an example. In vascular plants, ground tissue that makes up most of the primary plant body, supports plant parts, and stores food.
crypt of Lieberkuhn tubular glands at the base of the villi.
cytokinesis cytoplasmic division; the splitting of a parental cell into daughter cells.
dark reaction (stage) part of photosynthesis reaction proceeds in the absence of light in the stroma of the chloroplast.
decomposers heterotrophs that obtain energy by chemically breaking down the remains, products, or wastes of other organisms. Their activities help cycle nutrients back to producers. Certain fungi and bacteria are examples.
degassed when all air is removed.
dendrite a short, slender extension from the cell body of a neurone.
dichogamy a flower in which the stamen and the stigmas ripen at different times.
diffusion net movement of like molecules (or ions) down their concentration gradient.
diploid state cell nucleus containing two sets of chromosomes.
disaccharides a type of simple carbohydrate, of the class called oligosaccharides; two monosaccharides covalently bonded.
distal convoluted tubules the tubular section of a nephron most distant from the glomerulus; a major site of water and sodium reabsorption.
dormant resting condition e.g. in seeds.
dorsal of the back.
double circulation in mammals where the blood returns to the heart twice in each cycle.
double fertilization process characteristic of angiosperms in which two male nuclei enter the embryosac. One fuses with the egg cell nucleus to form the zygote which develops in the embryo, the other fuses with the two polar nuclei to form a triploid nucleus from which the endosperm develops.
duodenum first part of the small intestine.
dura mater outer most membrane of the meninges.
ecosystem a natural unit of biotic (living) and abiotic (non-living) components.
edaphic factors factors influenced by the soil.
efferent 'coming away from'.
elastin rubber-like material arranged as fibres and discontinuous sheets found in connective tissue.
electrophoresis technique used for separation of charged particles such as protein, under an electric field.
electron micrographs (EM) photographic images of electron microscopy.

electro-osmosis passage of water across a charged membrane.

embryo sac the female gametophyte of flowering plants.

endocrine gland ductless gland that secretes hormones into interstitial fluid, after which they are distributed via the bloodstream.

endocytosis movement of a substance into cells via phagocytosis; the substance becomes enclosed by a patch of plasma membrane that sinks into the cytoplasm, then forms a vesicle around it.

endosperm nutritive tissue that surrounds and serves as food for a flowering plant embryo and, later, for the germinating seedling.

endothelium diverse group of tissue lining all body surfaces, cavities and tubes.

enzymes one of a class of proteins that greatly speeds up (catalyse) reactions between specific substances, usually at their functional groups.

eosinophil fast-acting, phagocytic white blood cell that takes part in inflammation.

epicotyle stem of the embryo plant occurring above the cotyledon.

epigeal germination germination in which the cotyledons are carried above the ground.

epithelium sheet of cells bound together covering both external and internal organs.

epigynous flower in which the stamen and the perianth appear to stand on top of the ovary.

erythrocyte red blood cell.

essential amino acid any of eight amino acids which are not synthesised by the body and have to be obtained from the diet.

essential fatty acid any of the fatty acids that certain animals cannot synthesise for themselves and must obtain from food.

eukaryotic cell cell with a well defined nucleus enclosed within a nuclear membrane.

exine the outer coat of the pollen grain.

exocrine glands a gland whose secretion is released via a duct.

exocytosis movement of a substance out of a cell by means of a transport vesicle, the membrane of which fuses with the plasma membrane, so that the vesicle's contents are released outside.

exodermis layer of cells just inside the root epidermis of most flowering plants; helps control the uptake of water and solutes.

extrapolation co-ordinates determined by extending the line of the graph.

facilitated diffusion diffusion across a membrane facilitated by a carrier protein.

faeces the remains of undigested food.

fermentation anaerobic breakdown of glucose with the production of ethanol and carbon dioxide or lactic acid.

filament a thin stalk which supports the anther.

flaccid state of tissue (usually plant) lacking in water, as in wilting.

florets one of many flowers compressed on a capitulum, or in an inflorescence.

follicle in a mammalian ovary, a primary oocyte (immature egg) together with the surrounding layer of cells, see Graffian follicle.

food chain a straight-line sequence of who eats whom in an ecosystem, starting from the autotrophes.

food webs a network of cross-connecting, interlinked food chains, encompassing primary producers and an array of consumers, detritivores, and decomposers.

gamete sex cell.

ganglia a cluster (functional group) of cell bodies of neurones in regions other than the brain or spinal cord.

gaseous exchange exchange of respiratory gases oxygen and carbon dioxide between cell/ organisms and the environment.

gastric glands glands related to stomach.

gastric pits the region at the base of two villi.

geotropism a tropic response by plants to gravity.

gills a localised extension of the body surface of many aquatic animals, specialised for gas exchange.

gland a secretory cell or multicellular structure derived from epithelium and often connected to it.

Glisson's capsule tough connective tissue surrounding the liver.

glomerular filtrate filterate formed by ultrafiltration in the renal capsule.

glomerulus a mass of capillaries surrounded by the Bowman's capsule, where water and solutes are filtered from blood.

glucagon hormone that stimulates conversion of glycogen and amino acids to glucose; secreted by alpha cells of the pancreas when the flow of glucose decreases; an antagonistic hormone to insulin.

glumes the lowest two cataphylls (leaf blades) in grasses.

glycogen extensively branched glucose storage polysaccharide found in the liver and muscle of animals , that is a main food reserve; can be readily broken down into glucose subunits.

glycoprotein compound of protein and polysaccharide, such as those found in the cell membrane.

goblet cells mucus-secreting cells of the epithelium.

Graffian follicles mature follicle in the ovary, containing an ovum.

grana within chloroplasts, any of the stacks of flattened, membranous compartments with chlorophyll and other light-trapping pigments and reaction sites for ATP formation.

granulocyte (polymorphs) three of the five types of white blood cells; *neutrophils, eosinophils* and *basophils*, with granular cytoplasm.

guard cells a specialised epidermal plant cell that forms the boundaries of the stomata.

gynaecium the female reproductive organs of the flower.

haemocytometer a special microscope slide used to count cells.

haploid state cells having one set of chromosomes.

Haversian system the arrangement of bone cells and canaliculi in compact bone.
hilium a scar on the testa of a seed, where the seed was attached to the plant.
hepatic artery blood vessel which supplies oxygenated blood to the liver from the aorta.
hepatic portal vein blood vessel between intestine and the liver.
hepatocytes liver cell.
histology the study of the structure of tissue.
homologous chromosomes chromosome pairs of the same length, centromere position, and staining pattern that possess genes for the same traits at corresponding loci. One homologous chromosome is inherited from the male, the other from the female.
hormone any of the signalling molecules secreted from endocrine glands, endocrine cells, and some neurones that the bloodstream distributes (any cell having receptors for that hormone), which co-ordinate the various parts of the organism by interacting with target cells.
hyaline cartilage commonest form of cartilage in man.
hyaluronic acid predominant glycosaminoglycan in the loose connective tissue.
hypertonic a more concentrated solution than that of the cell (with a higher osmotic pressure) suspended in it.
hypocotyl the part of the stem below the point of attachment of the cotyledons.
hypogeal germination germination in which the cotyledons remain below the ground.
hypogynous flower flower in which the recepticle is a slight enlargement of the pedicel.
hypotonic a less concentrated solution than that of the cell suspended in it.
H-band (zone) of skeletal muscle, (heller) band; a dark band that bisects a more dense M band. Bands formed due to arrangement of myofilaments in the sarcomere.
ileum part of the digestive system where digestion is completed; second part of the small intestine.
inflorescence a group of flowers arranged on a stem.
ingestion the taking in of food.
inoculation the introduction of pathogen to allow the body to build up immunity to the pathogen or of bacteria on to agar plates.
insulin a vertebrate hormone secreted by endocrine cells of the islets of Langerhans, in the pancreas. It lowers blood glucose levels by promoting the uptake of glucose by most body cells and the synthesis and storage of glycogen in the liver; also stimulates protein and fat synthesis.
integument wall or coat of the ovule.
intercalary meristem meristem between regions of mature tissues.
intercalated discs specialised transverse junctions between cardiac muscles.
internode in vascular plants, the segment of a plant stem between the points where leaves are attached.
interphase the period in the cell cycle when the cell is not dividing. The interval is different for different species.
interpolation estimations of values other than those actually plotted from a graph.
interspecific competition two-species interaction in which both species can be harmed due to overlapping niches.
interstitial fluid fluid between the cells.
intine the inner wall of the pollen grain.
intraspecific competition interaction among individuals of the same species that are competing for the same resources.
involuntary or smooth muscle muscle specialised for continuos contraction of relatively low force in a diffused rhythmic fashion, occurring independently of neurological intervention e.g. in the digestive system.
islets of Langerhans group of endocrine cells in the pancreas.
isoelectric point the pH at which the molecule of an amphoteric substance carries no charge.
isotonic being of the same osmotic concentration, and therefore of the same water potential.
jejunum the section between the duodenum and the ileum in the small intestine.
juxtamedullary nephrons nephrons which have their renal corpusles close to the cortex and medulla.
keel of the pea flower, fusion of two of the lowest petal forms a structure in which the reproductive structures are enclosed.
keratin a tough, water-insoluble protein manufactured by most epidermal cells.
Kupffer cells phagocytic cell of the liver which remove spent RBCs and other debris.
lacteals intestinal lymphatics, involved in fat digestion.
lacuna a cavity, as in the Haversian canals in compact bone.
lamellae thin plate as in spongy bone or in 'gills' of fungi.
lamina the blade of a leaf.
large intestine last part of the digestive tract.
lateral roots of taproot systems, a lateral branching from the first, primary root.
legume a dry fruit also known as a pod which splits to release seeds. Any plant belonging to pea or bean family.
lemma lower of the two bracts in the grass florets.
lenticle pore in the bark of the tree that permits gaseous exchange to take place.
leucocyte a white blood cell; typically functions in immunity, such as phagocytosis or antibody production.
Leydig cells endocrine cells in the testis that secrete testosterone.
ligament strong fibrous elastic tissue connecting movable bones.
ligand a molecule that binds specifically to a receptor site of another molecule.
lignin a substance that strengthens and waterproofs

cellulose cell walls of vascular plants, an important adaptation for support in terrestrial species.

lipid one of a family of compounds, including fats, phospholipids, and steroids, that are insoluble in water.

lipoprotein a protein bonded to a lipid; includes the low-density lipoproteins (LDLs) and high-density lipproteins (HDLs) that transport fats and cholesterol in blood.

loop of Henle the hairpin-shaped, tubular region of a nephron that functions in re-absorption of water and solutes.

lumen internal space of a tube/vessel.

lung the invaginated respiratory surfaces of terrestrial vertebrates and land snails in the shape of a cavity or sac, connected to the atmosphere by narrow tubes.

lymph the tissue fluid, derived from interstitial fluid, in the lymphatic system of vertebrate animals.

lymphocyte any of various white blood cells which take part in non-specific and specific (immune) defence. Those that complete their development in the bone marrow are called B cells, and those that mature in the thymus are called T cells.

maceration process of chemically softening woody tissues to separate cells and vessels for observation.

Malpighian corpuscle glomerulus and renal capsule of mammalian nephron.

matrix ground substance of connective tissue or bone; innermost part of the mitrochondrion.

marrow tissue soft material forming the inside of the bone; consists mainly of fat cells.

mast cells cells found in the connective tissue.

meiosis a two-stage type of cell division in sexually reproducing organisms that results in gametes with half the chromosome number of the original cell.

melanin a pigment, (dark brown or black) occurring in hair and skin.

meristem plant tissue capable of dividing to give new cells.

meninges in vertebrates the three membranes covering the brain and the spinal cord.

menstrual cycle monthly cycle of ovulation and menstruation in human females.

mesophyll the ground tissue of a leaf parenchyma sandwiched between the upper and lower epidermis, specialised for photosynthesis.

metabolic pathway one of many orderly sequences of enzyme-mediated reactions by which cells normally maintain, increase, or decrease the concentrations of substances. Different pathways are linear or circular, and often interconnected.

metaphase of mitosis or meiosis II, the stage when each duplicated chromosome has become positioned at the midpoint of the microtubular spindle, with its two sister chromatids attached to microtubules from opposite spindle poles. Of meiosis I, the stage when all pairs of homologous chromosomes are positioned at the spindle's midpoint, with the two members of each pair attached to opposite spindle poles.

metaphloem latter-formed primary phloem.

metaxylem latter-formed primary xylem.

Michelis constant a measure of the affinity of an enzyme for its substrate.

micropyle a small hole in the seed coat; site of passage of the pollen tube into an ovule prior to fertilisation.

microtome an instrument to cut thin sections for microscopic examination.

microvilli tiny projections of the plasma membrane which make up the 'brush borders'.

mitosis a process of cell division in eukaryotic cells that maintains the parental chromosome number for daughter cells. It is the basis of bodily growth and, asexual reproduction in many species.

molality is the term used to express concentration of a solute relative to its mass of solvent i.e. mol kg^{-1}.

molecular mass this is the sum of the molar masses of its component atomic elements.

monocotyledons class of angiosperms having embryos with single cotyledon.

monocytes one of five types of white blood cells, with clear cytoplasm.

monosaccharide the simplest carbohydrate, with only one sugar unit. Also known as simple sugars, the molecular formulas of monosaccharides are generally some multiple of CH_2O. Glucose is an example.

morphology form and general structure of an organism

motor end plate the point of termination of an axon in a voluntary muscle fibre.

motor neurone nerve cells that carry impulses away from the CNS to an effector.

mouth an oral cavity; in human digestion, the site where polysaccharide breakdown begins.

mucosa the inner lining of the digestive system.

mucus a watery solution of glycoprotein with lubricating and protective properties.

mucin an important glycoprotein secreted by the Golgi apparatus, which forms mucus in solution.

murein a molecule consisting of polysaccharide chains cross-linked in a regular fashion by short peptide bonds.

muscularis mucosa smooth muscle fibres in sub-mucosa of gut wall.

mutalism a symbiotic relationship in which both the organisms benefit.

myelin sheath in a neurone, an insulating coat of cell membrane from Schwann cells that is interrupted by nodes of Ranvier.

myofibril the contractile filament consisting of actin, myosin and associate proteins within muscle cells.

myogenic rhythmic contractions arise from within the tissue itself, independent of nervous system.

myosin a type of protein filament that interacts with actin filaments to cause cell contraction.

nectary a gland in flowers which secretes a sweet juice called nectar.

nephron the tubular excretory unit of the vertebrate

kidney in which water and solutes filtered from blood, are selectively reabsorbed and in which urine forms.

neutrophil fast-acting, phagocytic white blood cell that takes part in inflammatory responses against bacteria.

Nissl's granules dark granular aggregation of rough endoplasmic reticulum found in cytoplasm of neurone cell body.

node in vascular plants, a point on a stem where one or more leaves are attached.

nodes of Ranvier the small gaps in the myelin sheath along the axon of a neurone; also, the site of high concentration of voltage-gated ion channels.

noradrenalin transmitter substance found in sympathetic nervous system.

nucellus initial uniform mass of cells of the ovule in plants.

nucleic acid a long, single or double-stranded biological molecule (such as RNA or DNA) that allows organisms to reproduce. Composed of four different kinds of monomers called nucleotides.

nucleotides the building block of a nucleic acid, consisting of a five-carbon sugar covalently bonded to a nitrogenous base and a phosphate group.

oogenesis the process in the ovary that results in the production of female gametes.

oogonia germ cells of the female.

organ a structure of definite form and function that is composed of several different types of tissues.

osmosis the diffusion of water across a selectively permeable membrane.

osmotic pressure a measure of the tendency of a solution to take up water when separated from pure water by a selectively permeable membrane.

osteoblasts immature bone cells responsible for secretion and synthesis of extracellular matrix of bone called osteoid.

osteoclasts multinucleate cells which are involved in resorption and continuos remodelling of the bone.

osteocytes when osteoblasts become trapped in the ground matrix they are referred to as osteocytes.

osteoid extracellular matrix of bone.

osteon one Haversian system of the bone.

ovum in animals, female gamete.

ovarian stroma ground substance of the ovary consisting of spindle-shaped cells and reticular fibres.

ovary in female animals, the structure that produces gametes and reproductive hormones. In seed-bearing plants, the portion of a carpel in which the egg-containing ovules develop.

ovule a structure that develops in the plant ovary and contains the female gametophyte.

ovum a mature female gamete (egg).

palea or pale a bracteole in grasses.

palisade tissue main photosynthetic tissue of the plant, in the upper part of the leaf mesophyll.

pancreas gland that secretes enzymes and bicarbonate into the small intestine during digestion, and that also secretes the hormones insulin and glucagon.

papillae apices of kidney pyramids.

parasite an organism living on or in another organism, obtaining all its food from the host and usually harming it.

parenchyma most abundant unspecialised simple tissues found throughout the whole plant. Its cells function in photosynthesis, storage, secretion, and develops into more differentiated cell types.

parietal (oxyntic) cells hydrochloric acid secreting cells of the stomach, found along the length of gastric gland.

pedicel a stem on which the flower is built.

pelvis of the kidney, expanded origin of the ureter.

pepsinogen inactive precursor to pepsin produced by the ribosomes.

perianth the accessory part of the flower; usually the sepals and the petals

pericardium fibrous case surrounding the heart.

perichondrium a zone of condensed connective tissue at the periphery of mature cartilage.

pericycle a layer, one or more layer thick, of ground tissue at the periphery of cell stele, next to the endodermis, present in roots.

perigynous flower which shows lateral expansion of the recepticle.

periosteum dense fibrous connective tissue layer on the external surface of the bone.

petaloid coloured sepals, resembling petals.

petals of the flower, inner whorl of leaf-like coloured structures inside the sepals.

petiole the stalk of a leaf, which joins the leaf to a node of the stem.

phaeophytin a grey pigment found in plants.

phagocytosis 'cellular eating' ingestion of cells or particles which involves wrapping around of the cytoplasm and cell membrane around it.

phloem the portion of the vascular system in plants consisting of tissue with living cells that interconnect and form the tubes through which transport of sugar and other organic nutrients are conducted.

phospholipid molecules that constitute the inner bi-layer of biological membranes, having a polar, hydrophilic head and a non-polar, hydrophobic tail.

phosphorus cycle movement of phosphorus from rock or soil through organisms, then back to soil.

photosynthesis the main biosynthetic pathway by which energy and carbon enter the web of life by conversion of light energy to chemical energy (ATP, NADPH, or both), followed by synthesis of sugar phosphates that is stored in glucose or other organic compounds; occurs in plants, algae, and certain prokaryotes.

photosynthometer an apparatus used to measure evolution of oxygen from plants.

phototropism growth of a plant shoot toward or away from light.

pia mater in vertebrates the innermost membrane of the three membranes surrounding the brain and the spinal cord.

piliferous layer the epidermis bearing the root hairs of a young root.

pinocytosis 'cellular drinking', a type of endocytosis in which the cell ingests extracellular fluid and its dissolved solutes by wrapping around cell membrane and cytoplasm.

pistil another name for carpel or gynaecium.

pith the core of the central vascular cylinder of monocot roots, consisting of parenchyma cells.

plasma liquid component of blood; consists of water, various proteins, ions, sugars, dissolved gases, and other substances in which the cells are suspended.

plasma membrane the bounding membrane of cells which controls the entry of molecules and the interaction of cells with the environment.

plasma cell of immune systems, a derivative of B cells that secretes antibodies.

plasmolysis in cells in which the cytoplasm shrinks and the plasma membrane pulls away from the cell wall when the cell loses water to a hypertonic environment.

platelet tiny cell fragments in blood derived from large cells in the bone marrow that release substances necessary in blood clotting.

pleomorphic varying in shape according to growth conditions/culture age.

plumule the part of the embryo which grows to form the main stem of a new plant.

podocyte cells of the inner layer of the Bowman's capsule.

polar nuclei two of the eight nuclei involved in plant fertilisation, eventually forming the endosperm.

pollen the microspores of seed plants.

polyacrylamide gel transparent cross linked acrylamide gel used in separation of proteins and nucleic acids.

polysaccharide a group of complex carbohydrates such as starch and cellulose.

population a group of individuals of the same species that live in a particular geographic area.

porphyrin belongs to a class of organic compounds to which haem belongs.

potometer an apparatus used to measure the rate of transpiration.

predation a two-species interaction in which one species (the predator) directly harms the other (its prey).

pressure potential of the cell, pressure due to the cell wall or the turgidity of the cell.

primary endosperm nucleus in plants, formed by fusion of one of the male nucleus and both of the polar nuclei (see *double fertilization*).

primary producer an autotroph, which collectively make up the trophic level of an ecosystem that ultimately supports all other levels; usually a photosynthetic organism.

primary structure of proteins, the level of protein structure referring to the specific sequence of amino acids.

primordial germ cells oogonia.

procambial the cells of primary meristem which differentiate into primary xylem and phloem and in some cases cambium.

prokaryotic major division of organisms which do not have a distinct nucleus e.g. bacteria.

prophase of mitosis, the stage when each duplicated chromosome starts to condense, microtubules form a spindle apparatus, and the nuclear envelope starts to break up.

prop-root adventitious root arising on a stem above soil level, growing into soil and serving as additional support for the stem.

prorennin an enzyme secreted by zymogen or chief (peptic) cells.

prosthetic groups non-proteinaceous entity essential for an enzyme's activity, functionally equivalent to co-enzyme and differs only in being tightly bound to its protein.

protandrous a flower in which the pollen opens before the stigma is mature.

protein large three-dimensional organic compound constructed from a set of 20 different monomers called amino acids held together by peptide bonds.

protogynous a flower in which the stigma ripens before the anther opens.

protophloem the first formed primary phloem.

protoxylem the first formed primary xylem.

proximal tubule of a nephron, the tubular region that receives water and solutes filtered from the blood.

Purkinji cells branched large pear-shaped cells found in the cerebellum.

pyramidal cells pyramid shaped cells found in the cerebral cortex.

pyramids formed by grouping together of collecting ducts and blood vessels in the kidney medulla.

quaternary structure of protein the particular shape of a complex, aggregate protein, defined by the characteristic three-dimensional arrangement of its constituent subunits, each a polypeptide.

rachilla the central axis (stem) on grass inflorescence.

receptacle the top of the flower stalk.

receptor-mediated endocytosis the movement of specific molecules into a cell by the inward budding of membranous vesicles containing proteins with receptor sites specific to the molecules being taken in; enables a cell to acquire bulk quantities of specific substances.

recombination reassortment of genes in combination different to what they were in the parents.

red blood cell (erythrocyte) an oxygen-transporting cell in blood.

redox reaction a chemical reaction involving the transfer of one or more electrons from one reaction to another, also called oxidation-reduction reaction.

reducing agent electron donor in a redox reaction.

reduction gaining of electrons by a substance involved in a redox reaction.

reflex action a simple automatic, involuntary and stereotype response to some stimulus (e.g. an eye blink).

reflex arc the simplest functional unit of the nervous system, consisting of an afferent sensory neurone conveying nerve impulses from a receptor to the CNS, generally the spinal cord.

Reinke crystals elongated crystals found only in man, Leydig cells, function not known.

renal cortex outer region of the kidney.

renal medulla the region inside the cortex in the kidney.

renal pelvis funnel shaped structures from which urine is conducted to the bladder.

resolution the ability of an imaging system to differentiate between two closely spaced objects.

respiratory quotient (RQ) the ratio of moles CO_2 evolved to moles O_2 absorbed in respiration; unity (1) when the substrate is carbohydrate, lower when the substrate is fat or protein.

respiratory surface an organ system involved in gaseous exchange in respiration.

respiratory tract respiratory organs.

respirometer apparatus used to measure the rate of respiration reflecting the demand for oxygen by the organism.

reticulate thickening secondary wall deposition in the form of irregular network in tracheids or vessel elements of metaxylem.

reticulo-endothelial system a term used to describe a system of cells with an ability to take up certain dyes and particles, now replaced with **mononuclear phagocytic system.**

R_f **value** of chromatography, relative front is the distance moved by the solvent divided by the distance moved by the solvent front.

root pressure pressure exerted by the roots for the movement of water from soil to vascular tissues aided by osmosis and active transport.

salt an ionic compound formed when an acid reacts with a base.

saprotrophic feed on dead organic material.

sarcolemma plasma membrane that binds the muscle fibre.

sarcomere arrangement of the contractile proteins on a muscle fiber which gives rise to the appearance of prominent cross-striations, along the fiber is called sarcomere.

sarcoplasm cytoplasm of the muscle fiber.

scalariform basic pattern of lignification in the metaxylem.

scanning electron microscope (SEM) type of electron microscope.

Schwann cell specialised neuroglial cells that grow around neurone axons, forming a myelin sheath.

sclerenchyma one of the simple tissues of flowering plants, generally with cells having thick, lignin-impregnated walls. It supports mature plant parts and often protects seeds.

scleried a short, irregular sclerenchyma cell in nutshells and seed coats and scattered through the parenchyma of some plants e.g. pears.

scurvy deficiency diseases caused by lack of vitamin C.

secondary cortex cork cambium which divides tangentially to form secondary cortex to the inside and cork cells to the outside.

secondary growth the increase in girth of the stems and roots of many plants, especially woody, perennial dicots.

secondary parenchyma parenchyma tissue formed between adjacent vascular bundles.

secondary phloem cambium, divides to form secondary xylem to the inside and secondary phloem to the outside.

secondary structure of proteins the localised, repetitive folding of the polypeptide backbone of a protein due to hydrogen bond formation between peptide linkages.

secondary xylem cambium, divide to form secondary xylem to the inside and secondary phloem to the outside.

seminiferous tubules highly coiled tubes in the testis in which sperm are produced.

sepal a whorl of modified leaves in angiosperms that encloses and protects the flower bud before it opens.

serosa the region of adventia exposed to the abdominal cavity.

Sertoli cells or **nurse cells** non-spermatogenic cells which support and nourish the developing spermatozoa in the testis.

SI units The System International d'United, is an internationally recognised form of measurement and represents the accepted scientific convention for measurement of physical quantities.

sieve plate the end wall between adjacent cells of phloem, which has characteristic pores.

sieve tube elements cells present in the phloem formed by the end-to-end fusion of cells.

sino-atrial node (pacemaker) a region of the heart which initiates the heartbeat.

skeletal muscle muscles connected to the skeletal system with powerful rapid contraction, under control of voluntary nervous system.

smooth muscle specialised for continuos contraction of relatively low force in a diffused rhythmic fashion, occurring independently of neurological intervention, under direct control of CNS.

solute potential osmotic concentration of the cell sap, same as osmotic potential.

solvent front highest point reached by the solvent in chromatography.

spermatids a cell formed by division of a secondary spermatocyte, and developing into a spermatazoon without further division.

spermatocytes a stage in the development of the male germ cells, arising by growth of spermatogonium or by division of another spermatocyte and giving rise to a spermatid.

spikelets inflorescence consisting of distinct units in grasses.

spinal cord of central nervous systems, the portion threading through a canal inside the vertebral column and providing direct reflex connections between sensory and motor neurones as well as communication lines to and from the brain.

spindle an assemblage of microtubules that orchestrates chromosome movement during eukaryotic cell division.

spindle apparatus a type of bi-polar structure that forms during mitosis or meiosis and that moves the chromosomes. It consists of two sets of microtubules that extend from the opposite poles and overlaps at the spindle's equator.

spirometer instrument used to measure change in lung volume during human breathing.

spongy mesophyll in the upper layers of leaves, loosely packed photosynthetic cells which carry out photosynthesis.

spore a reproductive cell, with a wall around it, formed by certain plants especially ferns and fungi.

squamous epithelium simple epithelia, found in lining regions where its thinness permits ease of diffusion e.g. Bowman's capsule, lung.

stamen the pollen-producing male reproductive organ of a flower, consisting of an anther and filament.

starch a storage polysaccharide in plants consisting entirely of glucose.

steroid a class of lipids characterised by a carbon skeleton consisting of four rings with various functional groups attached.

stigma of many flowering plants, the sticky or hairy surface tissue on the upper portion of the ovary that captures pollen grains and favours their germination.

stomach a muscular, stretchable sac that receives ingested food; of vertebrates, an organ between the oesophagus and intestine in which considerable protein digestion occurs.

stomata a microscopic pore surrounded by guard cells in the epidermis of leaves and stems that allows gas exchange between the environment and the interior of the plant.

stomium a line of weakness where the seed pod will rupture.

stroma of chloroplasts, the semi-fluid interior between the thylakoid membrane system and the two outer membranes; involved in the synthesis of organic molecules from carbon dioxide and water.

submucosa connective tissue layer which connects the mucosa to the underlying structures.

subrin an impermeable material similar to cuticle, deposited in cork formation by phellum.

surfactant a detergent like lipoprotein secreted by giant alveolar cell in the alveolus.

symbiosis a form of mutualism in which organisms of different species cannot grow and reproduce unless they spend their entire lives together in intimate interdependency. A mycorrhiza is an example.

sympathetic nerve of the autonomic nervous system, any of the nerves generally concerned with increasing overall body activities during times of heightened awareness, excitement, or danger; also work continually in opposition with parasympathetic nerves to bring about minor adjustments in internal organs.

symplast in plants, the continuum of cytoplasm connected by plasmodesmata between cells.

synapse the precise point where one nerve cell connects with another.

syncarpous ovary with several carpels fused together.

syncytium multinucleate cells e.g. skeletal muscle.

synecology study of ecosystem involving communities.

synergids in flowering plants two of the three non-functional cells which degenerate, the remaining third is the ovum.

tapetum nutritive tissue inside the anther which supplies the developing pollen.

tap root main root in herbaceous plants.

target organs organs on which hormones act.

telophase a phase in cell division when the daughter nuclei form.

tendon fibrous connective tissue which connects muscles to the bone.

terminal bud bud at the apex of the stem.

tertiary structure of protein non-uniform folding of the α-helical chain into compact shape due to interactions of side chains in the protein molecule.

testa outer seed coat.

testis male reproductive organ.

testestrone the main male sex hormone.

thalamus receptacle of a flower. One of two integrating centres of the vertebrate forebrain.

theca a protective covering around an organ such as the ovary.

thylakoid membrane system of the chloroplast.

thyroid gland an endocrine gland found in the neck of vertebrates, site of production of thyroxine.

thyroxin a hormone produced by the thyroid gland.

thyroglobulin throxine conjugated with protein.

tissue of multicellular organism, a group of cells and intercellular substances that function together in one or more specialised tasks.

tissue fluid fluid bathing all cell, plasma minus proteins.

tonoplast membrane separating the vacuole from the cytoplasm.

topography the delineation of the natural and artificial features of an area.

trabeculae sheets of strands of bone, forming spongy bone.

trachea the windpipe, an air-conducting tube that functions in respiration; of land vertebrates, which carries air between the larynx and bronchi.

tracheids water and dissolved minerals conducting and supportive element of xylem vessels in plants.

tetrad a group of four.

tracheal system a gas exchange system of branched, chitin-lined tubes that infiltrate the body and carry oxygen directly to cells in insects.

translocation of vascular plants, conduction of organic compounds through the plant body via the phloem. Of cells, a change in a chromosome's structure following the insertion of part of a non-homologous chromosome into it.
Transmission electron microscopy (TEM) type of electron microscope in which electrons are focussed through the specimen.
transect an arbitrary line selected through a habitat, to sample a community.
transitional epithelium epithelium lining in mammals urinary tract.
transpiration loss of water through the leaves of the plant.
transpiration stream the driving force for water movement from the roots to the leaves.
triglycerides components of fats and oils.
tricuspid valve right atrio-ventricular valve of the heart
tunica body wall or outer covering.
tunica adventitia of the circulatory system, outer connective tissue layer.
tunica intima of the circulatory system, an inner lining of endothelium supported by basement membrane and connective tissue.
tunica media of the circulatory system, intermediate muscular layer.
turgid having high internal pressure.
ultracentrifugation centrifugation at very high speeds, such as 100 000 x gravity.
ultrafilterate filtrate through the glomerulus into the Bowman's capsule.
ultrastructure the fine structure of the cells revealed by the electron microscope.
ureter a duct for urine flow between the kidney and urinary bladder.
urethra a duct for urine flow between the urinary bladder and an opening at the body surface.
vacuole large fluid-filled space in the cytoplasm in plant cells.
vagus nerve tenth cranial nerve, supplying many internal organs.
vasa recta capillary loops supplying the loop of Henle
vasa vasorum (i.e.' vessels of vessels') group of small blood vessels ranifying in the external coats of arteries and veins.
vascular bundle of xylem and phloem tissue in plants in which transport of food and water takes place.
vascular tissue plant tissue consisting of cells joined into tubes that transport water and nutrients throughout the plant body.
vein of the circulatory system, any of the large-diameter vessels that returns blood to the heart; of leaves, one of the vascular bundles that thread through photosynthetic tissues.
vena cava in vertebrates (except fish) the main vein entering the heart.
venous system the part of blood circulation in which the blood is returned to the heart, consisting of veins
ventral the underside of the body.
vegetative parts parts not involved in reproduction.
ventricles chamber of the brain or the lower chambers of the heart.
venule a small blood vessel that accepts blood from capillaries and delivers it to a vein.
vessels water-conducting tubes of plants.
vessel element a specialised short, wide cell in angiosperms; arranged end to end, which form continuous tubes for water transport.
vexillum the upper petal in pea plant, also called standard.
vibrio comma-shaped bacteria, e.g. *Vibrio cholerae* causes cholera.
villus (*pl. villi*) small finger-like projections on the wall of the small intestine.
viruses extremely small intercellular parasitic particle consisting of protein and nucleic acid.
vitamins any of more than one dozen organic substances that animals require in small amounts for normal cell metabolism but generally cannot synthesise for themselves, and obtain from the diet.
voluntary or striated muscle muscle responsible for movement of the skeleton and organs.
water potential the tendency of water molecules to enter or leave a solution via osmosis.
white blood cells see leucocytes.
white matter nerve fibres wrapped in myline sheath.
wood the hard part of the stem formed from impregnation of lignin in the cellulose cell wall.
xanthophyll a yellow pigment found in plant.
Xerophyte plants adapted to withstand drought.
xylem water conducting vessels of plants.
zwitterion amphoteric amino acid at its isoelectric point
zygomorphic irregularly shaped flower.
zymogen or chief (peptic) cells cells of gastric gland secreting pepsinogen.

GUIDE FOR TEACHERS AND TECHNICIANS

Practical 1 – Making an Aqueous Solution of Known Concentration
5 x 100cm^3 beakers
4 x 200cm^3 beakers
5 x test tubes in rack
1 x 10cm^3 pipette
1 x 1cm^3 pipette
100cm^3 volumetric flask or measuring cylinder
250cm^3 measuring cylinder
Pasture pipettes (teat pipettes)
100cm^3 reagent bottle
Balance
Spatula
Filter paper
Glass rods
Markers
Sodium Chloride (NaCl) salt 10g
Distilled water

Practical 2 – The Compound Microscope
Compound microscope, with x 10 and x 40 objective lenses
Prepared slides: *ameoba, paramesium, algae,* blood and other plant and animal tissues.
Lens tissue and/or lint-free soft duster
Immersion oil

Practical 3 – Observing Transparent Microscopic Specimens
Microscope
Immersion oil
Lens tissue/lint-free soft duster
Transparent ruler
Stage micrometer slide
Eyepiece graticule
Prepared slides of bacteria
Yeast cell culture

Practical 4 – Measuring Microscopic Objects
Microscope
Lens tissue and/or lint-free soft duster
Hand lens
Eyepiece graticule
Stage micrometer slide
A selection of prepared slides of animal and plant tissues such as: *Amoeba, paramecium,* Stem, Capillary, Red blood cell, Xylem tissue, yeast cells

Practical 5 – Observing Cell Structure
Microscope
Microscope slides
Coverslips
White tile
Sharp knife/scalpel
Fine forceps
Spatula
Box of cotton buds
Filter paper
Two mounted needles
Onion bulb
Moss plants (*minium sp.*)
Staminal hairs from the flower of *Tradescantia*
Absolute ethanol or disinfectant for sterilisation
1-% methylene blue
Glycerol in dropping bottle
Iodine solution

Practical 6 – Using the Haemocytometer to Count Cells
Haemocytometer, with a clean and dry coverslip
Hand lens
Microscope
Lens tissue
Marker pens
Pasture pipette (teat pipettes)
Distilled water wash-bottle
Small bottle of propanone/ethanol
Yeast suspension 1-2% or sample of culture solution of unicellular non-motile organisms, such as Chlorella
If the cell culture requires (serial) dilution, students will also require:
Test tubes in a stand, 1 cm^3 pipette, 10 cm^3 graduated pipette

Practical 7 – Observing Bacterial Cells
Sheets of lining paper for students' work table
Microscope with high-power and oil-immersion objectives
Stage micrometer slide
Eyepiece graticule
Glass slides
Wire inoculating loop
Bunsen burner
Large forceps
Slide-holders
Blotting paper or filter paper discs
Fresh box of tooth picks
Immersion oil
Lens tissues
Distilled water
Natural yoghurt
Nigrosin in dropping bottles
Crystal violet stain in dropping bottles
Sterilising solution (1% hypochlorite solution or other suitable disinfectant)

Practical 8 – Cells and Osmosis
Microscope
Microscope slide
Lens tissue/lint-free cloth
Cover slip
Pipettes x 6
Filter paper
Clock or stop watch
Onion bulb
Leaves of *Tradescantia virginiana*
Filamentous algae *Cladophora*
Distilled water
1.0 mol dm^{-3} sucrose solution 2cm^3
1.0 mol dm^{-3} potassium nitrate 2cm^3
1.0 mol dm^{-3} sodium chloride 2cm^3
Defibrinated blood (10cm^3) Leave a glass rod in the whole blood, a clot will form around the glass rod. Remove the glass rod carefully, twisting it as you take it out, so as to remove the clot with it.

Practical 9 – Effect of Temperature on Cell Membrane
12 x test tubes in rack
12 x 100 cm^3 beakers
10 cm^3 syringe or pipette
250cm^3 measuring cylinder
250cm^3 beaker
Marker pen
Bunsen burner, tripod and gauze
White tile,
Razor blade/scalpel
Thermometer
Stop watch
Forceps
Ruler (mm)
Distilled water
Colorimeter (if available) with tubes or cuvettes, and blue filter
12 cylinders of beetroot, cut with cork borer (0.5 x 3cm) or chip cutter to obtain cylinders of uniform thickness. Wash the cylinders overnight

in running tap water. Transfer them to a beaker of water before the practical.

Practical 10 (a) – Movement of Ions Through the Cell Membrane
Microscope
Glass slides
Coverslip
Distilled water
Red cabbage
1.0 mol dm^{-3} ammonium chloride solution $2cm^3$

Practical 10 (b) – The Water Potential of Cells of an Inflorescence Stalk
Ruler (mm)
10 cm^3 graduated pipettes
Test tubes in rack x 10
Stopwatch
Petri dishes
Scalpel
Tile
Clock/stop watch
1.0 mol dm^{-3} Sucrose solution
Distilled water
Hollow stalks of dandelion *Taraxacum officinale* (kakronda)

Practical 11 – Osmotic Fragility of Red Blood Cells
Microscope
Haemocytometer
Test tubes in rack x 10
Micropipette or $1cm^3$ graduated pipette
Glass slides and coverslips
Glass rod
Marker pen
Stop watch
10 x centrifuge tubes in racks
Bench centrifuge
Colorimeter with tubes or cuvettes
$20cm^3$ Sodium chloride solution (1.0 %)
Defibrinated blood ($10cm^3$) Leave a glass rod in the whole blood, a clot will form around the glass rod. Remove the glass rod carefully, twisting it as you take it out, so as to remove the clot with it.

Practical 12 – Water Potential of Plant Cells
6 x Petri dishes
10 cm^3 graduated pipettes
Ruler (mm)
Potato tuber
Marker pen
Razor blades/scalpel
Filter paper
Sensitive balance
Distilled water
Cork borer (0.5 x 1cm) or chip cutter to obtain cylinders of uniform thickness.
0.5 mol dm^{-3} sucrose solutions $100cm^3$

Practical 13 – Examining Bacteria in Milk
Please read 'Caution' on page 31
Boiling water bath or large beakers to melt agar
Bunsen burners, tripod, wire gauze
Sterilised Petri Dishes x 8
Sterilised $1cm^3$ and $10cm^3$ pipettes x 2
Sterilised test tubes (mouth covered with aluminium foil) in a rack x 5
Adhesive tape
30°C incubator
Markers pens
Prepare the nutrient agar and peptone agar ($200cm^3$/student) in conical flasks plugged with cotton wool and the mouth covered with aluminium foil.
Fresh, unboiled milk $1cm^3$
Boiled milk, (kept in an ordinary refrigerator) $1cm^3$
Stale milk (left at room temperature overnight) $1cm^3$
It is suggested that if an autoclave is not available, all glassware be boiled for at least 30 minutes, and then kept in a hot oven, until required.
If a camera with colour film is available, use this to record the appearance of the plates.

Practical 14 – Microscopic Examination of Bacteria
Please read 'Caution' on page 31
Microscopes
Coverslips
Microscope slides
Bunsen burner
Marker pen
Pasteur pipettes
Inoculation wire loop
Immersion oil
Acetone
Stop watch
Absolute ethanol/Disinfectant
Sterilised distilled water
Safranin aqueous in dropping bottles
Gram Stain in dropping bottles
Crystal violet solution in dropping bottles
Grams' iodine solution in dropping bottles
Copper sulphate solution in dropping bottles
Culture of Escherichia coli or Bacillus subtitles or Micrococcus luteus, or cultures from previous investigation or yogurt

Practical 15 – Bacterial Growth in the Presence of Antibiotics
Please read 'Caution' on page 31
Beaker
Tripod
Gauze
Bunsen burner
Boiling water bath
Clear adhesive tape
Forceps
Inoculation wire loop
Access to incubator at 30°C, if available
10 x Sterile plastic or glass Petri dish
200 cm^3 Sterilized nutrient agar
Access to the autoclave, (or pressure cooker).
Filter disc with antibiotics (cut discs with a paper punch or cork borer, soak in antibiotic solutions easily available from pharmacies).
If camera with colour film is available, use this to record the appearance of the plates.

Practical 16 – Testing for the Presence of Carbohydrates
Glass slides
Coverslips
Microscope
White tile
Blades
Scalpel
Boiling water bath
$10cm^3$ pipettes x 4
Pestle and mortar
Test tubes in rack x 10
Hand lens
Centrifuge and tubes
Bunsen burner
Distilled water
Iodine solution
Various types of foods to test specially grains such as rice, wheat, barley and potato, orange, apple, peas and flour.

Practical 17 – Testing for the Presence of Sugars
Microscope
Glass slides
Coverslips
White tile
Spatula
Pestle and mortar
Test tubes in rack
Blades/scalpel

Hand lens
Centrifuge and tubes
Bunsen burner
Boiling water bath/large beaker
Glucose powder
Sodium hydrogencarbonate
Colorimeter, tubes or cuvettes and filters
pH paper
Distilled water
Benedict's reagent in dropping bottles
Fehling's solution in dropping bottles
1% glucose solution in dropping bottles
1% sucrose solution in dropping bottles
1% lactose solution in dropping bottles
1% fructose solution in dropping bottles
Dilute hydrochloric acid in dropping bottles
Variety of plant and tissues, such as potato, apple, peas, liver, kidney, meat etc.

Cellulose stains purple with Schultz' solution
Microscope
Microscope slides
Razors
Tile
Watch glass
Cotton wool
Schultz' solution
Various plant tissues, such as stem, leaves, roots etc.

Lignin (wood) stains red with acidified phloroglucinol.
Watch glass
Razor
Microscope slides
Tile
Microscope
Phloroglucinol
Woody plant tissues
Match sticks
Conc. HCl

Practical 18 (a) – Testing for the Presence of Lipids
Microscope
Pestle and mortar
Spatula
Distilled water
Sudan III
Absolute ethanol
Bunsen burner, tripod, gauze
Watch glass
Teat tubes
Test tube rack
Filter paper
70% ethanol
Caster oil seeds, peanuts, sunflower seeds, linseed
Olive oil or corn oil

Practical 18 (b) – Testing for the Presence of Proteins
Microscope
Watch glass
Pasture pepettes
Test tubes in rack x 10
Bunsen burner, tripod, gauze
5% potassium hydroxide solution in dropping bottles
1% copper (II) sulphate solution in dropping bottles
Million's reagent, (harmful!) in dropping bottles
Dilute potassium hydroxide in dropping bottles
Egg albumin, peas, apple, orange, potato, meat, chicken

Practical 19 – Analysis of Amino Acids by Paper Chromatography
Breaking down the protein (takes about 48-72 hrs).
To 2g of egg white or 5.0 cm^3 of albumen add about $5cm^3$-trypsin solution (2g trypsin in 100 cm^3 of 1% sodium hydrogencarbonate). Add a crystal of thymol to kill any bacteria. Leave the mixture to incubate at 37°C for 48-72 hours.

Pencil
Ruler
Large test tubes
Clear adhesive tape
10 cm^3 measuring cylinder
30 cm^3 glass jar with a lid or a 500 cm^3 measuring cylinder covered with aluminium foil
Strips of chromatography paper (40 cm x 20 cm)
Capillary tubes or dropping pippetes drawn to a fine point
Ninhydrin spray, (or 1% ninhydrin in butanol)
1% solutions of a range of amino acids, preferably with a large difference in R_f values (see table on page 61).
Solvent (200 cm^3 solvent/student)
4 parts butanol, 1 part glacial ethanoic acid, 1 part distilled water.
Trypsin digested egg white

Practical 20 – Design an Investigation to show that: Tetrazolium Chloride is a Redox Indicator
Water baths (10°–70°C) or large beakers
Thermometer
Stop watch
Test tubes in rack x 10
$1cm^3$ and $10cm^3$ pipettes x 2
Bunsen burner, tripod, gauze
1% tetrazolium chloride (TTC) solution $20cm^3$
10% yeast solution $100cm^3$
Crushed ice
Adjust requirements as demanded by students

Practical 21 – Vitamin C Content of a Lemon
DCPIP (dichlorophenolindophenol) solution $5cm^3$
$500cm^3$, 100 cm^3 beakers
Measuring cylinder (large enough to hold a lemon)
1 cm^3 and 10 cm^3 pipette x 10
Test tubes x 5
Spatula
Knife
Distilled water
Fresh lemon juice 1 cm^3
0.1% ascorbic acid Vitamin C (0.1% aqueous solution)
Fresh whole lemon x 1

Practical 22 – Digestion of Starch by Salivary Amylase
Boiling water bath or large beaker to use as water bath
Bunsen burner, tripod, gauze
Test tubes x 15 in rack
50 cm^3 measuring cylinder
Marker pen
10 cm^3 graduated pipettes x 5
Paraffin wax
1% Starch suspension 50 cm^3
1% Dextrose (glucose) 10 cm^3
Benedict's solution in dropping bottles
1.0 mol dm^{-3} hydrochloric acid in dropping bottles
Iodine solution in dropping bottles

Practical 23 – Effect of Temperature on Catalase Activity
Test tubes in a rack x 10
Clock
Thermometer
Scalpels
Glass rod
White tile
Scissors
Forceps
Watch glasses x 2
Water baths set at 40°, 60°, 70°, 80° and 100°C
Hydrogen peroxide solution
Fresh or soaked dried peas
Small pieces of liver, meat, kidney

Practical 24 – Effect of pH on Enzyme Activity

Water bath at 38°C
Bunsen burner
Test tubes in rack x 20
Test tube holder
10 cm^3 graduated pipettes x 5
1 cm^3 graduated pippete x 5
Thermometer
Stop watch
Distilled water
Stock solution of saliva
Benedicts reagent
Buffer solutions at pH 3, 5, 7, 9, 11, 10cm^3 **(see page 219)**
1% starch solution 10cm^3

Practical 25 – Digestion of Egg White

Boiling tubes x 10 in rack
Marker pens
Incubator at 37°C
pH paper/(Universal indicator paper)
Pipettes or syringes (for measuring 10 cm^3) x 3
Pipettes or syringes (for measuring 1.0 cm^3) x 3
Trypsin solution (25 cm^3 1% solution)
Pepsin solution (25 cm^3 1% solution)
Hydrocholoric acid (5 cm^3, 0.1 mol dm^{-3})
Sodium carbonate (5 cm^3, 0.2 mol dm^{-3})
Boiled egg albumin of one egg
Distilled water
Iodine solution

Practical 26 – Design an Investigation to Observe the Effect of pH on Proteases

As required by students
Test tubes in racks
Water bath at 40°C
Marker pen
Stop watch
Graduated pipette or 5 cm^3 syringe
10 cm^3 1% pepsin solution
10 cm^3 1% trypsin solution
100 cm^3 citric acid/phosphate buffer solutions pH 2, 3, 4, 5, 6, 7, 8 **(see page 219)**
Each group of students require (or requires access to):
100 cm^3 albumen suspension prepared as follows:
Crush sufficient albumin flakes to make an adequate volume of 1% solution, allow to dissolve in cold water with stirring, (takes time) then heat and filter through glass fibre or scouring kitchen pad to remove large particles.

Practical 27 – Effect of Bead Size on the Activity of Immobilised Yeast

Sodium aliginate 1g/student
Clamps and stand
250 cm^3 beakers x 4
Tea strainer
Marker pens
Glass rods
Plastic syringe 10 cm^3 or pippetes x 5
Droppers and glass tubes of various appertures
Microscope
Ruler (mm)
Distilled water
Dried yeast 1g/student
500 cm^3 calcium chloride solution 1.4% (7g/500cm^3)
750 cm^3 3% sucrose solution
Fermentation apparatus (x3) as in **Fig. 7.2, page 72**, consisting of 250 cm^3 conical flask, rubber bung, delivery tube and 100 cm^3 measuring cylinder and two troughs as water baths.
Prepare spare delivery tubes, in case of accidents.

Practical 28 – Effect of Temperature on the Action of an Enzyme

Test tubes x 5 in rack
Marker pen
10 cm^3 pipettes x 5
White tile
Glass rods x 6
Iodine solution
25 cm^3 1% Di stase solution
25 cm^3 1% starch solution
Water baths maintained at 25°, 40°, 60°, 80° and 100°C

Practical 29 – The Effect of Substrate Concentration on Enzyme Action

Pestle and mortar
Muslin filter
Scissors
Cork fitted with rubber seal **(Fig. 7.4, page 74)**
10 cm^3 measuring cylinder
250 cm^3 measuring cylinder
250 cm^3 beaker
250 cm^3 Bucchner (side arm) flask
2 cm^3 hypodermic syringe with needle
100 cm^3 gas syringe
Piece of fresh liver
Clean sand
20 volume hydrogen peroxide (labelled corrosive) **see page 220**
pH 7 buffer **see page 219**
Preparation of enzyme extract
Homogenise the liver (liquidise if a food processor is available, or use pestle and mortar with a small amount of clean sand) in 10 cm^3 of buffer. Filter through several layers of muslin and make up to 200 cm^3 with buffer.

Practical 30 – Hydrolysis of Sucrose by Sucrase

Test tubes in racks x 10
Stop watch
Syringes or pipettes 1 cm^3 x 10, 10 cm^3 x 2
Marker pens
Measuring cylinder
Benedict's reagent in dropping bottles
1% sucrase (invertase solution) 12 cm^3
Distilled water
2% sucrose solution 20 cm^3
Water baths maintained at 38, and 50°C, with test tube racks

Practical 31 – Observing Cell Division

Mitosis in onion root tips
(this requires setting up two to three weeks in advance, to allow prolific root growth).
An onion bulb (or garlic) standing on a small beaker containing water, with the base of onion immersed in water

Alternatively, broad beans can be used. The beans should be germinated in damp peat or leaf compost 10 days before. When the radicle is 12 cm long, cut off the tip to promote lateral roots.

Microscope
Bunsen burner, tripod, gauze
Microscope slides
Coverslips
Filter paper
Fine forceps
Two mounted needles
Fine scissors
One beaker (250 cm^3) with a watch glass that fits across the top
Conc. hydrochloric acid, (corrosive!) in dropping bottles
Aceto-orcein stain in dropping bottles
Prepared slide of a thin section of an onion root tip taken through the apical meristem stained to show chromosomes and nuclei.

Preparation of anther squashes to observe stages in mitosis

White tile
Filter paper
Two mounted needles
Fine scissors
Bunsen burner
Microscope
Scalpel

Aceto-orcein in dropping bottles
A flowering plant of *Tradescantia virginiana*
Prepared slides showing meiosis

Practical 32 – Factors Affecting Photosynthesis
Destarching a Plant
Leave a well-watered plant in the dark for 24-48 hours. Test to see that destarching is complete before beginning any investigation
Suitable plants Geranium (*Pelargonium*), dahlia

To Test a Leaf for Starch **(see page 86)**
Leaf to be tested
Test tube
Forceps
White tile
100cm^3 beaker
Pasture pepettes
Hot water bath
90% ethanol
Iodine solution in dropping bottles

To investigate the need for light
Destarched leafy plant such as potted geranium (*Pelargonium*). Leave the plant in dark for 24-48 hours (see page 86)
Light source such as a bench lamp,
Black paper or metal foil
Leaf to be tested
Test tube
Forceps
Paper clips or adhesive tape
White tile
Hot water bath
90% ethanol
Iodine solution

To investigate the need for carbon dioxide
Destarched leafy plant such as potted geranium (*Pelargonium*) (see page 86)
Light source such as a bench lamp
Cotton wool
Small Petri dishes x 2
Clear plastic bags x 2
Rubber bands x 2
250 cm^3 conical flask
Clamp and clamp stand
Soda lime
20% potassium hydroxide solution
Sodium hydrogencarbonate
Starch test materials–iodine solution, white tile, Pasture pippet

To investigate the need for chlorophyll
Plant with variegated leaves such as Bougainvillea *glabra* 'Variegata' *cholorophyto* variegated ivy, geranium (*Pelargonium*)
Test tubes
Tracing paper
Forceps
White tile
Hot water bath
90% ethanol
Starch test materials–iodine solution, white tile, Pasture pippet

To investigate evolution of oxygen
Canadian pond weed (*Elodea*), or *Hydrilla*
Test-tube
Glass funnel
Plasticine
400 cm^3 beaker
Wooden splint
Light source such as a bench lamp
Sodium hydrogencarbonate

Practical 33 – Effect of Light Intensity on the Rate of Photosynthesis
Apparatus for collecting gas **Fig...** ***(make spare set as the glass tubing is fragile)***
Test tube
500 cm^3 beaker
Thermometer
Mercury vapour lamp
Sodium hydrogencarbonate
Meter ruler
Scissors
Stop watch
Bench lamp
Detergent (dish washing liquid)
Canadian pondweed *(Elodea* or *Hydrilla)* previously well illuminated for several hours kept in pond water

Practical 34 – Design an Investigation: To Test the Effect of Carbon Dioxide Concentration on the Rate of Photosynthesis
As required by students
20 cm^3 glass gas syringe (greased plunger) attached to a capillary tube, **(Fig. 9.7, page 89)**
10 cm^3 pipettes
Test tubes in rack
Beaker
Clamp and stand
Ruler
Graph paper
Pipettes
Lamp
Distilled water
0.1 mol dm^{-3} sodium hydrogencarbonate, ($NaHCO_3$)
Healthy pondweed (*Elodea* or *Hydrilla)* in pond water
Further investigation: analysis of gas
As for above and:
40% Potassium hydroxide solution
Pyrogallo, pyrogallic acid (Benzene 1, 2, 3-triol)

Practical 35 – Nutrient Requirements for Healthy Plant Growth
A large number of germinating chick peas, peas or broad beans (about 50/set up).
10 boiling tubes
20 cm^3 pipettes
Distilled water
Marker pens
Fine paint brush
Hand lens
Petri dishes
(i) 100 cm^3 complete culture medium:

$CaSO_42H_2O$	0.25g	$Ca(H_2PO_4)_2H_2O$	0.25g
$MgSO_47H_2O$	0.25g	NaCl	0.08g
KNO_3	0.70g	$FeCl_36H_2O$	0.005g

All dissolved in distilled water and made upto 1dm^3.
Access to labelled bottles (100 cm^3) with specific elements missing (potassium, calcium, iron, nitrogen, phosphorus and sulphur), made from the complete culture medium.
(ii) Minus nitrogen: replace with 0.52g KCl
(iii) Minus sulphur: replace $CaSO_42H_2O$ with 0.16g $CaCl_2$ and $MgSO_47H_2O$ with 0.21g $MgCl_2$
(iv) Minus phosphorus: replace Ca $(H_2PO_4)_2$ H_2O with 0.16 $CaNO_3$
(v) Minus potassium: replace KNO_3 with 0.59g $NaNO_3$
(vi) Minus calcium: replace $Ca_2SO_42H_2O$ with 0.20g of K_2SO_4, and Ca $(H_2PO_4)_2$ H_2O with 0.71g $Na_2HPO_412H_2O$
(vii) Minus iron: omit iron (III) chloride

Practical 36 – Photosynthetic Pigments (chlorophyll)
Extraction of photosynthetic pigment
1. Dip about 10–15g fresh spinach, grass, green cabbage or nettle leaves into boiling water.
2. Chop the leaves finely, removing the midribs and petioles and grind them with clean sand in 20cm^3 propanone in a pestle and mortar, or liquidised in a food processor.
3. Filter the extract through several layers of muslin. If available, centrifuge briefly.

4. Store in the dark in a stoppered test tube on ice.
5. Once extracted, the chlorophylls are quite unstable and need to be kept on ice in the dark.
6. Extract flower pigments as above, but instead of propanone use acidified methanol. Flowers such as geranium, chrysanthemum, roses etc. can be used.

For the demonstration of fluorescence:

For the measurement of the absorption spectrum:

Colorimeter with a set of filters, with manufacturer's filter chart
Projector set up in a darkened corner of a laboratory (or darkroom)
Teat pipette to charge the cuvettes with solvent/solution
Colorimeter
Identical glass cuvettes to fit colorimeter or glass colorimeter tubes

Separation of Chlorophyll by Chromatography

Chlorophyll extract
Large boiling tube with two bungs to fit in a rack
Chromatography, filter paper or TLC (thin layer chromatography plates)
Scissors to cut out an appropriate strip chromatogram
Glass rods
Hair dryer (if available)
Fine glass capillary tube or Pasture pipettes drawn to a fine point
Adhesive tape
Pencil
Ruler

Solvent A

30 cm^3 of solvent, consisting of nine parts petroleum ether (bp. 100-120°C) to one part of 90% aqueous propanone (acetone) labelled flammable.

Solvent B

Mixture of glacial ethanoic acid, hydrochloric acid and water

Practical 37 – The Hill's Reaction

Extraction of chlorophyll (see practical 36)

Test tubes in a rack x 10
Distilled water
Aluminium foil
1 cm^3 and 10 cm^3 pipettes
Lamp with 150W bulb
Colorimeter
Cuvettes
Green filter
Stop watch
Chloroplast suspension in ice bath, 50 cm^3
100 cm^3 phosphate buffer (**see page 219**)
10 cm^3 of 0.1% DCPIP solution

Practical 38 – The Synthesis of Starch

Extraction of starch phosphorylase

1. Peel a good-sized potato and chop it into tiny pieces.
2. Grind them to pulp using a blender (or a pestle and mortar).
3. Squeeze the juice through several layers of muslin.
4. Centrifuge the juice extracted for a few minutes at 5000 rpm, to remove suspended starch grains and all other solids.
5. Test the supernatant for the presence of starch, **if it tests positive re-centrifuge to make sure all the starch is removed.**
6. Decant the supernatant to a clean tube labelled starch phosphorylase in an ice bath.

For the extract:

Large potato, sharp knife
White tile
Blender or pestle and mortar
250 cm^3 beaker, muslin
Centrifuge, centrifuge tubes

Starch phosphorylase (potato extract) 25 cm^3

Test tubes in rack x 5
Marker pens
Distilled water
10 cm^3 pipettes,
5 cm^3 3% glucose (w/v) 10 cm^3
3% w/v glucose-1-phosphate (w/v) 10 cm^3
3% w/v maltose (w/v) 10 cm^3

Practical 39 – Formation of Starch in the Green Leaf

Place a healthy potted plant of geranium *Pelargonium*, in the dark for at least 48-72 hours to destarch it completely. Test for the presence of starch, prior to experiment (see page 86).

Bunsen buner, tripod, gauze
Forceps
Lamp
White tile
20 cm^3 syringe
Forceps
Cork borer of 0.5-1.0 cm diameter
Strong light source
6 x 100 cm^3 beakers with Petri dishes or watch glass as covers
Hypochlorite solution labelled **irritant!**
25 cm^3 of 1% sodium chlorate (I) in petri dishes
50 cm^3 of 3% (w/v) degassed glucose solution,
150 cm^3 of sodium hydrogen carbonate solution made as follows: 7.0g sodium hydrogen carbonate dissolved in 400cm^3 distilled/deionised water. Add 2 drops of liquid detergent using a Pasture pipette.
100 cm^3 distilled deionised water from which all air has been expelled by boiling for 15 minutes, and cooled in a stoppered flask, with 2 drops of liquid detergent using a Pasture pipette.
Iodine solution

Practical 40 – Gaseous Exchange in Leaves

4 x test tubes in rack
Forceps
White tile
2 cm^3 syringe
Aluminium foil
Unbleached cotton wool
Water bath
Bench lamp
Clamps and stand
Hydrogencarbonate indicator **see page 220**
Marker pens
Freshly picked **young leaves** *(Ficus)*
50cm^3 3% glucose (de-gassed)
Distilled water (de-gassed)
50cm^3 sodium hydrogencarbonate solution (de-gassed)
To degas a solution place it in a stoppered Buchner flask (side arm) and attach the side arm to a suction pump.
If suction pump is not available prepare solution in boiled water, avoid stirring

Modification of this Investigation

Philip Harris oxygen sensor meter, oxygen electrode, DL Plus 32 (Datalogger), Datadisc PRO linked to desktop computer. The software and the set up is available from Philip Harris (UK).

Further investigations

Young and old leaves of the same plant
Leaves from top of the plant and from low down deep inside the plant,
Variegated leaves
Leaves from different species
Water plants such as *Hydrilla, or Elodea* thoroughly washed
Colorimeter with tubes or cuvettes

Practical 41 – Multiplication of Yeast Cells in Aerobic and Anaerobic Conditions

***Pre-incubation* (one week before)**

Label three conical flasks of the following sizes 50 cm^3, 150 cm^3, and 500 cm^3. Pour 50 cm^3 of cider or clear apple juice into each flask. (If optical density is to be recorded, keep some apple juice to use as blank, to adjust the colorimeter to zero.) Mix the suspension of yeast thoroughly to ensure even distribution of cells, and add a drop of yeast suspension to each flask. Cover the flasks with four layers of muslin, and leave in a cupboard for one week.

Yeast suspension
Dried yeast (*Sacharomyces cereviside*) is usually available as granules consisting of dormant cells bound with inert filler (normally starch). In suitable conditions, the cells begin to be metabolically active in a matter of 30 minutes or so.
Add 10g of dried yeast (*Sacharomyces cereviside*) to 100cm^3 warm water in a conical flask. Add 3g glucose, and place a loose cotton wool plug. Leave in a 37°C water bath for about an hour.

For the yeast suspension:
Conical flasks (50, 150 and 500 cm^3)
Muslin
Measuring cylinder 50 cm^3
Rich culture of brewer's yeast
Cider or clear apple juice

Microscope
Haemocytometer
Pasture pipettes
Colorimeter with tubes or cuvettes
Glass rods

Practical 42 – Respiration in Yeast and the Effect of Temperature
Pre-incubation of yeast
Add 3g of dried yeast (*Sacharomyces cereviside*) to 100cm^3 warm water in a conical flask. Add 3g glucose, and place a loose cotton wool plug. Leave in a 37°C water bath for about an hour.
100 cm^3 yeast suspension prepared as above
Thermometers (0-100°C) x 5
Stop watch
Test tubes x 5
Water bath set at 10°, 20°, 30°, 40° and 50°C or large beakers with a supply of hot water
10cm^3 graduated pipette x 5
Waterproof marker pens
Pasture pipettes or teat pipettes
Fermentation tubes x 5
Rulers
Bunsen burners, tripod, gauze beakers to heat water

Practical 43 – The Effect of Temperature on the Rate of Respiration
Respirometers set up as shown in **Fig. 10.3**
Manometer
Manometer fluid
1 cm^3 syringe
2 x boiling tubes
Clamps and stands
Cotton wool
Soda lime
Vaseline or plaster of Paris (to seal leaks)
2 pieces of zinc gauze (to fit the diameter of a boiling tube)
Germinating seeds such as beans, peas, chick peas or small invertebrates such as woodlice or blow-fly larvae. Boiled seeds or glass beads (or any equivalent non-absorbent material of equal volume to the living organisms).
Water baths or large beakers and supply of hot water
Thermometer
Stop watch
Graph paper
Marker pens
Pipette filler
Crushed ice

Practical 44 – Design an Investigation to Measure the Respiratory Quotient of Germinating Broad Beans
Broad beans:
Soaked in water for 48 hours;
Soaked for 42 hours and exposed to air for 6 hours;
Soaked for 36 hours and exposed to air for 12 hours.
Respirometer set up as **Fig. 10.3 (see practical 43)**
Large beakers used as water baths
Thermometers
Hot and cold water supply
Glass beads or other innert material if invertebrates are being used
Vaseline

Practical 45 – General Structure of a Flowering Plant
Microscope
Dicotyledonous such as Geranium (*Pelargonium*) sunflower (*Helianthus*), tomato (*Lycopersicon esculentum*)
Fine forceps
Elder pith, carrot or potato tuber
Slides and coverslips
Dish for sections
Fine brush
Stiff razor blade
Iodine solution in dropping bottles
Fabil stain in dropping bottles
Dilute glycerine (25% aqueous) in dropping bottles
Macerated stem tissue/or 5% chromic acid (labelled highly corrosive)
Entire plant with leaves and axillary buds
Stem of sunflower (*Helianthus*) and marrow (*Cucurbita*, fresh or in 70 per cent ethanol)
Stem of monocotyledon, e.g. maize, iris
Prepared slides of dicotyledon TS and LS *Helianthus and Cucurbita*, TS monocotyledon e.g. maize, lily

Stem tissue macerated as follows:
(Franklin's method): Cut stem into small pieces about the size of half a matchstick. Immerse in a mixture of glacial ethanoic acid and 20 vol. hydrogen peroxide in equal parts. Maintain at 60°C for 24 hours or boil under reflux for 1 hour. Tissues should then disintegrate with vigorous shaking or stirring. Wash by decantation, neutralise with a little ammonium hydroxide, and store in 70 per cent ethanol.

Practical 46 – Structure of Roots
Germinating maize, wheat, mustard, peas or mung beans (*moong*)
Primary root of buttercup or broad bean
Microscope
Slides and cover slips
Elder pith or carrot tuber
Dish for sections
Fine brush
Razor blade
Phloroglucinol (benzenel 1, 3, 5-triol) in dropping bottles
Conc. hydrochloric acid in dropping bottles
FABIL in dropping bottles
Iodine solution in dropping bottles

Practical 47 – Structure of the Flower
Inflorascence such as Verbena (*Verbenae??*), Lupin (*Leguminosae*), Salvia (*Ladiatae*), Snapdragon (*Antirrium*)
Compositae flower such as sunflower (*Helianthus*), dandelion (*Taraxacum*), daisy (*bellis*)
Monocot flowers such as lily, grasses
Dicot flowers such as buttercup
Microscope
Scalpel
Glass slides

Practical 48 – Microscopic Structure of Stamen and Carpel
Prepared slides of flower bud of lily, anther of lily, pollen grains and ovary
Microscope

Practical 49 – Germination
Dry and soaked beans of caster oil, sunflower and maize
Germinating seeds of monocots and dicots
Glass slides
Coverslip
Microscope
Fine forceps
Hand lens
Food test material to test for starch in fat and protein **(see pages 56–59).**

Practical 50 – Rate of Translocation of Sucrose in a Stolon of Potato

Dig up potato tubers with their living stems attached.
Balance
Cotton wool
Microscope with high power
Stage micrometer slide
Eyepiece graticule
Microscope slides
Coverslips
Safety razor blade
Phosroglucinol (Benzene-1, 3, 5-triol) in dropping bottles
Conc. Hydrochloric acid (labelled highly corrosive)

Practical 51 – Structure of Leaves

Miscroscope
Slides and coverslips
Dish for sections
Fine brush
Small forceps
Safety razor blade
Elder pith and/or carrot tuber
Micrograph of chloroplast
Iodine solution
Distilled water
FABIL
Sudan III
Selection of leaves dicotyledoonous, monocotyledonous, such as:
Fresh young leaves of (evergreen–which stay on the tree for most of the year) e.g. *Ficus religiosa* (Peepul), Eucalyptus, Holly *(Ilex)* and deciduous such as Dahlia, Morus (*Moracae nigra*) Mulberry or shehtoot, Buddelia sp.(*Fallium alba)* (Din ka Raja) and monocotyledon leaves, e.g. *Tradescantia pallida*, (Spiderwort), Daffodil *(Narcissus)* grasses *(Poaceae)*, lily *(Lilium)*, iris *(Iridaceae)*

Practical 52 – Internal Structure of the Leaf

Super glue (Elfi), wide Scotch tape or the transparent adhesive covering used to cover books with a 'peel' off backing can be used.
Young leaves of Ficus *religiosa* (Peepul) Dahlia, and Mulberry (*Moracae nigra)* shehtoot
Microscope
Microscope slides
Coverslips
Lens tissue
Fine forceps
Pointer or mounted needle
Marker pens
Razor blades or sharp scalpels
Toluidine blue stain in dropping bottles
Prepared slides of leaf section and lower epidermis

Practical 53 – Distribution of Water in the Broad Bean Plant

2 x healthy transpiring shoots of broad bean *(Vicia faba)* at least 4 weeks old, growing in soil.
Microscope
Glass slides and coverslips
Test tubes x 2 in rack
Large beaker
Scalpel or razor blade
White tile
Paper
Lens
Stain (75 cm^3, a mixture or equal volume of 0.1% aqueous rose Bengal and 0.1% aqueous eosin)

Practical 54 – Distribution of Stomata in a Leaf

Selection of leaves such as *Eucalyptus* (Safaida), Silver Oak (*Grevillia robusta*), as well as xerophytes such as Yucca, *Sansevieria trifasciata* (Mother-in law tongue), *Euphorbia* (Spurge or Milkweed).
Leaves from the top of the tree (exposed) and leaves from deep within the tree (shaded)
Clear nail varnish
Fine forceps
Microscope
Microscope slides
Coverslips
Transparent plastic ruler
Eyepiece graticule
Stage micrometer slide

Practical 55 – Water Loss from Leaves of a Plant

Fine electric balance
Clamp, stand x 2
Hair dryer or fan
String/thread
Ruler
Fuse wire
Graph paper
Tissue paper
Glass slide
Elastic bands or paper clips
Marker pens
Transparent ruler
Vaseline or silicon grease
Anhydrous cobalt chloride paper or cobalt thiocyanate paper **see page 145**
Large quantity of leaves with their petioles still attached from evergreen deciduous plants such as *Eucalyptus* (Safaida), Silver Oak (*Grevillia robusta*), as well as xerophytes such as Yucca, *Sansevieria trifasciata* (Mother-in law tongue), *Euphorbia* (Spurge or Milkweed).

Two pieces of blue cobalt chloride paper 10 x 10 mm supplied in a sealed container (such as a small specimen tube) with a little silica gel
Scissors
Forceps
Broad sticky tape (transparent book covering material is almost as flexible and easier to distribute to a class).
Two plants - shoots of privet (*Ligustrum sp.*) are suitable, kept in water, (cover a specimen tube of water with clingfilm, strip the leaves off a portion of the plant stem and insert it through the film.) Keep one in a dark but dry place for at least an hour before use, and the other in a well-lit place enclosed in a transparent plastic bag to provide high humidity. They should be appropriately labelled for the class.

Practical 56 – Factors Affecting the Rate of Transpiration

Potometer set up as shown in **Fig. 12.60**
Large container such as a plastic bowl
Pasture pipette
Electric fan
Polythene bag
Graph paper
Vaseline
Plaster of Paris
Leafy shoot (cut under water and kept submerged) or intact plant

Practical 57 Structure of Muscle

Microscope and prepared slides of skeletal muscle in tongue, stomach, heart etc.

Practical 58 Microscopic Structure of the Nervous Tissue

Microscope and prepared slides of the nervous tissues such as the spinal cord, neurones, synapse, sections of the brain

Practical 59 – Microscopic Structure of the Endocrine System

Microscope and prepared slides of adrenal gland, thyroid gland and pituitary gland

Practical 60 – Microscopic Structure of the Pancreas

Microscope and prepared slides of pancreas

Practical 61 – Structure of the Mammalian Heart

Sheep or cow heart, preferably with atria, arteries and veins intact
Dissection kit
Dissection tray
Rubber tube, attached to cold water tap
Microscope
Prepared heart tissue and blood vessel slides

Practical 62 – Structure and Properties of the Cardiac Muscle
Microscope
Stop watch
Prepared slides of cardiac muscle
Electron micrographs of cardiac and skeletal muscle

Practical 63 – Microscopic Structure of Blood Vessels
Microscope
Micrometer slide
Graticule
Prepared slides of arteries, veins, capillaries
Arteries, veins and capillaries can be found in other tissues such as lung, liver and kidney etc.
A live tadpole or young fish if available
Electron micrograph of capillary

Practical 64 – Observing Red Blood Cells in Human Blood
Microscope
Lens tissue
Micrometer eyepiece and scale
Slides and cover slip
Elastic band
Sterile lancet
Ethanol
Cotton wool
Slide of human blood and frog's blood
Electron micrograph of red blood cells

Practical 65 – Observing White Blood Cells in Human Blood
Cotton wool
Sterilised lancets
Ethanol
Filter paper
Microscope
Glass slides
Graph paper
Coverslip
Lens tissue
Canada balsam
Leishman's or Wright's stain
Acidified ethanol
Distilled water

Practical 66 – Estimating the Number of White Bood Cells in Human Blood
Haemocytometer (slide, coverslip, pipette and rubber tubing)
Microscope
Sterile lancet
Ethanol
Cotton wool
Distilled water
Filter paper
Ethanoic acid
Lens tissue
Acetone
Sodium chloride solution 0.9%
Turk's solution **see page 221**

Practical 67 – Structure of the Mammalian Respiratory Apparatus
Microscope
Prepared slides of:
Tracheal epithelium, lung, bronchioles etc.

Practical 68 – Microscopic Structure of the Gasterointestinal Tract
Microscope
Prepared slides of:
Ileum, duodenum, stomach, villi, gastric gland, oesophagus, electron micrograph of sections of gastric tract

Practical 69 – Microscopic Structure of the Liver
Microscope
Prepared slides of human and pig's liver
Electron micrograph of liver cells

Practical 70 – Examination of the Mammalian Renal System
Freshly dissected mammal to show urinary system and/or fresh mammalian kidney
Liquid latex, preferably in red, blue and yellow colours, if not available use white.
Microscope
Dissection kit
Dissection board or tray
Thread
5 cm^3 syringes
Saline solution (1% NaCl)
Water bath
Prepared slides of kidney, tubules

Practical 71 – Microscopic Structure of the Mammalian Kidney
Microscope and prepared slides of kidney and its tubules from various regions

Practical 72 – Microscopic Structure of the Ovary and the Testis
Microscope
Prepared slides of:
Ovary, Graffian, follicle, corpus, leuteum, testis, seminefrerous tubules, epididymus

---

Preparation of Stains and Reagents

Acetic orcein
Dissolve 3.3g of orcein in 100 cm^3 of glacial ethanoic acid by gently boiling under reflux for about six hours. Filter. Dilute this stock solution when required 10cm^3 stock, 12cm^3 distilled water. The diluted solution deteriorates quickly.

Benedicts' reagent
Is available commercially. To prepare dissolve 173g of hydrated sodium citrate and 100g hydrated sodium carbonate in 800 cm^3 warm distilled water. Filter and make it up to 850 cm^3. This is solution A. Then dissolve 17.3g of hydrated copper sulphate in 100 cm^3 distilled water. This is solution B. Add A to B and make up to 1dm^3 with distilled water.

Buffer Solutions
Citrate-phosphate buffer (ph range 2.2–8.0)
Prepare 100 cm^3 from stock solutions of 0.2 mol dm^{-3} Na_2HPO_4 and 0.1 mol dm^{-3} citric acid as follows:

pH	phosphate	citric acid
2.2	2.0	98.0
3.0	20.5	79.5
4.0	38.5	61.5
5.0	51.5	48.5
5.6	58.0	42.0
6.0	63.2	36.8
7.0	82.4	17.6
7.6	93.6	6.4
8.0	97.2	2.8

Phosphate buffer (pH range 5.0–8.0)
Prepare 100 cm^3 from stock solutions of 0.15 mol dm^{-3} K2HPO4 and 0.15 mol dm^{-3} kH_2PO_4 as follows:

pH	K_2HPO_4	KH_2PO_4
5.0	2.0	98.0
5.5	6.0	94.0
6.0	17.0	83.0
6.5	38.0	62.0
7.0	67.0	33.0
7.5	86.0	14.0
8.0	95.0	5.0

Chromic Acid
Chromic trioxide 10g dissolved in 90 cm^3 distilled water.
Or
Potassium dichromate 10g made up to 100cm^3 with distilled water. Add 10 cm^3 conc. H_2SO_4

Cobalt chloride paper
Dip a strip of filter paper, into 5% solution of cobalt chloride. Dry and keep desiccated or in sealed plastic bags.

Cobalt thiocyanate paper
Dip strips of filter paper in 25% solution of cobalt thiocyanate. Dry and keep desiccated or in sealed plastic bags.

Copper Sulphate for Biuret Test
1g copper sulphate in 99 cm^3 distilled water.

Crystal Violet
(a) 2g crystal violet in 20 cm3 95% ethanol.
(b) 0.8g ammonium oxalate in 80 cm^3 distilled water.
Mix the two solutions together.

Dichlorophenolindophenol (DCPIP)
0.1% aqueous solution, dilute to 0.01% for use for REDOX reactions.

Eosin (alcoholic)
Dissolve 1g of alcohol soluble eosin in 100 cm^3 90% ethanol.
Eosin (aqueous)
1% aqueous solution.

Fabil
The following solutions are required:
Lactophenol: phenol (crystals), glycerol, lactic acid, and distilled water in equal parts by weight.
A Aniline blue: 0.5% in lactophenol.
B Basic fushin: 0.5% in lactophenol.
C Iodine 3g; potassium iodide 6g; lactophenol 1 dm^3.
To make up mix stock solutions in following proportions:
A, 4: **B**, 1: **C**, 5.
Allow to stand for 12 hours, then filter. Keeps indefinitely.

Fehling's A
34.64g cupric sulphate ($CuSO_4$ $5H_2O$) in 500 cm^3 distilled water. Heat if necessary.

Fehling's B
176g sodium potassium tartrate (Na K C_4 H_6 $4H_2O$), 77g sodium Hydroxide in 500 cm^3 distilled water.

Formalin
Dilute commercial formalin, 90 cm^3 water to 10 cm^3 formalin.

Grams' iodine solution (2g KI, and 1g I_2 in 300 cm^3 water),

Glycerine
Use 5% solution for mounting.

Haemotoxylin
Available commercially from suppliers.
To prepare:–
Solution A: 2g Haemotoxylin in 100 cm^3 absolute alcohol.
Solution B: 3g aluminium potassium sulphate to 100 cm^3 glycerole, 100 cm^3 distilled water and 10 cm^3 ethanoic acid (glacial acetic acid). Mix A to B and leave exposed to light for 2-3 weeks until it is dark red.

Hydrogen Carbonate Indicator
Solution A: Dissolve 0.2g thymol blue and 0.1g cresol red in 20cm^3 ethanol (dye solution)
Solution B: Dissolve 0.8g sodium hydrogen carbonate in 900 cm^3 distilled deionised water.
Add A to B and adjust the volume to 1 litre.
Working solution: Dilute stock solution 1 in 10.

Bubble air from outside the lab into the soution for 1 minute, solution will turn dark red – small sample in a test tube appears orange red.
Colour change increase in acidity turns yellow.
Decrease in acidity (increase in alkalinity) turns cherry red then purple.

Hydrogen Peroxide
Hydrogen peroxide is commercially available as 35%, or 20 vol. solution.
To make 1 dm^3 1M solution from a 35% solution:
35 cm^3 H_2O_2 make up to 1 dm^3.
To make 1 dm^3 1M solution from 20 vol. solution.
100 cm^3 H_2O_2 + 900 $H_2O \rightarrow$ 1M solution of H_2O_2

Iodine
1g iodine and 2g potassium iodide in 300cm^3 distilled water.

Lactophenol
Dissolve 100g of phenol in 100 cm^3 distilled water without heating. Add 100 cm^3 of lactic acid and 200 cm^3 of glycerine. Store in dark brown bottle.

Leishmans' or Wrights' stain
Leishman's stain 0.15g
Methyl alcohol (acetone free)

If Leishman's stain unavailable:
Dissolve 1g methylene blue in 100 cm^3 distilled water
Then dissolve 0.5g sodium carbonate in 100 cm^3 distilled water.
Mix the two solutions and heat to 65°C for 12 hours. Allow to stand for 10-12 days.
Add 2g eosin dissolved in 100 cm^3 distilled water.
Allow to stand for 6-12 hours. Filter, wash the ppt. until it is clear. Dry. This is Leishman's stain.

Methyline blue
Mix 1g methyline blue, 0. 6g sodium chloride in 100 cm^3 distilled water.

Million's Reagent
Commercially available.
To prepare:–
In a fume cupboard dissolve 1cm^3 of mercury in 9 cm^3 of conc. nitric acid. Dilute with 10 cm^3 of distilled water.

Nigrosine
10 % w/v aqueous.

Ninhydrin
0.2g ninhydrin in 200 cm^3 propanone

Phloroglucin (benzene-1, 2, 3-triol)
Dissolve 2-5 g of phloroglucine in 100 cm^3 of 90% ethanol. Acidify with conc. HCl before use.

Potassium Oxalate (prevents blood from clotting)
1g potassium oxalate dissolved in 99 cm^3 water

Potassium Pyrogallate
Dissolve 5g pyrogellel in 95 cm^3 distilled water. Add 25g KOH to 15 cm^3 distilled water. Mix the two together, use at once.

Safranin
Dissolve 1g of safranin in 100 cm^3 of 50 % ethanol.

Saline (physiological)
0.9% NaCl solution.

Schultz solution (chlor-zinc iodide)
Dissolve 110g of zinc in 300 cm^3 of hydrochloric acid and evaporate to half the volume, in an evaporating dish over a low flame.
In the course of evaporation add a little more zinc to ensure complete neutralisation of acid. Dissolve 10 g of potassium iodide in the least

possible quantity of water and add 0.15 g of iodine crystals. Mix thoroughly, and filter through glass wool. Store in tightly screwed bottle in the dark.

Sudan III
Sudan III saturated solution in 70% alcohol.

Triphenyl tetrazolium chloride (TTC)
0.5-1.0% is usually required for REDOX reactions, must be made just prior to using distilled deionised water.

Thymol
3g thymol in 97 cm^3 90% ethanol

Turks' solution
Mix 100cm^3 distilled water, 1cm^3 glacial ethanoic acid, 1 cm^3 I % gentian violet solution.

Wright's solution
See Leishman's Stain.

Reagents and Stains

Reagent and stains	Suitable for:	Final colour
Acetic – orcein	Stains chromosomes	Red – purple
Analine blue in lactophenol	Fungal hyphae and spores	Blue
Benedicts reagent	Sugars, reducing and non-reducing	Green → yellow Brick red precipitate
Biuret test	-CONH—gps. As in proteins	
Borax carmine	Nuclei	Pink
Dichlorophenolindophenol (DCPIP)	REDOX	Blue → colourless
Eosine	Cytoplasm Cellulose	Pink Red
FABIL	Xylem elements Sclerenchyma Cellulose Cytoplasm Nuclei, starch.	Brown Pink Pale blue Dark blue Black
Fehling's test	Test for carbohydrates	Green → Yellow → Brick red
Feulgen's stain	DNA	Blue
Gram	Bacteria Gram positive (+ive) or Gram negative (-ive)	Violet/purple Red/pink
Haematoxilin	Nuclei cytoplasm	Dark blue Light blue
Iodine solution	Starch	Blue black
Leishman's stain	White blood cells nuclei	Red-pink
Light green or fast green	Cytoplasm cellulose	Green
Neutral red	Living cells (pH<7) used to determine cell viability, or plant protoplasts in plasmolysis	Pink
Methylene blue	Nuclei (redox indicator), living cells decolourise, dead cells stain blue	Blue
Million's regent	Insoluble proteins	Brick red ppt.
Phloroglucin + conc. HCl	Lignin	Red
Safranin	Nuclei, lignin, suberin, used for plant sections and counter stain for cytoplasm	Red
Schultz solution	Lignin, cutin, suberin, protein Starch Cellulose	Yellow Blue Blue or violet
Sudan III	Test for oils	Red
Triphenyl tetrazolium chloride (TTC)	Redox reactions	Reduced from colourless to red compd.
Toludine blue	Lignified cell walls Cellulose cell walls	Blue Purple
Turk's solution	White blood cells	
Wright's solution	White blood cells	

Suggested Slides for Study of Histology

Prepared slides of plant tissue showing:
Different tissue types such as: Parenchyma, sclerenchyma, collenchyma
Vascular tissue: Xylem and phloem, tracheids, vessels
Meristematic tissue of root and shoot
TS, LS dicot and monocot stem
TS, LS dicot and monocot root
TS leaf, sun and shade, hydrophytes, xerophytes
Flower bud of lily, ovary, anther, pollen grains

Prepared slides of Animal tissues showing various epithelia; Squamous, Cuboidal, Columnar, Ciliated, Stratified, Transitional, Glandular
Connective tissues: Aerolar, White fibrous, Yellow elastic, Adipose
Skeletal tissue: Hayline cartilage, Yellow elastic cartilage, White elastic cartilage, Bone, Blood
Muscular tissue: Striated, Smooth, Cardiac
Sections of ovary and testis
Sections from digestive system: Small intestine, Stomach, Large intestine, Rectum etc.

Guide to Names of Plants and Flowers

Common English Name	Botanical Name	Local Urdu Name
arum lily	(*Arum zentedeschia*)	elephantaria
bougainvillea	(*Nyctaginaceae*)	bougainvillea
bryophyllum	(*Bryophyllum*)	pather chat
buddelia	(*Loganiaceae*)	din-ka-raja
buttercup	(*Ranunculus*)	crow foot
butterfly orchid	(*Orchidaceae*)	orchid
daffodil	(*Narcissus*)	nargis
daisy	(*Bellis*)	daisy
dandelion	(*Taraxacum*)	kakronda
deadnettle	(*Lamium*)	
delphinium	(*Ranunculaceae*)	sungleam
eucalyptus	(*Myrtaceae*)	eucalyptus
eucalyptus	(*Myrtaceae*)	safada
foxglove	(*digitalis*)	digitalis
geranium	(*Pelargonium*)	geranium
grasses	(*Poaceae*)	grass
hibiscus	(*Malvaceae*)	shoe flower
holly	(*Ilex*)	holly
honey-suckle	(*Lonicera*)	honey-suckle
horsechestnut	(*Aesulus*)	horsechestnut
iris	(*Iridaceae*)	iris
ivy	(*Hedera*)	ivy
lily	(*Lilium*)	lily
lily	(*Lilium*)	nargis
lupin	(*Leguminosae*)	lupin
marram grass	(*Ammophil*)	grass
mulberry	(*Moracae nigra*)	shehtoot
nastertuim	(*Tropaeolum*)	winter herb
night-scented stock	(*Matthiola*)	raat ki rani
oak	(*Quercus*)	shah baloot
orchid	(*Orchidaceae*)	orchid
papaya	(*papaw*)	papitta
pea	(*Pisum sativum*)	mutter
peepul	(*Ficus religiosa*)	peepul
petunia	(*Solanaceae*)	petunia
plantain	(*Musa paradisiaca*)	kela
prickly pear	(*Opuntia*)	naag phun
privet	(*Ligustrum vulgre*)	privet
sage	(*Salvia officinatis*)	sage
salvia	(*Labiatae*)	salvia
silver Oak	(*Grevillia robusta*)	
snapdragon	(*Antirrhium*)	kutta phool
spiderwort	(*Tradescantia pallida*)	spiderwort
spurge or Milkweed	(*Euphorbia*)	spurge
sunflower	(*Helianthus*)	suraj mokhi
sweet pea	(*Lathyrus odoratus*)	muttery
sycamore	(*Acer pseudoplatanus*)	sycamore
verbena	(*Verbenaceae*)	verbena
water lily	(*Nymphaea*)	kanwal
willow	(*Salix*)	willow
yucca	(*Sansevieria trifasciata*)	mother-in law's tongue

INDEX

A

B

C

D

I

J

K

L

M

N

O

P

Q

R

U

V

W

X

Y

Z